CLINICAL
FOR THE FRC

To Madelaine

*Commissioning Editor*: Mike Parkinson
*Project Development Manager*: Sarah Keer-Keer
*Project Controller*: Frances Affleck
*Designer*: Erik Bigland

# CLINICAL NOTES FOR THE FRCA

**Second Edition**

## Charles D. Deakin MA MD MB BChir MRCP FRCA

Consultant Anaesthetist
Shackleton Department of Anaesthetics
Southampton General Hospital
Southampton, UK

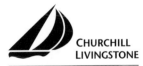
CHURCHILL
LIVINGSTONE

EDINBURGH LONDON NEW YORK PHILADELPHIA ST LOUIS SYDNEY TORONTO
2000

CHURCHILL LIVINGSTONE
An imprint of Harcourt Publishers Limited

First edition published 1996
Second edition published 2000

ISBN 0443 06403 2

**British Library Cataloguing in Publication Data**
A catalogue record for this book is available from the British Library

**Library of Congress Cataloging in Publication Data**
A catalog record for this book is available from the Library of Congress

**Note**
Medical knowledge is constantly changing. As new information becomes available, changes in treatment, procedures, equipment and the use of drugs become necessary. The author and the publishers have, as far as it is possible, taken care to ensure that the information given in this text is accurate and up-to-date. However, readers are strongly advised to confirm that the information, especially with regard to drug usage, complies with the latest legislation and standards of practice.

The publisher's policy is to use paper manufactured from sustainable forests

Printed in China
NPCC/01

# Preface

Over the past 4 years, there have been a large number of new developments in anaesthesia. In particular, several new drugs are now in regular clinical use, progress has been made in several fields related to anaesthesia, a plethora of new reports and guidelines have been published and the Royal College of Anaesthetists have published a new syllabus for the FRCA examination.

This second edition improves on the successful first edition by incorporating these changes and improving many areas of the original book. New chapters have been added on trauma management, major incident management, systemic inflammatory response syndrome, opioids, renal replacement therapy and ecstasy. Existing chapters have all been revised in terms of both their content and the references for further reading. Revisions have been made using all major anaesthetic and medical journals, reports and guidelines from official bodies and notes from current FRCA courses.

I hope this helps those sitting the FRCA exams. Good luck!

C.D.D.                                                                      January 2000

# Contents

# Abbreviations

| | | | |
|---|---|---|---|
| AAG | $\alpha_1$ acid glycoprotein | ECMO | Extracorporeal membrane oxygenation |
| ACTH | Adrenocorticotrophic hormone | EEG | Electroencephalogram |
| ADH | Antidiuretic hormone | ETT | Endotracheal tube |
| AIO | Ambulance incident officer | FEV$_1$ | Forced expiratory volume in 1 s |
| ANS | Autonomic nervous system | | |
| Ao | Aorta | FFP | Fresh frozen plasma |
| APTR | Activated partial thromboplastin time ratio | FRC | Functional residual capacity |
| ARDS | Acute respiratory distress syndrome | FSH | Follicle-stimulating hormone |
| ATLS | Advanced trauma life support | GA | General anaesthetic |
| A-V | Atrioventricular | GFR | Glomerular filtration rate |
| | | GH | Growth hormone |
| BBB | Blood–brain barrier | GI | Gastrointestinal |
| | | GTN | Glyceryl trinitrate |
| CCF | Congestive cardiac failure | | |
| CCS | Casualty clearing station | Hb | Haemoglobin |
| CO | Cardiac output | HbF | Fetal haemoglobin |
| CPAP | Continuous positive airway pressure | HT | Hydroxytryptamine |
| CPP | Coronary perfusion pressure | ICP | Intracranial pressure |
| | | IHD | Ischaemic heart disease |
| CVA | Cerebrovascular accident | i.m. | Intramuscular |
| CVP | Central venous pressure | INR | International normalised ratio |
| CVS | Cardiovascular system | | |
| CPR | Cardiopulmonary resuscitation | IPPV | Intermittent positive pressure ventilation |
| CXR | Chest X-ray | IUGR | Intrauterine growth retardation |
| DIC | Disseminated intravascular coagulation | i.v. | Intravenous |
| | | IVC | Inferior vena cava |
| DO$_2$ | Oxygen delivery | JESCC | Joint emergency services control centre |
| dTC | Tubocurarine | | |
| ECG | Electrocardiograph | JVP | Jugular venous pressure |

| | | | |
|---|---|---|---|
| LA | Local anaesthetic | PVP | Pulmonary vascular pressure |
| LA | Left atrium | | |
| LH | Luteinising hormone | PVR | Pulmonary vascular resistance |
| LMWH | Low-molecular-weight heparin | | |
| LPA | Left pulmonary artery | RA | Right atrium |
| LPV | Left pulmonary vein | RPA | Right pulmonary artery |
| LV | Left ventricle | RPV | Right pulmonary vein |
| LVEDP | Left ventricular end-diastolic pressure | RSD | Reflex sympathetic dystrophy |
| LVF | Left ventricular failure | RV | Right ventricle |
| | | RVP | Rendezvous point |
| MAC | Minimum alveolar concentration | SSEP | Somatosensory evoked potential |
| MAP | Mean arterial pressure | | |
| MH | Malignant hyperthermia | SIRS | Systemic inflammatory response syndrome |
| MI | Myocardial infarction | | |
| MIO | Medical incident officer | SNS | Sympathetic nervous system |
| MODS | Multiple organ dysfunction syndrome | | |
| | | STP | Standard temperature and pressure |
| NO | Nitric oxide | | |
| NSAID | Non-steroidal anti-inflammatory drug | SVC | Superior vena cava |
| | | SVR | Systemic vascular resistance |
| PA | Pulmonary artery | | |
| PAP | Pulmonary artery pressure | TIA | Transient ischaemic attack |
| PCA | Patient-controlled analgesia | TOE | Transoesophageal echocardiography |
| PCWP | Pulmonary capillary wedge pressure | TOF | Train of four |
| PDA | Patent ductus arteriosus | $V_D$ | Volume of distribution |
| PEFR | Peak expiratory flow rate | VF | Ventricular fibrillation |
| $P_{ET}CO_2$ | End-tidal carbon dioxide | $V_{O_2}$ | Oxygen consumption |
| PNS | Parasympathetic nervous system | VOC | Vaporizer outside the circle |
| PVC | Premature ventricular contraction | VIC | Vaporizer inside the circle |
| | | VT | Ventricular tachycardia |

# 1. Cardiovascular system

**New York Heart Association classification of cardiovascular disease**

- I   Normal cardiac output. Asymptomatic on heavy exertion
- II  Normal cardiac output. Symptomatic on exertion
- III Normal cardiac output. Symptomatic on mild exercise
- IV  Cardiac output reduced at rest. Symptomatic at rest

**ASSESSMENT OF RISK** – Predictors in non-cardiac surgery

**Goldman risk factors** (Goldman et al 1977)

Shown to be poor predictors in prospective studies. They fail to take into account the standard of anaesthetic care.

- History
  - age > 70 years                                         5
  - MI within 6 months                                    10
- Physical examination
  - signs of heart failure ($\uparrow$ JVP, S3)           11
  - aortic stenosis                                        3
- ECG
  - rhythm other than sinus                                7
  - greater than five PVCs/min                             7
- Poor general medical status
  - $\downarrow Po_2$, $\uparrow Pco_2$, $\downarrow K^+$, $\downarrow HCO_3^-$   3
  - emergency surgery                                      4
  - intrathoracic, GI or aortic surgery                    3

                                                   = 53 points

**Modified by Detsky et al (1986)**

In addition to Goldman's factors, Detsky et al included additional variables of MI at any time (i.e. > 6 months), unstable angina within 6 months and poor LV function. These have been shown to correlate better with perioperative morbidity.

- Coronary artery disease
  - — MI < 6 months                                   10
  - — MI > 6 months                                    5
  - — Canadian Cardiovascular Society angina
    - — Class 3                                        10
    - — Class 4                                        20
  - — Unstable angina within 6 months                 10
- Pulmonary oedema
  - — within 1 week                                    10
  - — ever                                              5
- Arrhythmias
  - — rhythm other than sinus                           5
  - — greater than five PVCs/min                        5
- Poor general medical status                           3
  - — age > 70 years                                    5
  - — emergency surgery                                 4
  - — critical aortic stenosis                         20

Goldman and Detsky indices may be useful in allocation of patients to a risk group but are not necessarily useful in predicting individual risk.

### ASA grade combined with Goldman's cardiac risk index

Combination of these two scores increases the accuracy of prediction of perioperative mortality (Prause et al 1997).

### Coronary Artery Surgery Study (Myers et al 1999)

Risk factors were:

- age, female sex
- raised PVP, raised LVEDP
- impaired LV wall motion, left main stem coronary artery stenosis.

### Risk of recurrent perioperative MI

Reduction in risk since 1972 (Table 1.1) may reflect improved anaesthetic and surgical techniques. Rao et al used preoperative optimization, aggressive invasive monitoring and prompt treatment of haemodynamic observations, which may also have contributed to improved results.

In a population of 323 patients at risk for perioperative MI (angina, previous MI, Q waves or angiographic evidence), 5.6% suffered perioperative MIs. Most occurred within 48 h, were painless and usually non-Q wave in nature (Badner et al 1998). Perioperative MIs have a 60% mortality rate.

**Table 1.1** Risk of recurrent perioperative MI

| Time since MI | Risk of recurrent MI (Tarhan et al 1972) | Risk of recurrent MI (Rao et al 1983) |
| --- | --- | --- |
| < 3 months | 37% | 5.7% |
| 4–6 months | 16% | 2.3% |
| > 6 months | 6% | 1.5% |

**Other important risk studies**

- Mahar et al (1978) — patients with IHD who undergo coronary artery bypass grafting (CABG) subsequently have a normal risk of perioperative MI.
- Slogoff & Keats (1986) — perioperative ischaemia increases the risk of postoperative MI.
- Shah et al (1990) — previous MI, active IHD and emergency surgery result in a high risk of perioperative infarction.
- Mangano et al (1990) — postoperative myocardial ischaemia is the most important predictor of adverse outcome. Risk increase × 9.2. (83% of ischaemic events are silent).

**Hypertension**

Diastolic blood pressure (BP) is a good indicator of the severity of vascular disease. Diastolic BP > 110 mmHg is associated with exaggerated swings in BP and an increased risk of perioperative complications. Severe (diastolic BP > 115 mmHg) or malignant (diastolic BP > 140 mmHg) hypertension should be treated before surgery. LV hypertrophy is associated with reduced ventricular compliance and these patients may benefit from perioperative monitoring of PCWP.

Perioperative hypertension doubles the risk of complications and is associated with increased silent ischaemia.

**Controversial risk factors**

These include age, angina, diabetes, ECG abnormalities and calcified aorta on CXR.

## INVESTIGATIONS

*Ambulatory ECG* using Holter monitor. Ischaemic events are a highly significant predictor of adverse postoperative cardiac events in patients with peripheral vascular disease in some studies.

*Exercise ECG* (Bruce protocol). Aim for target heart rate by stage 4. Good predictor of risk in patients with angina. Severe peripheral vascular disease limits exercising and may mask exercise-induced angina.

*ECHO.* Ejection fraction, wall motion and valve abnormalities.

*Thallium-201 scan.* $K^+$ analogue injected i.v. and taken up by well-perfused myocardium, showing underperfused areas as cold spots. Cold spots resolving by 4 h are areas of ischaemia; those persisting are infarcted tissue.

*Technetium-99m scan.* Similar to thallium scan but underperfused areas show as hot spots.

*Dipyridamole–thallium scan.* Dipyridamole causes coronary vasodilation to assess coronary stenosis. Similar effect with dobutamine which also increases myocardial work, i.e. pharmacological stress test. Good predictor of postoperative cardiac complications.

*Multiple uptake gated acquisition (MUGA) scan.* Red cells labelled with thallium. Evaluates myocardial function and measures ejection fraction (normal > 60%), amplitude and synchrony of contraction. Preoperative ejection fraction < 35% correlates with high risk of peri-operative infarction.

*Angiography.* Definitive investigation. Right coronary artery supplies sinoatrial node in 60% of patients and atrioventricular node in 50%.

## GENERAL ANAESTHESIA FOR NON-CARDIAC SURGERY

Choice of anaesthetic technique or volatile agent has no proven effect on cardiac outcome. Aim to optimize myocardial oxygen balance (Table 1.2).

**Table 1.2** Factors affecting oxygen supply and demand

| Supply | Demand |
|---|---|
| Coronary perfusion | Preload (LVEDP) |
| $O_2$ content | Afterload (SVR) |
| Heart rate | Heart rate |
|  | Contractility |

### Laplace's law

Wall tension (preload and afterload) determined by Laplace's law:

$$\text{Wall tension} \propto \frac{\text{pressure} \times \text{internal radius}}{\text{wall thickness}}$$

### Premedication

Continue all cardiac medication until the day of surgery. Heavy premedication reduces anxiety, which may otherwise cause tachycardia, hypertension and myocardial ischaemia. Consider $O_2$ after morphine premedication to avoid hypoxaemia from respiratory depression; the prevention of tachycardia results in less myocardial ischaemia overall. A single dose of β-blocker dampens the hypertensive response to intubation.

## Monitoring

*ECG.* Leads II and $V_5$ together detect 95% of myocardial ischaemic events. Leads II, $V_5$ and V4R together detect 100% of events. ST segment monitoring may be a more sensitive indicator.

*BP* (invasive/non-invasive). Invasive BP monitoring enables blood gases/acid–base and $K^+$ measurements.

*CVP.* Use right atrium (RA) as zero reference point (midaxillary line, 4th costal cartilage). Normal range with spontaneous respiration is 0–6 $cmH_2O$. The manubriosternal junction is 5–10 cm above the RA when the patient is supine. Ischaemia causes abnormal 'v' waves.

*Pulmonary artery catheter.* Good monitor of LV function but low sensitivity for detection of myocardial ischaemia (ischaemia causes ↑PCWP and ↑PAP). Rao et al (1983) showed increased reinfarction risk if preoperative PCWP was > 25 mmHg. Thus monitoring of PCWP and aggressive treatment with inotropes/vasodilators may reduce the risk of reinfarction. If ejection fraction > 0.50 and there is no dyssynergy, CVP is an accurate correlate of PCWP, and PAP monitoring may be unnecessary.

*Transoesophageal ECHO (TOE).* Myocardial wall motion abnormalities detected by TOE are a much more sensitive method than ECG in detecting myocardial ischaemia. However, wall motion abnormalities are not always due to ischaemia. Post-bypass TOE is a sensitive predictor of outcome (MI, LVF, cardiac death).

## Induction

Aimed at limiting hypotensive response to induction agent and hypertensive pressor response to intubation. High-dose opioid is a popular technique.

## Anaesthetic

Avoid CVS changes that precipitate ischaemia. Tachycardia and hypertension increase myocardial $O_2$ consumption and reduce diastolic coronary filling time. Hypotension reduces coronary perfusion pressure.

$N_2O$ is a sympathetic stimulant, but will decrease sympathetic outflow if the SNS is already stimulated, e.g. LVF. In the presence of an opioid, it may cause CVS instability.

*Volatiles.* Enflurane and halothane both decrease coronary blood flow, but isoflurane, sevoflurane and desflurane increase coronary blood flow in normotensive patients. Tachycardia with isoflurane increases myocardial work, but this is minimal with balanced anaesthesia. Isoflurane and desflurane maintain LV function better than enflurane or halothane.

*Relaxants.* Vecuronium combined with high-dose opioids tends towards bradycardia. Use of pancuronium avoids bradycardia.

### Epidural/spinal

Decreases afterload and may improve LV function. General anaesthetic combined with epidural may cause severe hypotension because of vasodilation of vessels that have constricted above the block. In animals, redistribution of blood from epicardial to endocardial vessels reduces MI size.

Blocks below $L_3$ have no effect on the SNS. Blocks above $T_{10}$ block sympathetic afferents to the adrenals and reduce catecholamine release. Blocks to $T_1$–$T_4$ interrupt cardioaccelerator fibres, preventing the coronary vasoconstrictive response to surgery, cause coronary vasodilation, decrease coronary perfusion pressure and decrease contractility and heart rate. Central hypovolaemia due to vasodilation causes a vagally mediated bradycardia which responds to fluid challenge.

Angina following spinal anaesthesia tends to occur at cessation of the block, probably due to increased pre- and afterload aggravated by volume loading.

### Coronary steal

Originally described by Becker in 1978, in a canine model. It occurs with coronary artery disease when dilatation of non-stenotic vessels reduces flow to myocardium supplied by collateral vessels (Fig. 1.1). Because isoflurane is a potent coronary artery vasodilator, Reiz et al (1983) suggested that it may induce ischaemia in some patients with steal-prone anatomy. Steal-prone anatomy was reported in 23% patients in the Coronary Artery Surgery Study (Myers et al 1999).

There is no evidence that isoflurane in humans increases myocardial ischaemia compared with other agents, even in the presence of steal-prone anatomy, and no evidence that isoflurane is detrimental to outcome in these patients (Slogoff et al 1991). In animal models, desflurane does not cause ischaemia in steal-prone anatomy. Isoflurane did not affect the outcome in 361 patients undergoing heart valve replacement when compared with other volatiles (Tuman et al 1989). Isoflurane increases flow in small endocardial vessels but does not vasodilate epicardial vessels.

## PACEMAKERS

### Nomenclature

The type of permanent pacemaker is denoted by three or four letters (Fig. 1.2).

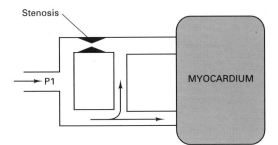

(A) P1 = perfusing pressure. Stenosis reduces flow to myocardium but adequate perfusion is achieved through collateral flow.

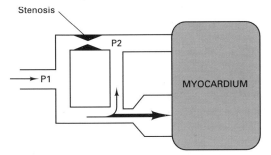

(B) Vasodilator increases run off, reducing pressure at P2 and therefore reducing perfusion pressure of myocardium.

**Fig. 1.1** A) Myocardial perfusion pressure (P1) reduced by stenosis. Adequate perfusion is achieved through collateral flow. B) Vasodilator increases run-off, reducing pressure at P2 and therefore reducing myocardial perfusion pressure distal to the stenosis.

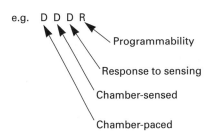

e.g.  D D D R

Programmability

Response to sensing

Chamber-sensed

Chamber-paced

**First and second letters**
O = None
A = Atrium
V = Ventricle
D = Dual (atrium and ventricle)

**Third letter**
I  = Inhibited
T = Triggered
D = Dual response

**Fourth letter**
O = None
P = Simple
M = Multi-programmable
R = Adaptive rate pacing

**Fig. 1.2** Pacemaker nomenclature. For example: DDDR = atrial and ventricular sensing and pacing with adaptive rate response; VVI = pacing wire triggers ventricular contraction. Any spontaneous electrical activity is sensed in the ventricle and inhibits pacemaker firing.

## Indications for perioperative pacing

- Acute anterior MI
- First-degree heart block combined with bifascicular block or left bundle branch block
- Acute MI with Mobitz type II
- Third-degree heart block
- Sick sinus syndrome
- Faulty permanent pacemaker.

### Intraoperative risks

Rate responsive pacemakers sense electrical activity or vibration around the pacing box and cause a tachycardia in response. Thus, shivering may cause a tachycardia. Fasciculations from suxamethonium are too transient to cause a tachycardia, but there is a case report of a pacemaker that stopped firing following administration of suxamethonium.

Pacemakers that sense blood temperature to control rate may trigger a tachycardia as a hypothermic patient is rewarmed. Those that measure respiratory rate by sensing thoracic impedance and adjust heart rate accordingly can also trigger a tachycardia if the ventilator is set at a high respiratory rate.

Risks associated with $K^+$ are:

- hypokalaemia – risk of loss of pacing capture
- hyperkalaemia – risk of VT or VF.

### Diathermy

Diathermy current risks reprogramming the pacemaker (not AOO, VOO), causing microshock and inducing VF.

Bipolar diathermy is the safest. If unipolar, mount the diathermy plate away from the pacemaker and use short bursts of minimum current. Do not use within 15 cm of pacing box.

Application of a magnet over a non-programmable ventricular-inhibited pacemaker (VVI) reverts it to asynchronous mode (VOO). Application of a magnet over a programmable pacemaker increases the risk of reprogramming, but it will remain in an asynchronous mode until the magnet is removed, when the reprogrammed mode will take over. Do not use any magnets unless the pacemaker reprograms during surgery.

## AUTOMATIC IMPLANTABLE CARDIOVERTER DEFIBRILLATORS (AICDs)

Implanted in patients with drug-resistant malignant ventricular arrhythmias.

Reduce 1-year mortality from 66 to 9%. AICDs consist of a lead electrode system for sensing, pacing and delivery of shocks for cardioversion/ defibrillation and a control unit consisting of a pulse generator, micro-processor and battery. Modern devices also act as DDD pacemakers.

- In general, all AICDs should be deactivated with a programming device before surgery. In modern AICDs, the anti-bradycardia function can be left activated. Effects of magnets are not consistent between devices, but newer AICDs are inhibited by a magnet.
- Electromagnetic interference, e.g. diathermy, can inhibit the AICD or cause shock discharge. If used, place the diathermy plate as far as possible from the generator. Bipolar diathermy generates less current and is therefore preferential.
- External defibrillation pads should be placed prior to surgery. External defibrillation does not damage an AICD. If an AICD discharges, only a mild electric shock will be felt by anyone touching the patient.

## ANAESTHETIC CONSIDERATIONS FOR VALVULAR HEART DISEASE

### Aortic stenosis

Becomes symptomatic when the normal valve area of 3 cm$^2$ is reduced by 25%. Gradient > 70 mmHg is severe (= 0.6 cm$^2$). There is a fixed output, dependent upon rate. Low CO and poorly compliant ventricle. Ischaemia occurs even with normal coronaries. Atrial contraction is important to fill a poorly compliant LV. Tachycardia is poorly tolerated because reduced time for LV filling reduces ejection time and diastolic time during which coronary perfusion occurs. Bradycardia reduces CO and therefore BP. Aortic diastolic pressure must be maintained to preserve coronary blood flow. Fall in SVR is poorly tolerated. Therefore, maintain both pre- and afterload and avoid regional techniques.

### Aortic regurgitation

Causes a dilated, overloaded and failing LV. Low aortic diastolic pressure impairs coronary perfusion. Slight tachycardia reduces regurgitant time and keeps LV small (Laplace's law), thereby improving LV efficiency. A slight reduction in SVR reduces regurgitation but may reduce coronary perfusion pressure.

### Mitral stenosis

A value area < 1 cm$^2$ is severe. Poor LV filling and a fixed output dependent upon rate. Low CO is worsened by tachydysrhythmia. Rapid heart rate reduces diastolic time for ventricular filling and thus reduces CO so bradycardia is beneficial. There is a high PVP (risk of pulmonary oedema, avoid overtransfusion) but keep the patient well filled. Fall in SVR is poorly tolerated. Consider inotropes and pulmonary vasodilators.

**Mitral regurgitation**

Often well tolerated; PVP remains low. Slight tachycardia and reduction in SVR reduce regurgitation. Ischaemia is not usually a problem. General anaesthesia is usually well tolerated unless pulmonary hypertension has developed, when inotropic support may also be indicated.

**Hypertrophic obstructive cardiomyopathy (HOCM)**

Autosomal dominant with variable penetrance. Variable subaortic obstruction and impaired diastolic function. Try to avoid drugs that depress LV function. Increase pre- and afterload, maintain sinus rhythm and avoid excessive tachy/bradycardia. Good LV function. Ventricular arrhythmias are common. Depression of myocardial contractility reduces outflow obstruction. β-agonists increase outflow obstruction.

**Shunts**

- *Right-to-left shunt* (Fallot's tetralogy, Eisenmenger's syndrome). Risk from microemboli, LVF and cyanosis. Shunt worsens with ↑ PVR or ↓ SVR. Keep lung inflation pressures low.
- *Left-to-right shunt* (ASD, VSD, PDA). Shunt worsens with ↓ PVR or ↑ SVR. IPPV increases PVR.

**Ischaemic heart disease**

Rate pressure product (RPP) = heart rate × systolic pressure. Aim to maintain value below 12 000.

Decrease preload (wall tension) and maintain afterload. Slight decrease in both contractility and rate can be beneficial by reducing work if there is good LV function. Myocardial depression may improve oxygenation unless severe IHD or aortic stenosis.

If ischaemia occurs, decrease heart rate (β-blockers, calcium-channel blockers), increase ventricular volume (GTN) and increase afterload.

## ENDOCARDITIS PROPHYLAXIS

### Indications

Not indicated for physiological, functional or innocent heart murmurs, rheumatic fever, pacemakers, dental procedures not likely to cause gingival bleeding or Caesarean section.

**INFECTIVE ENDOCARDITIS PROPHYLAXIS** Endocarditis Working Party of the British Society for Antimicrobial Chemotherapy 1997. As summarized in the *British National Formulary* 1999, No. 37 (5.1). For updates see subsequent editions.

*Dental procedures under GA*
Amoxycillin:   p.o. – 3 g 4 h preoperatively, then 3 g after procedure
i.v. – 1 g at induction, then 500 mg p.o. 6 h later.

*Special risk (patients with prosthetic valve or history of endocarditis)*
Amoxycillin 1 g i.v. + gentamicin 120 mg i.v. at induction, then amoxycillin 500 mg 6 h later.

*Penicillin-allergic patients*
Vancomycin 1 g i.v. 1 h preoperatively + gentamicin 120 mg i.v. at induction
*or*   clindamycin 300 mg i.v. 15 min preoperatively, then 150 mg i.v. 6 h later.

*Upper respiratory tract procedures*
As for dental procedures.

*Genitourinary/gastrointestinal/obstetric/gynaecological procedures*
As for special risk patients.

**References**

Badner N H, Knill R L, Brown J E, Novick T V, Gelb A W 1998 Myocardial infarction after noncardiac surgery. Anesthesiology 88: 572–578

Bloomfield P, Bowler G M R 1989 Anaesthetic management of the patient with a permanent pacemaker. Anaesthesia 44: 42–46

Boldt J 1998 Perioperative management of patients with impaired left ventricular function. Current Opinion in Anaesthesiology 11: 315–319

British National Formulary 1999 Infective endocarditis prophylaxis. BNF No. 37 (5.1)

Clarke M 1993 Cardiac pacemakers. Prescribers' Journal 33: 103–111

Coriat P 1998 Reducing cardiovascular risk in patients undergoing non-cardiac surgery. Current Opinion in Anaesthesiology 11: 311–314

Detsky A S, Abrams H B, McLaughlin J R 1986 Predicting cardiac complications in patients undergoing non-cardiac surgery. Journal of General Internal Medicine 1: 211–219

Edwards N D, Reilly C S 1994 Detection of perioperative myocardial ischaemia. Review. British Journal of Anaesthesia 72: 104–115

Goldman L 1995 Cardiac risk in noncardiac surgery: an update. Anesthesia and Analgesia 80: 810–820

Goldman L, Caldera D L, Nussbaum S R et al 1977 Multifactorial index of cardiac risk in non-cardiac surgical procedures. New England Journal of Medicine 297: 845–850

Juste R N, Lawson A D, Soni N 1996 Minimising cardiac anaesthetic risk: the tortoise or the hare? Anaesthesia 51: 255–262

Kam P C 1997 Anaesthetic management of a patient with an automatic implantable cardioverter defibrillator in situ. British Journal of Anaesthesia 78: 102–106

Khan S S, Denton T, Matloff J M 1994 Long-term survival after coronary artery bypass grafting. Current Opinion in Cardiology 9: 692–703

Mahar L J, Steen P A, Tinker J H, Vliestra R E, Smith H C, Pluth J R 1978 Perioperative myocardial infarction in patients with coronary artery disease with and without aorto-coronary bypass grafts. Thoracic and Cardiovascular Surgery 76: 533–537

Mangano D T, Browner W S, Hollenberg M, London M J, Tubau J F, Tateo I N 1990 Association of perioperative myocardial ischaemia with cardiac morbidity and mortality in men undergoing non-cardiac surgery. The study of the Perioperative Ischaemia Research Group. New England Journal of Medicine 323: 1781–1788

Myers W O, Blackstone E H, Davis K, Foster E D, Kaiser G C 1999 CASS registry: Long term surgical survival. Journal of the American College of Cardiology 33: 488–498

Prause G, Ratzenhofer-Comenda B, Pierer G, Smolle-Jüttner F, Glanzer H, Smolle J 1997 Can ASA grade or Goldman's cardiac risk index predict peri-operative mortality? A study of 16,227 patients. Anaesthesia 52: 203–206

Rao T L K, Jacobs K H, El-Etr A A 1983 Reinfarction following anesthesia in patients with myocardial infarction. Anesthesiology 59: 449–505

Reiz S, Balfors E, Sorensen M B, Ariola S, Friedman A, Truedsson H 1983 Isoflurane – a powerful coronary vasodilator in patients with coronary artery disease. Anesthesiology 59: 91–97

Shah K B, Kleinman B S, Rao T L K, Jacobs H K, Mestan K, Schaafsma M 1990 Angina and other risk factors in patients with cardiac diseases undergoing noncardiac operations. Anesthesia and Analgesia 70: 240–247

Slogoff S, Keats A S 1986 Does perioperative myocardial ischemia lead to postoperative myocardial infarction? Anesthesiology 62: 539–542

Slogoff S, Keats A S, Dear W E et al 1991 Steal-prone coronary anatomy and myocardial ischemia associated with four primary anesthetic agents in humans. Anesthesia and Analgesia 72: 22–27

Tarhan S, Moffitt E A, Taylor W F, Giuliani E R 1972 Myocardial infarction after general anesthesia. Journal of the American Medical Association 220: 1451–1454

Tuman K J, McCarthy R J, Spiess B D, DaValle M, Dabir R, Ivankovich A D 1989 Does choice of anesthetic agent significantly affect outcome after coronary artery surgery? Anesthesiology 70: 189–198

Walker J M, Cooper J 1993 Modern methods for assessing cardiac function. In: Kaufman L (ed) Anaesthesia Review 10. Churchill Livingstone, London, p 1–14

# CARDIAC SURGERY

## GENERAL

There are 20 000 cardiac operations per annum in the UK. Surgical mortality is only 1–2% for low-risk patients.

In uncomplicated cases, patients are generally rewarmed and extubated within 3–4 h of the completion of surgery (fast-tracking).

### Risk factors for major postoperative complications

- Previous heart surgery
- Low cardiac output
- Reduced LV ejection fraction
- Peripheral vascular disease
- Renal failure
- Preoperative IPPV
- Age.

New ischaemia occurring prior to cardiopulmonary bypass (CPB) increases the risk of perioperative MI in patients undergoing CABG (Slogoff 1985).

## CARDIOPULMONARY BYPASS

### Drug pharmacokinetics

- Haemodilution on bypass decreases plasma drug concentration but is counterbalanced by reduced total protein binding due to decreased plasma protein concentration.
- Decreased flow into peripheral vascular beds results in decreased drug uptake by peripheral tissues and decreased mobilization of previously stored drugs out of peripheral tissues.
- Decreased liver perfusion and decreased hepatic metabolism.

Therefore, there is little change in most drug concentrations during bypass. Neuromuscular blockers have a small $V_D$ and therefore are greatly diluted on bypass and additional perioperative doses may be needed.

Plasma levels of fentanyl rise on rewarming and after separation from CPB due to reperfusion of peripheral compartments and washout of drug bound in lung.

### Bypass circuit

A cardiopulmonary bypass circuit is illustrated in Figure 1.3.

### Advantages of membrane over bubble oxygenators

- Less blood trauma and complement activation
- Fewer microemboli
- Ability to regulate $O_2$ and $CO_2$ separately
- Less neuroendocrine stress response.

### Pump

Most centres now use non-pulsatile flow. However, pulsatile pumps cause less neuroendocrine stress response.

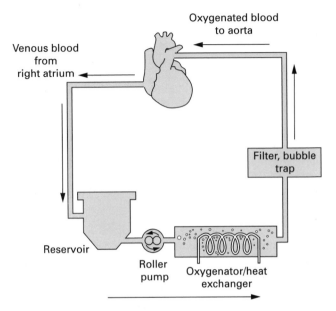

**Fig. 1.3** Membrane oxygenator circuit.

Lower bypass pressure results in less mechanical damage to blood, reduces aortic trauma at the clamp site and allows use of smaller arterial and venous catheters. However, higher pressures (60–90 mmHg) avoid loss of CNS autoregulation (occurs at < 50 mmHg) with less postoperative neurological dysfunction.

Pump flow rate is set at $2.4 \, 1/m^2$, pressure at 40–80 mmHg; 99% $O_2 \pm$ 1–5% $CO_2$.

Variable priming volume is 2 000 ml. Usually primed with crystalloid but blood is used for paediatric bypass. Priming without blood decreases haematocrit to 20–25%, which offsets the increase in viscosity caused by hypothermia.

### Cardioplegia solution

This solution contains 15–30 mEq/l $K^+$. It may also contain:

- citrate (to bind $Ca^{2+}$)
- GTN (improves distribution)
- glucose and insulin (energy for cells)
- mannitol (decreases cellular swelling)
- bicarbonate (increases intracellular shift of $K^+$).

## ANAESTHESIA FOR CARDIAC SURGERY

### Premedication

Benzodiazepines and opiates. (Anxiety increases endogenous catecholamines and causes coronary vasospasm.) Heavy premedication may cause hypoventilation and hypoxaemia so consider starting oxygen at time of premedication.

### Monitoring

*ECG.* Either CM5 or combinations including lead II (inferolateral wall) or posterior wall (oesophageal lead).

*BP.* Radial arterial line. Internal mammary artery dissection can dampen ipsilateral arterial line trace.

*CVP.* Monitoring through triple-lumen line.

*Pulmonary artery catheter.* Controversial but may improve outcome in selected patients.

*Other.* Urinary catheter and core temperature (nasopharyngeal, oesophageal, tympanic).

*TOE.* Detects wall motion abnormalities and is a more sensitive indicator of myocardial ischaemia than ECG or invasive pressure monitoring.

### Induction

Thiopentone, propofol, midazolam and etomidate have all been used safely. Propofol and thiopentone may cause more hypotension on induction, especially if there is poor LV function. High-dose opiate technique (50–100 $\mu$g/kg fentanyl) requires postoperative IPPV but improves perioperative cardiovascular stability.

### Intubation

Avoid pressor response which worsens ischaemia by the use of opiates, β-blockers, clonidine or lignocaine. Non-depolarizing relaxants reduce chest wall rigidity caused by high-dose opioids.

### Maintenance

Isoflurane/desflurane cause least myocardial depression. All volatiles decrease myocardial oxygen demand but also decrease coronary perfusion pressure. Unlike enflurane or halothane, isoflurane increases coronary blood flow if diastolic > 40 mmHg.

Vecuronium avoids CVS side-effects present in other neuromuscular blockers.

Sternotomy and aortic manipulation cause intense stimulation. Further increments of fentanyl may be needed.

If there is no CNS disease, a MAP of 35–40 mmHg is adequate when patient is hypothermic.

Avoid $N_2O$ because of risk of air bubble emboli expanding, especially dangerous with right-to-left shunt. Aim for a haematocrit of 20–30%.

### Anticoagulation

Use 3 mg/kg heparin (= 300 U/kg) which accelerates antithrombin III to neutralize clotting factors II, X, XI, XII and XIII. Aim for activated clotting time (ACT) > 400. (Celite in test tube at 37°C triggers clotting.) Normal ACT = 120–150 s. Half-life of heparin = 100 min.

Reverse heparin with protamine at 1 mg/100 U heparin. Protamine may increase PVR causing right ventricular failure. Also causes hypotension by binding to $Ca^{2+}$.

### Acid–base management

- *pH-stat approach* – arterial blood gases corrected for temperature
- *Alpha-stat approach* – arterial blood gases not corrected for temperature.

pH-stat results in relative hypercarbia and acidaemia which increases cerebral blood flow and may increase the risk of cerebral emboli. pH-stat management may be optimal for children undergoing deep hypothermic circulatory arrest, because it increases the rate of brain cooling and results in slower exhaustion of brain $O_2$ stores, providing better CNS protection. Alpha-stat management, however, may cause less CNS dysfunction in adults undergoing moderately hypothermic CPB because of the formation of fewer cerebral emboli.

### CABG patients

*Good LV function.* Main problem is hyperdynamic circulation. Avoid tachycardia and hypertension. Aim to decrease myocardial work, e.g. with volatiles, β-blockers.

*Poor LV function.* Main problem is cardiac failure. Avoid myocardial depression, i.e. high-dose opioids. Use volatiles sparingly and maintain myocardial performance. May require inotrope infusion to wean from bypass which is continued in the immediate postoperative period.

### Sequence of events in CABG surgery

*Anaesthesia.* Invasive monitoring and induction of general anaesthesia.

*Pre-bypass.* Surgical incision and sternal splitting. Disconnect ventilator during sternal splitting, allowing lungs to deflate, reducing risk of damage from the sternal saw.

Heparin is administered into a central vein and ACT checked prior to commencing CPB.

Pericardial stretching during cardiac manipulation may impair venous return and lower BP.

Nitrous oxide is discontinued to avoid enlargement of any air emboli (or not used at all).

*Establishment of bypass.* The aortic cannula is first inserted through a purse string suture into the ascending aorta to allow infusion of volume from the bypass reservoir if the BP drops. The venous cannula is then inserted into the right atrium or superior and inferior venae cavae.

CPB is then initiated. Ventilation is stopped when full bypass is established. The aorta is clamped proximal to the cannula and cardioplegia solution infused into the aortic root where it perfuses the coronary arteries causing asystole (Fig. 1.4).

Hypothermia to 30°C is achieved by cooling the blood through a heat exchanger to reduce myocardial and cerebral oxygen requirements.

*Coronary artery surgery.* The vein grafts are anastomosed to the diseased coronary arteries, the distal anastomosis being performed first to enable administration of cardioplegia solution distal to the stenosis.

Rewarming is begun once the final distal anastomosis is complete. The aorta is unclamped, which results in washout of cardioplegia solution from the myocardium. The proximal vein graft anastomoses are completed.

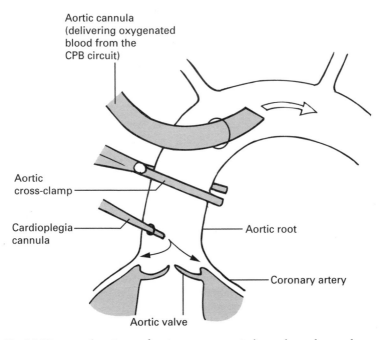

**Fig. 1.4** Diagram of aortic root showing arrangement of cannulae and cross-clamp for administration of cardioplegia.

*Weaning from bypass.* Once the heart is rewarmed, it begins to fibrillate. Internal paddles are used to defibrillate the heart if sinus rhythm has not begun spontaneously. Lungs are re-expanded to peak pressure of 30–40 cmH$_2$O with 100% O$_2$ and IPPV is commenced.

Flow through the venous cannulae is reduced to allow the heart to refill and spontaneous cardiac output subsequently increases. Once adequate filling and output are established, the venous and then arterial cannulae are clamped.

*Post-bypass management.* If the patient remains hypotensive, give fluid challenge in 50–100 ml increments from venous reservoir. Further fluid continues to be needed because of continued rewarming of vascular beds causing vasodilation, changing ventricular diastolic compliance and continued bleeding before heparin reversal. If hypotension persists despite adequate filling, inotropes may be required.

Once adequate output is established, venous and arterial cannulae are removed and the effects of heparin are reversed with protamine.

### Weaning from bypass

Difficulty occurs usually due to ischaemia following aortic cross-clamping or myocardial stunning.

Causes of failure to wean from cardiopulmonary bypass are:

- Ischaemia
  — graft failure – clot, air bubble, kink
  — inadequate coronary blood flow – coronary spasm, inadequate coronary perfusion pressure or flow
- Valve failure
- Inadequate gas exchange
  — low $F_iO_2$, bronchospasm, pulmonary oedema
- Hypovolaemia
- Reperfusion injury
- Electrolyte or acid–base imbalance
- Negatively inotropic drugs
- Pre-existing LV failure.

### Intra-aortic balloon-pump counterpulsation

This is used as a mechanical assist device for the failing myocardium. The intra-aortic balloon is placed in the aortic arch/early descending thoracic aorta via the femoral artery so that the tip lies distal to left subclavian artery, but is not occluding renal arteries (Fig. 1.5).

- *Diastolic effects.* Expands during diastole, increasing aortic diastolic pressure and therefore coronary perfusion pressure.
- *Systolic effects.* Sudden decrease in balloon volume prior to systole

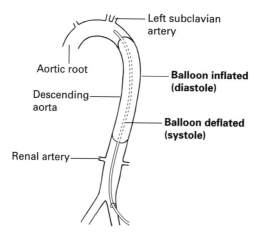

**Fig. 1.5** Intra-aortic balloon pump showing inflated and deflated position.

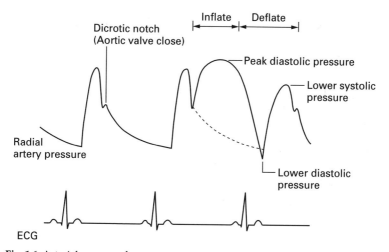

**Fig. 1.6** Arterial pressure changes using an intra-aortic balloon pump.

decreases systemic vascular resistance, afterload and myocardial work, and increases cardiac output, cerebral and renal perfusion (Fig. 1.6).

### Postoperative complications

*Cardiac.* Avoid postoperative hypertension, common in fit young patients with good LV function or those with pre-existing hypertension.

Worsened by inadequate analgesia/sedation and hypothermia. Often due to neuroendocrine responses to CPB (renin–angiotensin activation).

Low-output syndrome is associated with poor preoperative LV function, intraoperative damage and effects of bypass.

*Respiratory.* Infection and sputum retention are relatively common. Cardiogenic and non-cardiogenic pulmonary oedema may develop at any time in the postoperative period.

*Neurological.* 2–6% of patients have neurological damage following CPB. Usually slight (neuropsychiatric) rather than gross. Cause of subtle damage unknown but may include micro/macroemboli (particularly common at insertion of aortic cannula and initiation of bypass), air bubbles, effect of non-pulsatile flow, inadequate cerebral perfusion or hyperglycaemia during neuroischaemia. Known risk factors include age, prolonged bypass, severe atherosclerosis and hypertension.

*Renal.* Risk of prerenal failure and failure from direct tubular damage, e.g. myoglobin, antibiotics.

*Haematology.* Haemorrhage is a major complication, usually due to platelet dysfunction. Antifibrinolytic agents (e.g. aprotinin, tranexamic acid, aminocaproic acid) preserve the adhesive capacity of platelets which are altered by circulation through the CPB circuit, and may reduce postoperative blood loss. Platelet transfusions and FFP may be needed if bleeding persists.


## NEUROLOGICAL MONITORING AND PROTECTION

### Monitoring

*Unmodified EEG.* Some evidence for correlation with outcome.

*Processed EEG.* Easier to interpret.

*Transcranial Doppler.* Research tool. Correlates with neuroinsults.

*Jugular bulb $O_2$ saturation.* Desaturation is common but significance is not known.

*Regional cerebral blood flow.* Research tool.

*Cerebral oximetry.* Non-invasive and only monitors small region.


### Protection

*Physiological.* Pulsatile flow, hypothermia, alpha-stat management, euglycaemia, filtration of arterial blood to remove microemboli.

*Pharmacological.*

Barbiturates – may protect in high doses (> 30 mg/kg) but conflicting studies.

Steroids – no evidence for benefit.

Free radical scavengers (e.g. superoxide dysmutase) and calcium channel blockers remain experimental.

### References

Doolan L, Georghi S 1994 Fast track recovery after cardiac surgery. Current Opinion in Anaesthesiology 7: 73–79

Goldsack C, Berridge J C 1996 Acid-base management during cardiopulmonary bypass. Current trends in the United Kingdom. Anaesthesia 51: 396–398

Hensley F A, Martin D E (eds) 1990 The practice of cardiac anaesthesia. Little, Brown, Boston

Kingsley C 1995 Cardiac anaesthesia. Current Opinion in Anaesthesiology 8: 33–67

Lampa M, Ramsay J 1999 Anesthetic implications of new surgical approaches to myocardial revascularization. Current Opinion in Anaesthesiology 12: 3–8

Rady M Y, Ryan T, Starr N J 1998 Perioperative determinants of morbidity and mortality in elderly patients undergoing cardiac surgery. Critical Care Medicine 26: 225–235

Slogoff S, Keats A S 1985 Does perioperative myocardial ischemia lead to postopertive myocardial infarction? Anesthesiology 62: 107–114

Urzua J, Lema G, Canessa R et al 1999 Cardiopulmonary bypass: new strategies for weaning from cardiopulmonary bypass. Current Opinion in Anaesthesiology 12: 21–27

# MAJOR VASCULAR SURGERY

## ABDOMINAL AORTIC ANEURYSM

### Pathogenesis

Destruction of elastin in the media results in abnormal widening of all three layers of the vessel wall. Genetic predisposition, acquired risk factors (smoking, hypertension, atherosclerosis), defective and decreased elastin. If > 6 cm, 50% rupture in 10 years.

Associated pathology common:

- hypertension (50%)
- COAD (30%)
- diabetes (10%)
- chronic renal failure (10%).

### Mortality

- Elective: < 5%
- Emergency: > 50%.

### Anaesthetic aims

- Maintain cardiovascular stability
- Blood replacement

- Maintain renal function
- Temperature control.

## Anaesthetic management

*Preoperative.* Mostly elderly patients. Full cardiac work-up for elective patients. Assess severity and treat other coexisting diseases. Systolic BP at presentation is the most important predictor of survival.

*Fluid resuscitation.* There is some evidence that aggressive preoperative fluid resuscitation may increase mortality by accelerating bleeding, increasing the risk of clot dislodgement and causing a dilutional coagulopathy. Bleeding makes surgery more difficult and distended veins (IVC and left renal vein) are at greater risk of rupture. It is suggested that the MAP should be maintained at ≈ 65 mmHg until the aorta has been clamped, after which blood, FFP and platelets should be given to restore haemodynamic parameters. All fluids should be warmed.

*Preparation.* Prepare and drape the patient in the operating theatre. Induction may result in cardiovascular collapse as the tamponading effect of abdominal muscle tone is lost and surgeons must therefore be ready to start immediately.

Adequate analgesia with small doses of i.v. opioids prevents hyperventilation, hypertension, increased endocrine stress response and increased oxygen consumption.

*Induction.* Ketamine may be of benefit with severe haemorrhagic shock but increases cardiac work, possibly precipitating ischaemia. Induction with combined opioid (e.g. fentanyl) and hypnotic (e.g. midazolam) provides the best CVS stability. Thiopentone and propofol may cause CVS collapse if the patient is haemodynamically unstable.

Commence GTN infusion if known IHD or ischaemic ECG changes.

*Maintenance of anaesthesia.*

*General anaesthesia.* Nitrous oxide–oxygen–relaxant technique and nitrous oxide–oxygen–relaxant–volatile technique alone are associated with depressed ventricular performance and hyperdynamic circulation. Addition of high-dose fentanyl maintains cardiac function and is not associated with hyperdynamic changes; however, it requires postoperative ventilation. Isoflurane is relatively stable on the cardiovascular system and has been shown to maintain a higher GFR than halothane during aneurysm surgery.

*Combined regional and general anaesthesia.* Regional anaesthesia combined with a light GA may reduce operative mortality and postoperative morbidity. Epidural followed by heparinization does not increase the risk of epidural haematoma. May vasodilate stenotic coronary arteries. It improves regional blood flow and maintains GFR although there is no evidence for improved postoperative creatinine clearance. Increases perioperative fluid requirements in elective surgery by 25–50%.

### Haemodynamic changes

*Mesenteric traction syndrome.* Causes flushing, hypotension and tachycardia due to prostacyclin and $PGF_{1\alpha}$ release. Treat with fluids and vasoconstrictors. Abolished if patient on NSAIDs.

*Aortic cross-clamping.* Location of clamp determines degree of cardiovascular stress and increase in MAP. Increased afterload increases myocardial wall tension and may worsen LV function. Infrarenal clamping reduces stroke volume by 15–35%, increases SVR by 40% and reduces renal cortical blood flow. There is increased perfusion proximal to the clamp and anaerobic metabolism distal to the clamp.

Decrease afterload with vasodilators. Nitroglycerine infusion at 0.25–5 $\mu$g/kg per min reduces myocardial wall tension by reducing pre- and afterload, and may maintain normal myocardial blood flow, decrease arterial blood pressure, lower SVR and reduce myocardial oxygen consumption.

Lumbar epidurals attenuate the increased SVR occurring with cross-clamping.

*Declamping.* Hypoxic vasodilation, sequestration of blood in pelvic and lower limb capacitance vessels, hypovolaemia and release of vasoactive and myocardial depressant metabolites (lactate, $K^+$) cause hypotension. Severity of hypotension is related to cross-clamp time and the speed at which the clamp is released. Fluid loading until PCWP is 3–5 mmHg above preoperative value prior to declamping reduces hypotension. Severe hypotension may necessitate partial reclamping. Epidurals may exaggerate hypotension after declamping but tend to produce greater CVS stability.

*Postoperative.* Ventilate until warm, well-filled and cardiovascularly stable. Correct any clotting abnormalities. Monitor renal function closely. Good analgesia is important. Postoperative complications are common and include MI (40%), respiratory failure (40%), renal failure (35%), bleeding (15%) and stroke (5%).

## Arterial supply to the spinal cord

The major arterial supply to the spinal cord is a single anterior spinal artery lying in the anterior median fissure of the cord and two posterior spinal arteries located just medial to the dorsal roots. The anterior spinal artery is fed from several sources (Figs 1.7 and 1.8):

- $C_1$–$T_4$: vertebral, thyrocervical and costocervical arteries
- $T_4$–$T_9$: intercostal arterial branches
- below $T_9$: artery of Adamkiewicz which arises from the aorta between $T_9$ and $L_2$.

The anterior spinal artery supplies the anterior two-thirds of the cord and anastomoses with both posterior spinal arteries.

*Spinal cord injury.* Impaired flow in this vessel from cross-clamping results in cord ischaemia and paraplegia. Motor damage is greater than sensory damage. Poor recovery. There is a 40% incidence of paraplegia

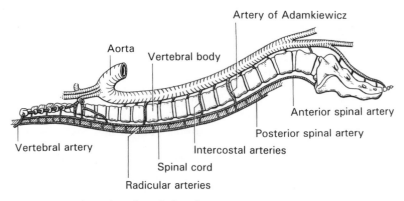

Fig. 1.7 Arterial supply to the spinal cord.

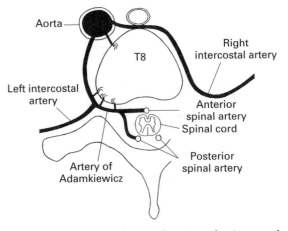

Fig. 1.8 Cross-section of the spine showing the relationship between the artery of Adamkiewicz and the anterior spinal artery. (Reproduced from Djurberg & Haddad 1995.)

following emergency repair of a dissecting aneurysm compared with 0.1% for elective infrarenal procedures. Attempts to protect cord function include:

- Avoiding glucose-containing solutions
- Monitoring of cord function with SSEPs
- Maintaining distal aortic pressure with shunts
- 3 ml 1% preservative-free epidural papaverine has been shown to protect the cord during prolonged aortic cross-clamping by dilating anterior spinal arteries
- Cross-clamping causes increased CSF pressure, further decreasing cord

perfusion. Lumbar drain insertion in an attempt to decrease CSF pressure has shown variable results in reducing cord damage
- Steroids, barbiturates and superoxide dismutase.

### Renal function

There is a high risk of renal failure due to hypovolaemia, renal atherosclerosis, changes in renal perfusion with cross-clamping and nephrotoxic drugs.

Optimize fluid and electrolyte balance and consider mannitol, frusemide and renal-dose dopamine. Prophylactic administration of mannitol (25–50 ml 25% solution) prior to cross-clamping may protect against renal cortical ischaemia by several mechanisms:

- osmotic diuresis
- volume expansion, increasing renal blood flow and GFR
- haemodilution
- free radical scavenger activity
- atrial expansion, suppressing renin release
- reducing endothelial cell swelling.

## CAROTID ARTERY SURGERY

Patients with severe carotid artery stenosis (> 70%) have a better outcome with surgery. Benefits for moderate stenosis (30–69%) are unclear. Surgery for carotid artery obstruction may be carried out if patient is having transient ischaemic attacks:

- 80% TIAs from carotid territory
- 20% TIAs from vertebrobasilar territory.

Vessels distal to a stenosis are maximally dilated and further flow can only come via collaterals from the Circle of Willis. Thus, these patients are extremely sensitive to hypotension. If non-diseased areas vasodilate, a 'reverse steal' may occur, reducing collateral flow to poststenotic areas.

### Preoperative

A detailed preoperative neurological examination is needed to enable assessment of the postoperative neurological state. Also examine the cardiovascular system to assess the degree of atherosclerosis. Diabetes and hypertension are common. Stop smoking.

### Anaesthetic techniques

*Premedication.* Short-acting only to prevent prolonged postoperative somnolence and allow early assessment of neurological function. Short-acting benzodiazepine is suitable.

*Monitoring*

*CVS.* Potential for large swings in heart rate and BP due to manipulation of carotid baroreceptors. Consider invasive BP monitoring.

*Neurological.* The awake patient allows continuous assessment of multiple levels of neurological function, but this is less sensitive if the patient is sedated. Also consider EEG, SSEPs, transcranial Doppler or intracarotid xenon washout curve to measure cerebral blood flow (CBF), and internal carotid artery distal stump pressure > 50 mmHg (but poor correlation with regional CBF).

*Regional technique ($C_2$–$C_4$).* Deep and superficial cervical plexus block or cervical extradural anaesthesia. Provides excellent haemodynamic stability resulting in a very low incidence of perioperative MI. However, oxygenation and ventilation are poorly controlled and hypoxaemia/hypercarbia may necessitate intubation during surgery.

*General anaesthesia.* No specific technique has been shown to be of any advantage. Pre-oxygenate. Induction with thiopentone followed by vecuronium or atracurium. Avoid pressor response to intubation (topical/ i.v. lignocaine, opioids, esmolol, nitroprusside etc). Oxygen–air mixture + isoflurane may provide more EEG depression than halothane or enflurane for a given blood flow. Animals pretreated with barbiturates show protection from ischaemia, but there is no evidence suggesting thiopentone protects in humans.

Swings in BP are best treated with changes in volatile concentration, because use of short-acting haemodynamic drugs (nitroprusside, nitroglycerine, adrenaline etc.) is associated with greater myocardial ischaemia.

Hyperglycaemia during ischaemia may worsen the neurological outcome by increasing anaerobic metabolism. Patients with poorly controlled blood glucose following a stroke have a worse outcome. Therefore, although no outcome studies have proven the risks of hyperglycaemia in carotid artery surgery, maintain tight control of perioperative glucose in diabetic patients.

## Postoperative

Avoid postoperative hypertension and hypercapnia, which increase risk of cerebral oedema and haemorrhage because maximally vasodilated areas are unable to autoregulate. Hypocapnia may cause cerebral ischaemia.

Wound haematoma may cause airway obstruction. Laryngeal and hypoglossal nerve injury has been documented. Myocardial infarction is the commonest cause of perioperative mortality.

### References

Brimacombe J, Berry A 1993 A review of anaesthesia for ruptured abdominal aortic aneurysm with special emphasis on preclamping fluid resuscitation. Anaesthesia and Intensive Care 21: 311–323

Colombo J A, Tuman K J 1998 Peripheral vascular surgery: does anesthetic management affect outcome? Current Opinion in Anaesthesiology 11: 23–27

Djurberg H, Haddad M 1995 Anterior spinal artery syndrome. Anaesthesia 50: 345–348

Garrioch M A, Fitch W 1993 Anaesthesia for carotid artery surgery. British Journal of Anaesthesia 71: 569–579

Leigh J, Manara A R 1992 Vascular surgery. Current Anaesthesia and Critical Care 3: 207–211

Lineberger C K, Lubarsky D A 1998 Anesthesia for carotid endarterectomy. Current Opinion in Anaesthesiology 11: 479–484

Sansome A, Norman J 1999 Monitoring spinal cord function during aortic surgery: can we reduce the risks? British Journal of Anaesthesia 82: 315–318

# HYPOTENSIVE ANAESTHESIA

This was first described by Gardner in 1946 who used controlled haemorrhage to induce hypotension. It was introduced clinically by Griffiths & Gillie in 1948 and Enderby in 1950. There was initial concern over high morbidity and mortality, but recent studies suggest that when carefully performed, the technique is reasonably safe. East Grinstead reported a mortality rate of 1 in 4 128 cases.

## Benefits

- Improves surgical field, e.g. ENT, maxillofacial and plastic surgery
- Reduces blood loss
- Reduces risk of cerebral aneurysm rupture during clipping.

## Contraindications

- Hypertension – BP may be extremely labile
- Ischaemic heart disease – hypotension reduces myocardial perfusion
- Severe cerebrovascular disease
- Respiratory disease – vasodilating drugs abolish hypoxic pulmonary vasoconstriction, making shunting worse. Reversible airways obstruction may be made worse by the use of β-blockers or ganglion-blocking drugs
- Diabetes – ganglion blockade impairs stress-induced gluconeogenesis. β-blockers potentiate hypoglycaemia
- Hypovolaemia, anaemia
- Renal and hepatic disease
- Pregnancy.

## EFFECTS OF HYPOTENSION

*CVS.* Reduced diastolic pressure reduces coronary perfusion pressure.

*Respiratory.* Greatly increased physiological dead space, $\uparrow$ V/Q (ventilation/perfusion) mismatch and $\downarrow$ FRC. Volatile agents may further impair hypoxic pulmonary vasoconstriction. May need $F_iO_2 > 0.3$ to maintain arterial saturation.

*CNS.* Loss of cerebral autoregulation < 50 mmHg. Risk of ischaemia in the presence of hypocapnia.

*Renal.* Poor GFR below 50 mmHg with risk of renal failure.

## TECHNIQUES OF INDUCED HYPOTENSION

### Pre-medication

Avoid atropine. Ensure patient is well sedated. Consider droperidol/ chlorpromazine.

### Induction

Spray cords. Thiopentone, fentanyl and neuromuscular blocker (not pancuronium which causes tachycardia – tubocurare is often used because of its hypotensive effects). Maintenance with isoflurane/$N_2O$ and a high $F_iO_2$.

### Posture

Head-up tilt reduces arterial and venous pressure in tissues higher than the heart.

### IPPV

Positive intrathoracic pressure reduces venous return and thus cardiac output. Reflex vasoconstriction then normally maintains the BP but ganglion blockade or $\beta$-blockers may abolish this compensatory reflex. Positive end-expiratory pressure (PEEP) produces a further reduction in venous return and BP. Hyperventilation augments hypotension.

### Volatiles

Halothane > enflurane causes peripheral vasodilation and myocardial depression. Isoflurane has little effect on myocardial contractility and hypotension is a result of peripheral vasodilation. Increasing doses cause CNS depression, which limits any reflex tachycardia. Isoflurane has the advantage that its cardiovascular effects can be altered with a change in inspired concentration faster than enflurane or halothane and it has less effect on intracranial pressure.

### Sympathetic ganglion blockade

Trimetaphan (3–4 mg/min) blocks nicotinic receptors at PNS and SNS ganglia. The SNS block reduces myocardial contractility but the PNS block results in tachycardia which may impair the degree of hypotension. Tachyphylaxis is marked.

### Non-depolarizing neuromuscular blockers

Alcuronium and d-tubocurarine induce hypotension through histamine release. Mild ganglionic blockade also contributes to the hypotensive effect.

### Alpha-adrenoceptor blockade

Phentolamine (5–10 mg i.v.), phenoxybenzamine, chlorpromazine and droperidol all produce competitive blockade of sympathetic postsynaptic noradrenergic receptors. Phentolamine is short-acting whereas phenoxybenzamine is usually used preoperatively for chronic vascular expansion. Droperidol and chlorpromazine are useful additions to the premedication.

### Beta-adrenoceptor blockade

Reduces cardiac output and heart rate. Labetolol (50 mg i.v. over 1 min, max. 200 mg) is short-acting and also has some α-blocking action. Esmolol (100–300 μg/min) is a short-acting drug which may be suitable for intraoperative i.v. use. Preoperative oral administration of β-blockers, e.g. propanolol, may prevent wide fluctuations in BP.

### Direct-acting vasodilators

The very short half-life of sodium nitroprusside (SNP) enables rapid reduction in BP and equally rapid restoration (2–4 min). It dilates resistance

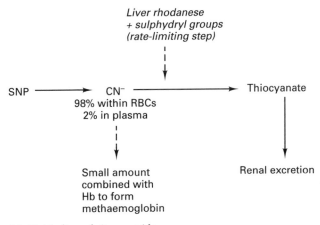

**Fig. 1.9** Metabolism of nitroprusside.

and capacitance vessels. Vasodilation causes raised intracranial pressure and SNP should not be used in neurosurgery until the cranium has been opened. SNP increases aortic flow, increasing shearing pressure; therefore β-blockers may need to be used in addition. Start at 0.3 $\mu$g/kg per min to limit cyanide toxicity (max. 8 $\mu$g/kg per min). Base deficit > –7 mmol/l is suggestive of CN⁻ toxicity. Sodium thiosulphate reduces CN⁻ levels by providing sulphydryl groups at the rate-limiting step (Fig. 1.9).

Glyceryl trinitrate (0.25–5.0 $\mu$g/kg per min) causes a slower reduction and recovery in BP (10–20 min) than SNP, with a greater effect on the systolic than on the diastolic BP. Dilates capacitance vessels with little effect on resistance vessels. Maintains coronary perfusion pressure more effectively than SNP but may raise intracranial pressure even more. Degree of hypotension achievable may be limited. Hydralazine (5–10 mg i.v. slowly) is also suitable for rapid control of BP.

### Regional anaesthesia

Spinal and epidural anaesthesia with blocks extending to thoracic levels will produce hypotension by arterial and venous dilatation. Blocks extending to cardioaccelerator fibres (T2–T4) augment the hypotension further by preventing a compensatory tachycardia.

### References

Simpson P J 1992 Hypotensive anaesthesia. Current Anaesthesia and Critical Care 3: 90–97

Sorkun F 1996 Comparison of propofol with isoflurane during hypotensive anaesthesia for middle ear surgery. Acta Anaesthesiologica Italica 47: 287–293

# 2. Respiratory system

During routine anaesthesia, the incidence of difficult tracheal intubation has been estimated as 3–15%. Tracheal intubation is best achieved with the neck flexed and the atlantoaxial joint extended ('sniffing the morning air'). Factors affecting this position may result in difficult intubation.

## HISTORY AND EXAMINATION

Remember to check anaesthetic notes for previous difficulties and ask the patient if he or she is aware of any anaesthetic problems.

### Visual inspection

The following features suggest a difficult intubation: obesity, large breasts, short muscular neck, full dentition, limited neck flexion or head extension, receding jaw, prominent upper incisors, limited mouth opening, high arched palate.

### Cormack & Lehane grading (1984)

Used to grade the view at laryngoscopy (Fig. 2.1):

- grade I – visualization of the entire laryngeal aperture
- grade II – visualization of the posterior part of the laryngeal aperture

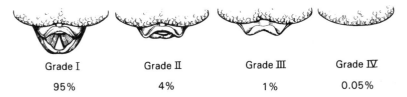

| Grade I | Grade II | Grade III | Grade IV |
| --- | --- | --- | --- |
| 95% | 4% | 1% | 0.05% |

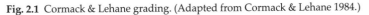

**Fig. 2.1** Cormack & Lehane grading. (Adapted from Cormack & Lehane 1984.)

- grade III – visualization of epiglottis only
- grade IV – not even the epiglottis is visible.

Recent reclassification has subdivided grade II view further:

- grade IIa – only part of the glottis is visible
- grade IIb – only the arytenoids or the very posterior origin of the cords are visible.

## PREDICTIVE TESTS

### Mallampati classification (Mallampati et al 1985)

The patient sits upright with the head in the neutral position and the mouth open as wide as possible, with the tongue extended to maximum. The following structures are visible (Fig. 2.2):

- class I    – hard palate, soft palate, uvula, tonsillar pillars
- class II   – hard palate, soft palate, uvula
- class III  – hard palate, soft palate
- class IV  – hard palate.

Class I view is grade I intubation > 99% of the time. Class IV view is grade III or IV intubation 100% of the time.

This classification may fail to predict > 50% of difficult intubations.

### Thyromental distance (Patil et al 1983)

Measure from the upper edge of thyroid cartilage to tip of jaw with the head fully extended. A short thyromental distance equates with an anterior larynx which is at a more acute angle and also results in less space for the tongue to be compressed into by the laryngoscope blade. This is a relatively unreliable test unless combined with other tests:

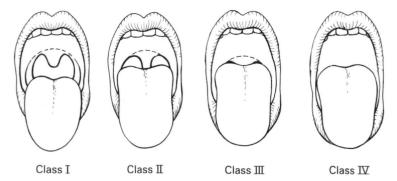

Class I          Class II          Class III          Class IV

**Fig. 2.2** Mallampati classification. (Reproduced from Mallampati et al 1985.)

- Thyromental distance > 6.5 cm = easy intubation
- Thyromental distance < 6.0 cm = difficult intubation.

### Sternomental distance (Savva 1994)

Measure from the sternum to the tip of the mandible with the head extended. A sternomental distance of ≤ 12.5 cm predicts difficult intubation.

### Horizontal length of mandible

Horizontal mandibular length > 9 cm is suggestive of a good laryngoscopic view.

### Mandibulohyoid distance (Chou & Wu 1993)

This is the vertical distance between the anterior edge of the hyoid and the mandible vertically above measured by lateral X-ray. A distance greater than 6 cm is suggestive of difficult intubation. A longer distance results in more of the tongue being present in the hypopharynx, which must be displaced to view the vocal cords.

### Cervical spine movements

The effect of mobility of the atlanto-occipital and atlantoaxial joints on ease of intubation is probably underestimated. May be best assessed by asking patients to extend their head whilst their neck is in full flexion. Extension of the head with atlantoaxial joint immobility results in greater cervical spine convexity which pushes the larynx anteriorly and impairs the laryngoscopic view.

### Prayer sign

Inability to place both palms flat together suggests difficult intubation. It is probably a reflection of generalized joint and cartilage immobility limiting atlantoaxial and cervical extension. May be particularly common in diabetics.

### Wilson risk score (Wilson 1993; see Table 2.1)

A total of 3 predicts 75% of difficult intubations, whilst a total of 4 predicts 90%. However, the test has a poor specificity and may fail to predict > 50% of difficult intubations. Many of the measurements are subjective.

## RADIOGRAPHIC PREDICTORS OF DIFFICULT INTUBATION

These have the disadvantage of X-ray exposure and thus cannot be performed as routine tests.

**Table 2.1** Wilson Risk Score

| Parameter | Risk level |
|---|---|
| Weight | 0–2 (e.g. > 90 kg = 1; > 110 kg = 2) |
| Head and neck movement | 0–2 |
| Jaw movement | 0–2 |
| Receding mandible | 0–2 |
| Buck teeth | 0–2 |
| Maximum | 10 points |

**Cass et al (1956)** (absolute measurements not given)

- Incisor tooth to posterior border of ramus
- Alveolar margin to lower border of the mandible
- Angle of the mandible.

### White & Kander (1975)

- Increased length of mandible
- Increased depth of mandible
- Reduced distance between occiput and spinous process of $C_1$ or reduced distance between $C_1$–$C_2$ interspinous gap.

### Nichol & Zuck (1983)

These authors stressed the importance of a reduced atlanto-occipital distance as a predictor of ability to extend the head during laryngoscopy.

## COMBINED INDICATORS

By combining prognostic indicators, a greater specificity for predicting difficult intubation may be achieved.

- Freck (1991) found that a thyromental distance of 7 cm in patients with Mallampati class III/IV predicts a grade IV intubation. The test has high sensitivity and specificity.
- Benumof (1991) suggested that a combination of relative tongue/pharyngeal size, atlantoaxial joint extension and anterior mandibular space provides a good predictor of difficult intubation and that the tests are quick and easy to perform.
- Best multifactorial index scores the following criteria to give sensitivity and specificity > 90% in prediction of difficult intubation (Arné et al 1998):
  1. previous history of difficult intubation
  2. pathologies associated with difficult intubation
  3. clinical symptoms of a pathological airway
  4. inter-incisor gap

5. thyromental distance
6. head and neck movement
7. Mallampati's modified test.

### References

Arné J, Descoins P, Fusciardi J, Ingrand P, Ferrier B, Boudigues D, Ariès J 1998 Preoperative assessment for difficult intubation in general and ENT surgery: predictive value of a clinical multivariate risk index. British Journal of Anaesthesia 80: 140–146

Benumof J L 1991 Management of the difficult airway. Anesthesiology 75: 1087–1110

Bluman L G, Mosca L, Newman N, Simon D G L 1998 Preoperative smoking habits and postoperative pulmonary complications. Chest, Apr; 113(4): 883–889

Calder I 1992 Predicting difficult intubation. Anaesthesia 47: 528–529

Cass N M, James N R, Lines V 1956 Difficult laryngoscopy complicating intubation for anaesthesia. British Medical Journal 1: 488–489

Charters P 1996 What future is there for predicting difficult intubation? British Journal of Anaesthesia 77: 309–311

Chou H C, Wu T L 1993 Mandibulohyoid distance in difficult laryngoscopy. British Journal of Anaesthesia 71: 335–339

Cormack R S, Lehane J 1984 Difficult tracheal intubation in obstetrics. Anaesthesia 39: 1105–1111

Freck C M 1991 Predicting difficult intubation. Anaesthesia 46: 1005–1008

Mallampati S R, Gatt S P, Gugino L D, Desai S P, Waraksa B, Freiberger D, Liu P L 1985 A clinical sign to predict difficult intubation: a prospective study. Canadian Journal of Anaesthetics 32: 429–434

Nichol H L, Zuck D 1983 Difficult laryngoscopy – the 'anterior' larynx and the atlanto-occipital gap. British Journal of Anaesthesia 55: 141–143

Patil V U, Stehling L C, Zaunder H L 1983 Fibreoptic endoscopy in anaesthesia. Year Book Medical Publishers, Chicago

Savva D 1994 Prediction of difficult tracheal intubation. British Journal of Anaesthesia 73: 149–153

White A, Kander P L 1975 Anatomical factors in difficult direct laryngoscopy. British Journal of Anaesthesia 47: 468–474

Wilson M E 1993 Predicting difficult intubation. British Journal of Anaesthesia 71: 333–334

Yentis S M, Lee D J H 1998 Evaluation of an improved scoring system for the grading of direct laryngoscopy. Anaesthesia 53: 1041–1044

## ANAESTHESIA AND RESPIRATORY DISEASE

### SMOKING

#### Effects of smoking

- Increased oxygen demand through nicotine activation of the sympatho-adrenergic system ($\uparrow$HR, $\uparrow$BP and $\uparrow$SVR)

- Decreased oxygen supply via carboxyhaemoglobinaemia (HbCO) and raised coronary vascular resistance
- Increased airway reactivity with greater risk of laryngospasm
- Increased mucus production
- Decreased ciliary motility
- Increased closing capacity
- Impaired humoral and cell-mediated immunity ($\downarrow$ immunoglobulins and $\downarrow$ leucocyte activity)
- Increased risk of chest infection
- Impaired wound healing
- Cor pulmonale
- Lung cancer.

### Preoperative cessation of smoking

A study in patients undergoing CABG (Warner et al 1989) showed that in those stopping smoking, the incidence of postoperative pulmonary complications did not fall until at least 8 weeks had elapsed:

- current smokers – 33%
- ex-smokers < 8 weeks – 57%
- ex-smokers > 8 weeks – 15%.

A recent study found that postoperative pulmonary complications occurred in 22% of current smokers but only 5% of men who had never smoked. Again, complications were more common in patients who reduced their cigarette consumption before surgery compared with those who had smoked their usual quantity (Bluman et al 1998).

## CHRONIC BRONCHITIS

Chronic bronchitis is defined as productive cough > 3 months of the year for 2 or more years.

## POSTOPERATIVE PNEUMONIA

Predisposed by:

- decreased ciliary activity
- sputum retention
- poor cough
- lack of humidification.

## VIRAL UPPER RESPIRATORY TRACT INFECTION (VRTI)

This is common in paediatric ENT patients. Causes worsening of asthma and $\uparrow$ bronchial reactivity for up to 6 weeks following resolution of symptoms.

May be due to viral-mediated damage to vagus releasing acetylcholine and potentiating bronchoconstriction.

In children, there is a 2–7 fold increase in respiratory related adverse events, if intubated, an 11-fold increase in adverse events, and an increased risk of transient hypoxaemia in the postoperative period. In adults with URTI, upper airway reactivity is also increased by an amount related to severity of symptoms.

Therefore, postpone routine surgery at least 2–3 weeks. If anaesthesia is given during this period, consider topical anaesthesia to larynx to reduce vagally mediated reflexes and consider the use of atropine to block hyper-reactivity. Monitor $O_2$ saturation postoperatively.

## EFFECTS OF GENERAL ANAESTHESIA

- Central respiratory depression
- Reduced compliance
- Cranial shift of diaphragm, atelectasis, reduced tone of chest wall and reduced thoracic blood volume cause ↓ FRC (17%, 500 ml)
- FRC approaches and may exceed closing capacity (CC)
- Impaired $O_2$ and $CO_2$ exchange
- Increased shunt
- Increased $V/\dot{Q}$ scatter
- Hypoxic pulmonary vasoconstriction inhibited by up to 25% with volatiles but not by i.v. agents.

All these factors result in an increased A–a$O_2$ (difference in alveolar and arterial oxygen tensions), which persists for at least 1–2 h postoperatively. Postoperative wound pain, abdominal distension, pulmonary venous congestion and a supine posture all increase CC–FRC and result in further alveolar collapse.

## ANAESTHESIA FOR CHRONIC RESPIRATORY DISEASE

### Risk factors for postoperative pulmonary complications

- American Society of Anesthesiologists (ASA) classification
- Extremes of age
- Obesity (↓ compliance, ↓ FRC)
- Suboptimal respiratory therapy
- Smoking (need to stop > 8 weeks to be of benefit)
- Severe dyspnoea at rest
- Copious sputum production
- Respiratory failure ($P_aCO_2 > 6.7$ kPa)
- Pulmonary hypertension
- Surgery > 4 h duration
- Thoracic, upper > lower abdominal surgery (decreases postoperative $FEV_1$ and FVC by 50%)

- Midline > transverse incisions
- Bowel distension.

**Respiratory function tests predicting increased postoperative morbidity with chronic respiratory disease**

- $\dfrac{FEV_1}{FVC} < 50\%$ = high risk (obstructive pattern)

  ($FEV_1$ = forced expiratory volume in 1 s, FVC = forced vital capacity)

- $\dfrac{RV}{TLC} < 50\%$ = high risk (restrictive pattern)

  (RV = residual volume, TLC = total lung capacity)

  $FEV_1 < 1000$ ml or $< 50\%$ predicted

  FVC  $< 1500$ ml or $< 50\%$ predicted

- Maximum breathing capacity (MBC) $< 50\%$ predicted
  (MBC = PEFR $\times$ 0.25 or $FEV_1 \times 35$)

- Forced expiratory time :  $> 4$ s is abnormal
                           $> 10$ s indicates severe obstruction.

Morbidity of high-risk patients can be reduced by:

- pre- and postoperative physiotherapy
- humidified oxygen
- optimization of medication (antibiotics, bronchodilators, steroids etc.)
- optimization of nutritional status.

## ANAESTHETIC TECHNIQUES

### Aims

- Avoid bronchospasm (which causes autoPEEP)
- Avoid hypoxia or hypercapnia
- Minimize postoperative complications (e.g. pain relief reduces atelectasis)
- Avoid postoperative ventilation (reduces ciliary motility, acts as route for infection, causes bronchospasm).

Use either regional/local technique or maximal support approach with GA. Plan elective surgery for summer.

### Regional technique

Requires the patient to be able to lie flat for the duration of surgery and not cough. Avoid sedation which may precipitate respiratory failure. Can be combined with a light GA and spontaneous ventilation, but reactive airways are irritated by an endotracheal tube which may cause severe bronchospasm. Avoided by using local/regional technique.

### General anaesthetic

The technique of choice for patients with respiratory failure or upper abdominal/thoracic surgery. Light/no premedication. Use a heat and moisture exchanger or humidifier. Use drugs allowing rapid recovery. IPPV allows control of $O_2$ and $CO_2$ and enables airway suctioning and may need to be continued postoperatively. Use slow inspiratory flow to allow equilibration of fast and slow alveoli. A long expiratory time reduces air trapping. Avoid PEEP in patients with COAD. If there are high-frequency bullae, avoid $N_2O$ and consider double-lumen tube. Spontaneous respiration or jet ventilation (HFJV) may be appropriate with bullae.

At the end of surgery, ensure bowel is decompressed and drain any peritoneal air. Sit patient up postoperatively, which increases FRC. Epidurals also increase FRC (bupivacaine > morphine). Prior to extubation, ensure cardiovascular stability and fluid balance and ensure no residual effects of anaesthetic or neuromuscular blockade.

## ANAESTHESIA FOR ASTHMATICS

Asthma affects 4–5% of the population. There are 2000 deaths p.a. in the UK. Prevalence and mortality are increasing.

Avoid factors precipitating bronchospasm (differential diagnosis = aspiration, pulmonary oedema, endobronchial intubation, patient too light, mechanical obstruction of the tube).

### Preoperative

Assess severity: severe if patient unable to speak sentences, pulse >120/min, pulsus paradoxus > 20 mmHg, $FEV_1$ < 25%, $\uparrow P_a CO_2$. Consider bronchodilators, hydration, antibiotics and steroids. Measure baseline arterial blood gases (ABGs). Percussive physiotherapy is contraindicated because it exhausts the patient further.

### Premedication

Atropine limits vagal reflexes that cause bronchospasm. The small doses used for premedication do not cause bronchodilation but increase the viscosity of sputum. Consider nebulized salbutamol.

### Anaesthetic

Use of a regional or local technique avoids most precipitating factors. Induction with ketamine ($\uparrow$ secretions but is the best bronchodilator),

**Chart 2**

# Acute severe asthma in adults

---

## Recognition and assessment in hospital

### Features of acute severe asthma

- Peak expiratory flow (PEF) ≤ 50% of predicted or best
- Can't complete sentences in one breath
- Respirations ≥ 25 breaths/min
- Pulse > 110 beats/min

### Life threatening features

- PEF < 33% of predicted or best
- Silent chest, cyanosis, or feeble respiratory effort
- Bradycardia or hypotension
- Exhaustion, confusion, or coma

If $Sao_2$ < 92% or a patient has **any life threatening** features, measure arterial blood gases.

**Blood gas markers of a very severe, life threatening attack:**
- Normal (5–6 kPa, 36–45 mm Hg) or high $Paco_2$
- Severe hypoxia: $Pao_2$ < 8 kPa (60 mm Hg) irrespective of treatment with oxygen
- A low pH (or high H+)

No other investigations are needed for immediate management.

**Caution**
**Patients with severe or life threatening attacks may not be distressed and may not have all these abnormalities. The presence of any should alert the doctor**

---

### 1 Immediate treatment

- Oxygen 40–60% ($CO_2$ retention is not usually aggravated by oxygen therapy in asthma)
- Salbutamol 5 mg or terbutaline 10 mg via an oxygen driven nebuliser
- Prednisolone tablets 30–60 mg or intravenous hydrocortisone 200 mg or both if very ill
- No sedatives of any kind
- Chest radiograph to exclude pneumothorax

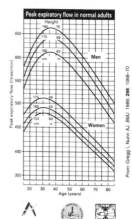

Peak expiratory flow in normal adults

*From: Gregg I, Nunn AJ. BMJ 1989; 298: 1068–70*

IF LIFE THREATENING FEATURES ARE PRESENT:

- Add ipratropium 0.5 mg to the nebulised β agonist
- Give intravenous aminophylline 250 mg over 20 minutes or salbutamol or terbutaline 250 µg over 10 minutes. Do not give bolus aminophylline to patients already taking oral theophyllines

### 2 Subsequent management

IF PATIENT IS IMPROVING CONTINUE:

- 40–60% oxygen
- Prednisolone 30–60 mg daily or intravenous hydrocortisone 200 mg 6 hourly
- Nebulised β agonist 4 hourly

IF PATIENT IS NOT IMPROVING AFTER 15–30 MINUTES:

- Continue oxygen and steroids
- Give nebulised β agonist more frequently, up to every 15–30 minutes
- Add ipratropium 0.5 mg to nebuliser and repeat 6 hourly until patient is improving

IF PATIENT IS STILL NOT IMPROVING GIVE:

- Aminophylline infusion (small patient 750 mg/24 hours, large patient 1500 mg/24 hours); monitor blood concentrations if it is continued for over 24 hours
- Salbutamol or terbutaline infusion as an alternative to aminophylline

### 3 Monitoring treatment

- Repeat measurement of PEF 15–30 minutes after starting treatment
- Oximetry: maintain $Sao_2$ > 92%
- Repeat blood gas measurements within 2 hours of starting treatment if

- initial $Pao_2$ < 8 kPa (60 mmHg) unless subsequent $Sao_2$ > 92%
- $Paco_2$ normal or raised
- patient deteriorates
- Chart PEF before and after giving nebulised or inhaled β agonists and at least 4 times daily throughout hospital stay

**Transfer patient to the intensive care unit accompanied by a doctor prepared to intubate if there is:**

- Deteriorating PEF, worsening or persisting hypoxia, or hypercapnia
- Exhaustion, feeble respirations, confusion or drowsiness
- Coma or respiratory arrest

### 4 When discharged from hospital, patients should have:*

- Been on discharge medication for 24 hours and *have had inhaler technique checked and recorded*
- PEF > 75% of predicted or best and PEF diurnal variability < 25% *unless discharge is agreed with respiratory physician*
- Treatment with *oral and inhaled steroids* in addition to bronchodilators
- Own PEF meter and *written self management plan*
- GP follow up arranged *within 1 week*
- Follow up appointment in respiratory clinic *within 4 weeks*

### Also

- Determine reason(s) for exacerbation and admission
- Send details of admission, discharge and potential best PEF to GP.

*Adapted from poster designed by Business Design Group*

NATIONAL **ASTHMA** CAMPAIGN

Working for Healthier Lungs

in association with the General Practitioner in Asthma Group, the British Association of Accident and Emergency Medicine, the British Paediatric Respiratory Society and the Royal College of Paediatrics and Child Health

**Fig. 2.3a** Acute severe asthma in adults. 1997 Guidelines of the British Thoracic Society. Thorax 52, Suppl. 1, Chart 2. Reproduced with permission from the BMJ Publishing Group.

**Chart 3**

# Acute severe asthma in those aged 5–15 years

---

### Recognition of acute severe asthma

- Too breathless to talk
- Too breathless to feed
- Respirations ≥ 40 breaths/min
- Pulse ≥ 120 beats/min
- PEF ≤ 50% predicted or best

No other investigations are needed for immediate management

Blood gas estimations are rarely helpful in deciding initial management in children

**Life threatening features**

- PEF < 33% predicted or best
- Cyanosis, silent chest, or poor respiratory effort
- Fatigue or exhaustion
- Agitation or reduced level of consciousness

**Caution:**
**Children with severe attacks may not appear distressed; assessment in the very young may be difficult. The presence of any of these features should alert the doctor.**

---

### Management of a severe asthma attack

**1 Immediate treatment**

- High flow oxygen via face mask
- Salbutamol 5 mg or terbutaline 10 mg via an oxygen driven nebuliser (half doses in very young children)
- Prednisolone 1–2 mg/kg body weight orally (maximum 40 mg)

IF LIFE THREATENING FEATURES ARE PRESENT:

- Give intravenous aminophylline 5 mg/kg over 20 minutes followed by maintenance infusion, 1 mg/kg/h; omit the loading dose if child already receiving oral theophyllines

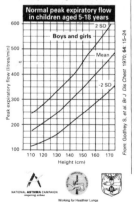

Normal peak expiratory flow in children aged 5-18 years

Boys and girls

2 SD

Mean

-2 SD

Peak expiratory flow (litres/min)

600, 500, 400, 300, 200, 100

110 120 130 140 150 160 170

Height (cm)

From: Godfrey S, et al. Br J Dis Chest 1970; 64: 15–24

- Give intravenous hydrocortisone 100 mg 6 hourly
- Add ipratropium 0.25 mg to nebulised β agonist (0.125 mg in very young children)
- Pulse oximetry is helpful in assessing response to treatment. An Sao$_2$ ≤ 92% may indicate the need for chest radiography.

**2 Subsequent management**

IF PATIENT IS IMPROVING CONTINUE:

- High flow oxygen
- Prednisolone 1–2 mg/kg daily (maximum 40 mg/day)
- Nebulised β agonist 4 hourly

IF PATIENT IS NOT IMPROVING AFTER 15–30 MINUTES:

- Continue oxygen and steroids
- Give nebulised β agonist more frequently, up to every 30 minutes
- Add ipratropium to nebuliser and repeat 6 hourly until improvement starts

IF PATIENT IS STILL NOT IMPROVING GIVE:

- Aminophylline infusion (1 mg/kg/h); monitor blood concentrations if continued for over 24 hours

**3 Monitoring treatment**

- Repeat PEF measurement 15–30 minutes after starting treatment (if appropriate)
- Oximetry: maintain Sao$_2$ > 92%
- Chart PEF if appropriate before and after the child inhales β agonists and at least 4 times daily throughout hospital stay

**4 Transfer to the intensive care unit accompanied by a doctor prepared to intubate if there is:**

- Deteriorating PEF, worsening or persisting hypoxia, or hypercapnia
- Exhaustion, feeble respirations, confusion or drowsiness
- Coma or respiratory arrest

**5 When discharged from hospital patients should have:**

- Been on discharge medication for 24 hours and have had inhaler technique checked and recorded
- If recorded, PEF > 75% of predicted or best and PEF diurnal variability < 25%
- Treatment with soluble steroid tablets and inhaled steroids in addition to bronchodilators
- Own PEF meter and if appropriate self management plan or written instructions for parents
- GP follow up arranged within 1 week
- Follow up appointment in clinic within 4 weeks

*Adapted from poster designed by Business Design Group*

NATIONAL ASTHMA CAMPAIGN
Working for Healthier Lungs

*In association with the General Practitioner in Asthma Group, the British Association of Accident and Emergency Medicine, the British Paediatric Respiratory Society and the Royal College of Paediatrics and Child Health*

**Fig. 2.3b** Acute severe asthma in those aged 5–15 years. 1997 Guidelines of the British Thoracic Society. Thorax 52, Suppl. 1, Chart 3. Reproduced with permission from the BMJ Publishing Group.

**Chart 8**

# Acute severe asthma in children under 5 years of age

### Recognition of acute severe asthma

**Remember:** • in preschool children there are other important causes of breathlessness and wheeze
• if you think a child has severe asthma, give β agonist at once

- Too breathless to talk
- Too breathless to feed
- Respirations > 50 breaths/min
- Pulse > 140 beats/min
- Use of accessory muscles of breathing

No other investigations are needed for immediate management; blood gas estimations are rarely helpful in deciding initial management in children

**Life threatening features**

- Cyanosis, silent chest, or poor respiratory effort
- Fatigue or exhaustion
- Agitation or reduced level of consciousness

**Caution:**
Children with severe attacks may not appear distressed; assessment in the very young may be difficult. The presence of any of these features should alert the doctor.

### Management of a severe asthma attack

**1 Immediate treatment**

- High flow oxygen via face mask
- Salbutamol 2.5–5 mg or terbutaline 5–10 mg via an oxygen driven nebuliser (half doses in children under 1) or similar doses by spacer device.
- Prednisolone < 1 year 1–2 mg/kg/day; 1–5 years 20 mg/day
- Pulse oximetry is helpful. Sao₂ <92% in air indicates the need for admission.

IF LIFE THREATENING FEATURES OR POOR BRONCHODILATOR RESPONSE:

- Give intravenous aminophylline 5 mg/kg over 20 minutes followed by maintenance infusion of 1 mg/kg/h; omit the loading dose if child already receiving oral theophyllines
- Give intravenous hydrocortisone 100 mg 6 hourly
- Add ipratropium 0.25 mg to nebulised β agonist (0.125 mg in very young children)

**2 Subsequent management**

IF THE PATIENT IS IMPROVING CONTINUE:

- Oxygen to maintain Sao₂ >92%
- Prednisolone daily
- Nebulised β agonist 1–4 hourly

IF PATIENT IS NOT IMPROVING AFTER 15–30 MINUTES

- Continue oxygen and steroids
- Give nebulised β agonist more frequently, up to every 30 minutes
- Add ipratropium to nebuliser and repeat 6 hourly until improvement starts
- Consider need for chest radiography

IF PATIENT IS STILL NOT IMPROVING GIVE:

- Aminophylline infusion after loading dose if not already given; monitor blood concentrations if continued for over 24 hours.

**3 Monitoring treatment**

- Oximetry: maintain Sao₂ >92% Note clinical features at appropriate intervals.

**4 Transfer to the intensive care unit accompanied by a doctor prepared to intubate if:**

- Worsening or persistent hypoxia or hypercapnia
- Exhaustion, feeble respirations, confusion or drowsiness
- Coma or respiratory arrest

**5 When discharged from hospital patients should have:**

- Been stable on discharge medication for 6–8 hours and have had inhaler technique checked and recorded
- Treatment with soluble steroid tablets for total of 1–3 days
- Self management plan or written instructions for parents
- GP or hospital follow up arranged, with direct readmission for any deterioration within 24 hours.

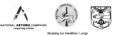

NATIONAL **ASTHMA** CAMPAIGN

Working for Healthier Lungs

in association with the General Practitioner in Asthma Group, the British Association of Accident and Emergency Medicine, the British Paediatric Respiratory Society and the Royal College of Paediatrics and Child Health

Adapted from poster designed by Business Design Group

**Fig. 2.3c** Acute severe asthma in children under 5 years of age. 1997 Guidelines of the British Thoracic Society. Thorax 52, Suppl. 1, Chart 8. Reproduced with permission from the BMJ Publishing Group.

**Chart 5** # Asthma in accident and emergency departments

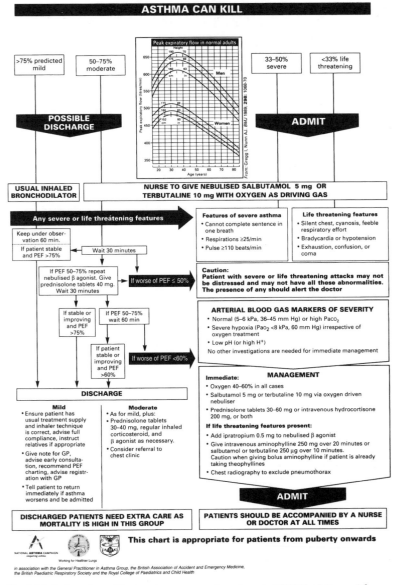

**Fig. 2.3d** Asthma in accident and emergency departments. 1997 Guidelines of the British Thoracic Society. Thorax 52, Suppl. 1, Chart 5. Reproduced with permission from the BMJ Publishing Group.

propofol, etomidate or benzodiazepines. Thiopentone causes histamine release and may cause bronchoconstriction.

Although suxamethonium causes histamine release, there is no evidence that it precipitates bronchospasm. Intubate deep to avoid stimulating reflexes which cause bronchospasm and avoid excessively light anaesthesia which may also cause endotracheal tube irritation and bronchoconstriction. Consider topical lignocaine or lignocaine 1.5 mg/kg i.v. pre-intubation.

Although halothane is a potent bronchodilator, it sensitizes the myocardium. Enflurane and isoflurane are equipotent bronchodilators. If theophylline infusion is running (6 mg/kg loading dose, 0.5 mg/kg per hour maintenance), halve the rate because general anaesthesia decreases liver blood flow. If the patient is ventilated, aim for slow inflation for optimal alveolar gas distribution. Slow exhalation reduces air trapping. There is little work on the effects of neuromuscular blockers on asthma. Avoid those that cause histamine release. Remember to give steroid supplements if the patient is taking steroids.

Perioperative complications (bronchospasm, laryngospasm) are more common in older patients (> 50 years) and those with active asthma.

### Reversal

Anticholinesterases cause bronchospasm, prevented by the addition of an anticholinergic.

## ANAESTHESIA FOR CYSTIC FIBROSIS

Cystic fibrosis is caused by an autosomal recessive gene localized to chromosome 7, occurring in 1:2000 births. It is the commonest fatal inherited disease. The prognosis is improving, with median life expectancy of 40 years. Gene encodes for cystic fibrosis transmembrane inductance regulator which is involved in chloride transport on epithelial cell membranes. Results in impaired chloride and sodium transport with increased electrolyte content of secretions.

Presents as meconium ileus, recurrent respiratory infections, steatorrhoea and failure to thrive. Diagnosed by sweat test with sweat sodium and chloride > 60 mmol/l.

Patients may present for heart–lung transplantation.

### Pathophysiology

*Cardiovascular.* Chronic hypoxaemia and pulmonary disease result in cor pulmonale. Left ventricular abnormalities and cardiomyopathy.

*Respiratory.* Chronic sinusitis, nasal polyps, turbinate hypertrophy, mucous plugging of airways, hyperinflation, bronchial hyperreactivity, bronchiectasis, chronic infection (*Staphlyococcus aureus, Haemophilus influenzae, Pseudomonas*), obstructive and restrictive defects.

*Gastrointestinal.* Gastro-oesophageal reflux, impaired liver function, biliary cirrhosis causing portal hypertension, insulin-dependent diabetes and malabsorption secondary to pancreatic insufficiency causing malnutrition.

*Other.* Anaemia of chronic disease, renal impairment secondary to aminoglycosides, diabetes and amyloidosis.

### Anaesthesia

*Preoperative.* Urea and electrolytes, liver function tests, glucose, full blood count, chest X-ray. Pulmonary function tests ($FEV_1$ < 30% = poor prognosis), arterial blood gases, exclusion of active infection, vigorous physiotherapy, good diabetic control.

*Premedication.* Sedatives and narcotics best avoided. Anticholinergics probably of little benefit. $H_2$ antagonists if reflux.

*Induction.* Gas induction slow due to $\dot{V}/\dot{Q}$ mismatch but may be unavoidable, particularly in children with poor venous access. Coughing and laryngospasm are common. Pre-oxygenate to avoid desaturation. Ketamine increases secretions and is relatively contraindicated. Aim to intubate for most procedures to allow tracheobronchial suctioning and control of ventilation. Ensure adequate depth of anaesthesia prior to intubation in view of bronchial hyperreactivity. Low airway pressures reduce the risk of pneumothorax.

*Maintenance.* Humidify inspiratory gases. Isoflurane allows rapid recovery permitting early physiotherapy. Long-acting muscle relaxants risk incomplete postoperative reversal. Aminoglycoside antibiotics may prolong neuromuscular blockade. Aim for early extubation.

*Postoperative.* Effective analgesia is essential to allow good coughing and regular physiotherapy. Maintain adequate hydration.

## PULMONARY HYPERTENSION

Tachycardia reduces filling time, causing ischaemia. Hypoxia causes pulmonary vasoconstriction and precipitates right heart failure. Pulmonary hypertension results in coronary filling during diastole rather than systole.

## LARYNGEAL MASK AIRWAY (LMA)

Designed by Brain in 1981 and released in the UK in 1988.

### Aspiration

6% of patients have a visible oesophagus when viewed through a fibreoptic scope placed down a LMA.

Of patients given methylene blue dye to swallow preoperatively, 25% had methylene blue inside the LMA postoperatively. This high percentage is in contrast to 5% aspiration found to occur when using mask and airway. There are two theories about this:

- LMA cuff sensed as bolus of food, causing decreased lower oesophageal sphincter tone
- there is increased resistance to breathing from LMA, causing more negative intrathoracic pressure.

LMA appears to provide a good seal from blood in the pharynx, although blood clots have been found on the underside following ENT procedures. A throat pack is therefore advisable.

### Failed intubation

LMA is also advocated in failed intubation combined with cricoid pressure, especially in obstetrics. Although risks regurgitation, rapid correction of hypoxia removes this major stimulus to aspiration. Most obstetric deaths are from failed intubation and not regurgitation. A 6 mm cuffed ETT can be passed down a size 4 LMA for blind intubation. Larger size tubes can be passed by first passing bougie through the LMA.

### Other

LMA is advocated for use in patients where pressor response to intubation would be detrimental. LMA also reduces coughing and stridor on removal, compared with ETT. Brain recommends leaving LMA in situ until pharyngeal reflexes are fully recovered and then removing it with the cuff inflated.

## OBSTRUCTIVE SLEEP APNOEA

Absence of air flow for at least 10 s and occurring > 30 times in 7 hours sleep. Either obstructive or central (no respiratory movements). Associated with obesity, hypertension and diabetes. Patients are at even greater risk with i.v. sedation.

Common symptoms are snoring, daytime somnolence, restless sleep.

Reduced activity of genioglossus muscle combined with negative pressure from the diaphragm causes pharyngeal obstruction, just posterior to the soft palate. Also impaired contractility of respiratory muscles.

Nasal CPAP abolishes sleep apnoea in most patients and improves the clinical symptoms. It improves daytime oxygenation by increasing FRC and hence alveolar ventilation and improves chronic CCF and LV function. Nocturnal $O_2$ may also be of benefit.

## POSTOPERATIVE HYPOXIA

Severity and incidence of arterial desaturation are closely related to the surgical site and are greatest for thoracoabdominal surgery, less for upper abdominal surgery and least for peripheral surgery.

*Early hypoxaemia.* One-third of patients being transferred from theatre to recovery room developed $O_2$ saturation < 90%, despite being given 100% $O_2$ for 5 min at the end of surgery. This early phase hypoxaemia is mostly due to upper airway obstruction, increased oxygen consumption, alveolar hypoventilation, atelectasis, $V/\dot{Q}$ mismatch, diffusion hypoxia, aspiration or central or obstructive apnoea.

*Late hypoxaemia* is due to impaired gas exchange (atelectasis), impaired control of breathing (sleep, analgesia), impaired diaphragmatic contractility and collapse of pharynx with negative inspiratory pressures and reduced muscle tone. Persists for up to 5 days. Related temporally to hypertension, tachycardia, myocardial ischaemia and arrhythmias. Some episodes of post-operative LVF and myocardial infarction are probably related to this ischaemia. Hypoxaemia may impair wound healing and promote bacterial infection.

Nasal oxygen delivery is more comfortable than a mask and does not require additional humidification, but 35% patients fail to keep $O_2$ on overnight. Intratracheal and nasopharyngeal catheters may be more effective.

Recent recommendations (Powell et al 1996) include:

- Use of pulse oximetry to monitor all postoperative patients in the recovery room
- Patients at risk of prolonged postoperative hypoxaemia need prolonged monitoring and oxygen supplementation (obese patients with BMI > 27–35 kg/m$^2$, upper abdominal surgery or thoracotomy, patients receiving opioids and those with respiratory disease)
- Patients with impaired $O_2$ delivery (hypovolaemia, anaemia, myocardial/cerebral ischaemia, sickle cell disease) all require postoperative oxygen therapy
- Oxygen should be continued until $S_aO_2$ exceeds 93% or reaches preoperative value.

### References

Berry A M, Brimacombe J R, Verghese C 1998 The laryngeal mask airway in emergency medicine, neonatal resuscitation, and intensive care medicine. International Anesthesiology Clinics 36: 91–109

Brimacombe J, Shorney N 1993 The laryngeal mask airway – a review. In: Kaufman L (ed) Anaesthesia review 10. Churchill Livingstone, London, p 183–202

Brimacombe J R, Berry A M, White P F 1998 The laryngeal mask airway: limitations and controversies. International Anesthesiology Clinics 36: 155–182

Hanning C D 1992 Editorial. Prolonged postoperative oxygen therapy. British Journal of Anaesthesia 69: 115–116

Kaufman L 1993 The respiratory system. In: Kaufman L (ed) Anaesthesia review 10. Churchill Livingstone, London, p 15–34

Mangat P S, Jones J G 1993 Perioperative hypoxaemia. In: Kaufman L (ed) Anaesthesia review 10. Churchill Livingstone, London, p 83–106

Nel M R, Morgan M 1996 Smoking and anaesthesia revisited. Anaesthesia 309–311

Peterfreund R A 1994 Pathophysiology and treatment of asthma. Current Opinion in Anaesthesiology 7: 284–292

Powell J F, Menon D K, Jones J G 1996 The effects of hypoxaemia and recommendations for postoperative oxygen therapy. Anaesthesia 51: 769–772

Walsh T S, Young C H 1995 Anaesthesia and cystic fibrosis. Anaesthesia 50: 614–622

Warner M A, Offord K P, Warner M E, Lennon R L, Conover M A, Jansson–Schumacher U 1989 Role of preoperative cessation of smoking and other factors in postoperative pulmonary complications: a blinded prospective study of coronary artery bypass patients. Mayo Clinic Proceedings 64: 609–616

Xue F S, Li B W, Zhang G S et al 1999 The influence of surgical sites on early
   postoperative hypoxemia in adults undergoing elective surgery. Anesthesia and
   Analgesia 88: 213–219

## THORACIC ANAESTHESIA

### ANAESTHESIA FOR THORACOTOMY

**Preoperative**

Full cardiovascular and respiratory work-up, including room air ABGs and
pulmonary function tests. Patient is often arteriopathic with end-organ
damage.

**Lung function tests**

1. Predicted postoperative $FEV_1$ and FVC as a percentage of preoperative
   values:
   - One lobe resection – 80%
   - Left lung – 60%
   - Right lung – 40%
2. Predicted postoperative $FEV_1$:
   - < 0.8 l – ventilator-dependent; therefore resection is contraindicated
   - < 1.0 l – sputum retention
3. $\% \dfrac{\text{preop. FVC}}{\text{postop. FVC}} + \% \dfrac{\text{preop. } FEV_1}{\text{postop. } FEV_1} < 100 \Rightarrow$ postoperative IPPV necessary
4. Postoperative maximum breathing capacity (MBC):
   - < 25 l/min – respiratory cripple
   - 25–50 l/min – severe respiratory impairment
   - > 60 l/min – normal (60–200)
5. Preoperative $FEV_1$ > 1.5 l is needed for pneumonectomy.

**Pulmonary artery pressure (PAP)**

High risk if mean PAP > 25 mmHg at rest. Mimic postoperative PAP with
balloon occlusion.

**Operative**

*Monitoring.* ECG, good venous access, CVP line on side of thoracotomy
for easier access, chest drain positioned on same side postoperatively
avoids risks of pneumothorax on opposite side to surgery. Arterial line
placed in contralateral radial artery. Wright's respirometer to measure
expired air volumes, pulse oximeter and capnograph.

*Positioning.* Take care with positioning because of risk of nerve injury (axillary rolls cause brachial plexus compression). Dependent pooling in head and legs reduces cardiac output. Worse with hypovolaemia.

*Intubation and ventilation.* Use bronchial blockers if patient is too small for a double-lumen tube.

Intubate with double-lumen tube and use fibreoptic scope if necessary to check position. Usually intubate left main bronchus unless this would interfere with surgery.

IPPV with muscle relaxation prevents coughing and high-volume IPPV ensures more even ventilation.

*Maintenance.* Use volatiles and high $F_iO_2$. Intravenous anaesthetic agents may suppress hypoxic pulmonary vasoconstriction less than volatiles.

*Reversal.* Inflate lungs to 40 $cmH_2O$ for 40 s to reverse atelectasis and check for leaks. Ensure complete reversal and return of protective reflexes before extubation.

### Postoperative analgesia

Pain pathways are:

- Visceral
  - PNS: vagus
  - SNS: $T_2$–$T_5$
- Somatic
  - diaphragm: $C_2$–$C_5$ (phrenic)
  - chest wall: $T_2$–$T_{12}$.

Pneumonectomy removes most of the visceral input.

Use thoracic epidural or intrathecal analgesia (misses vagus and phrenic nerves), intercostal nerve blocks, interpleural local anaesthetic or paravertebral blocks. Use systemic opioids sparingly.

## ANAESTHESIA FOR ONE-LUNG VENTILATION

### Physiology of spontaneous ventilation in lateral decubitus position

GA reduces compliance of both upper and lower lungs which is returned to normal values by the application of PEEP.

Weight of mediastinum and pressure of abdominal contents on diaphragm impair lower lung expansion and cause decreased FRC. However, greater curvature of the diaphragm results in more efficient contraction with greater expansion matching increased blood flow to dependent lung, i.e. V/Q̇ remains balanced.

During spontaneous ventilation, dependent diaphragm moves cephalad on expiration, pushing the mediastinum upwards, resulting in inefficient ventilation. This mediastinal shift causes sympathetic activation, reduces venous return and reduces cardiac output.

When the upper chest is opened during spontaneous ventilation, paradoxical respiration results. During inspiration, gases are drawn from upper lung, which collapses. During expiration, gases pass from lower into upper lung causing upper lung inflation. Mediastinal shift as a result of paradoxical respiration also generates more work.

## Physiology of two-lung IPPV in lateral decubitus position

IPPV results in most ventilation being directed to the upper rather than the lower lung, with perfusion remaining greatest in the lower lung, thus increasing the $V/\dot{Q}$ mismatch.

- High $F_iO_2$ (0.8–1.0) causes vasodilation and increases flow in the dependent lung.
- Aim for 10 ml/kg IPPV once on single-lung ventilation.
- Aim for $P_aCO_2$ of 6 kPa. Since the overall tidal volume is decreased by about 20%, respiratory rate may need to be increased by a similar amount to maintain minute volume.
- PEEP to dependent lung may improve oxygenation by recruiting closed alveoli and restoring compliance to normal, but may worsen oxygenation by compressing pulmonary vasculature and diverting more blood to the upper unventilated lung. Countered by upper lung CPAP.
- Blood flow through unventilated lung is the main determinant of $PO_2$.

  Maintain two-lung ventilation until pleura is opened.

## Hypoxia during single-lung IPPV

If this occurs:

- Check position of double-lumen tube. Suction down ETT
- Non-dependent lung CPAP (5–10 cmH$_2$O)
- Dependent lung PEEP
- Operative lung HFJV
- Intermittent IPPV to operative lung
- Clamp pulmonary artery.

## Postoperative

Any $V/\dot{Q}$ mismatch is improved by nursing the patient in a lateral position with the healthy lung lowermost if breathing spontaneously, or the healthy side uppermost if IPPV.

## Double-lumen tubes

Because of the wide variation in anatomical position of the right upper lobe bronchus, a left-sided tube is usually chosen unless surgery is to the left main bronchus (carina to left upper lobe = 5.0 cm; carina to right upper lobe = 2.5 cm). The presence of a carinal hook increases the stability of the tube but makes insertion more difficult.

The following are types of double-lumen tube:

- *Carlens* (left-sided) and *White* (right-sided) – carinal hook; four sizes
- *Robertshaw* – left/right; no carinal hook; small/medium/large
- *Gordon–Green* – single-lumen right-sided tube; carinal hook
- *Bryce–Smith* – left/right; no carinal hook.

Carlens and White tubes have lumens of a smaller diameter than the Robertshaw tubes. All double-lumen tubes are connected to a Cobb's connector.

### Indications
- Soiling below cuff (empyema, bronchiectasis, haemoptysis, tracheo-oesophageal fistula (TOF))
- Gas leak below cuff (TOF, bronchopleural fistula, ruptured cyst).

### Insertion of tube with carinal hook
1. Advance tip of tube through cords and then turn 180° so that hook is anterior.
2. Once hook is through cords, rotate to correct position and advance until resistance is felt.
3. Ventilate both lungs first; then inflate tracheal cuff and listen at the mouth for any air leak. Inflate endobronchial cuff and inflate single lung through endobronchial port. Check there are no air leaks via tracheal port. Inflate opposite lung via tracheal port and check there are no air leaks via endobronchial port. Measure expired air volumes to check for leaks.

### Complications
- Trauma to laryngeal cartilage and trachea during insertion
- Tube malposition resulting in hypoxia
- Surgical compression can displace tube and disrupt isolation of operative lung
- Tube displacement may result in ball valve effect with hypercapnia and prolonged expiratory flow.

## ANAESTHESIA FOR BRONCHOPLEURAL FISTULA

Fistula usually occurs after lung resection; also with abscess, tumour, bullae. There is a sudden onset of productive cough, worse at night.

It is diagnosed by fall in fluid level on CXR, failure of hemithorax to opacify, return of mediastinum to midline, and consolidation of healthy lung from overspill from infected lung.

Sit patient up, with the affected side lowermost and the fistula clear of pleural fluid. Give oxygen, resuscitate preoperatively. Carry out early endobronchial intubation to isolate fistula. Induction by:

- awake intubation, but risk of coughing and contamination
- rapid sequence induction, but trachea may be distorted following pneumonectomy
- deep volatile induction, but marked CVS depression in shocked patient.

Aim for early extubation to avoid pressure from IPPV on stump sutures.

## ANAESTHESIA FOR LUNG CYSTS/BULLAE

Lung cysts are often compliant and therefore preferentially ventilated. IPPV may deliver large volumes to the cyst, resulting in its rupture. Therefore aim for small tidal volumes, low inflation pressure, no PEEP and long expiratory phase. Spontaneous respiration until chest opening may avoid hyper-inflation.

A ball-valve effect may occur with mucous plugs, causing tensioning of the cyst. Avoid $N_2O$ which may rupture the cyst.

Consider spontaneous respiration or HFJV.

Good postoperative pain relief (e.g. epidural) allows quicker return of normal lung function.

## ANAESTHESIA FOR TRACHEAL RESECTION

A partially obstructed airway is at risk of complete obstruction. Therefore avoid sedative premedication and use gas induction in case a paralysed apnoeic patient cannot be ventilated. Airway obstruction will slow induction. Since ventilation may be dependent upon a patient's spontaneous respiratory effort, avoid neuromuscular blockers until obstruction resected.

When trachea is divided, surgeon places Tovell endotracheal tube in distal trachea to continue ventilation and the original tube is then withdrawn.

When trachea is reanastomosed, the neck is kept flexed to prevent strain on sutures. Aim to extubate as soon as possible to avoid high airway pressures on anastomosis.

## ANAESTHESIA FOR BRONCHOSCOPY

Methods of anaesthesia for bronchoscopy include:

- *Apnoeic oxygenation.* Apnoea with insufflation of $O_2$ via catheter placed at carina. Arterial $CO_2$ rises by 0.26–0.66 kPa/min, therefore use for short periods only.
- *Flexible fibreoptic bronchoscope.*
- *Ventilating (rigid) bronchoscope with sidearm.* Glass window opened for passage of instruments prevents effective ventilation.
- *Sanders injector.* Injection of $O_2$ at 4 bar through 16G cannula with entrainment of air by Venturi effect. $F_iO_2$ uncertain.

Complications include dental and laryngeal damage, tracheal rupture, haemorrhage and pneumothorax.

## LASER SURGERY

Carbon dioxide or Nd-Yag laser used for surgery to thoracic neoplasms. There is a risk of fire and explosion in the airway, risk of ignition of the endotracheal tube and risk to eyesight from laser beam.

Endotracheal tube must be shielded from the laser by coating of aluminium foil or use of a stainless steel tube. Use double cuff in case laser bursts upper cuff. Fill cuffs with water, which absorbs stray energy better than air. Both $O_2$ and $N_2O$ support combustion. Reduce risk of fire by keeping $F_iO_2 < 0.40$, adding helium and using laser for as short a burst as possible. Use saline-soaked swabs to protect surrounding tissue from laser.

Everyone in theatre should wear protective goggles.

### References

Conacher I D 1997 Anaesthesia for the surgery of emphysema. British Journal of Anaesthesia 79: 530–538

Plummer S, Hartley M, Vaughan R S 1998 Anaesthesia for telescopic procedures in the thorax. British Journal of Anaesthesia 80: 223–234

Prough D S, Marshall B E 1994 Thoracic anaesthesia. In: Nimmo W S, Rowbotham D J, Smith G (eds) Anaesthesia, 2nd edn. Blackwell Scientific Publications, Oxford, p 823–862

Tschernko E M, Kritzinger M, Gruber E M et al 1999 Lung volume reduction surgery: preoperative functional predictors for post-operative outcome. Anesthesia and Analgesia 88: 28–33

## MECHANICAL VENTILATION

### HISTORY

Mechanical ventilation was first described in the 16th century by Vesalius, who used bellows to ventilate a donkey. Advances in mechanical ventilation were encouraged by the 1952 polio epidemic in Copenhagen during which Lassen organized relays of medical students to ventilate hundreds of patients by hand for many weeks.

### AIMS OF INTUBATION

- Establish and maintain an upper airway
- Protect the lower airway
- Facilitate IPPV ± hyperventilation
- Reduce dead space
- Facilitate airway suctioning.

## RESPIRATORY FAILURE

### Definition

- $P_aO_2 < 8.0$ kPa
- $P_aCO_2 > 6.7$ kPa.

### Causes

*Ventilatory failure*
- Hypoventilation (lesion in medulla → spinal cord → lungs)
- ↑ dead space.

*Intrapulmonary shunt*
- True shunt (collapse, consolidation, pulmonary oedema etc.)

  Shunt equation $= \dfrac{Q_s}{Q_t} = \dfrac{C_cO_2 - C_aO_2}{C_cO_2 - C_vO_2}$
- ↑ V/$\dot{Q}$ scatter

  $\left(\text{normal } V/\dot{Q} = \dfrac{4000 \text{ ml/min}}{5000 \text{ ml/min}} = 0.8\right)$

### Indications for ventilation

*Subjective.* Clinical grounds, trends in condition, response to treatment, ability to cough etc.

*Objective*
- Respiratory rate > 40/min
- $V_t < 5$ ml/kg
- Vital capacity < 10–15 ml/kg
- ABGs: $P_aO_2 < 8$ kPa, $P_aCO_2 > 8$ kPa.

## TIME CONSTANTS

- Time constant = resistance ($cmH_2O$) × compliance (l/$cmH_2O$)
  = time for 63% of change in pressure to be distributed through lungs
- 5 time constants = complete equalization of pressure
- Short inspiratory time favours fast units (short time constant) with incomplete filling of slower units.

## MECHANICAL VENTILATION

### Ventilators

There are four main groups of ventilator:

- Minute volume dividers, e.g. Manley Pulmovent, Blease Brompton
- Bag squeezers, e.g. Cape Waine ventilator, Manley Servovent
- Thumb occluders, e.g. occlusion of T-piece outlet by thumb
- Intermittent blowers, e.g. Pneupac ventilator, Nuffield Penlon 200.

### Initiation of inspiration

- Time initiated – inspiratory mode begins after a set time
- Pressure initiated – inspiratory mode begins when pressure falls below the baseline pressure.

### Termination of inspiration

- Volume cycle – ends inspiration after a preset volume is delivered
- Pressure cycle – ends inspiration when circuit pressure reaches predetermined level
- Time cycle – ends inspiration after a set time. Commonest used trigger
- Flow cycle – ends inspiration when circuit flow diminishes to a predetermined level.

Infant ventilators are usually pressure-limited, time-cycled flow generators. Adult ventilators are usually volume-limited ventilators.

## VENTILATORY MODES

### Intermittent positive pressure ventilation (IPPV)

*Effects of IPPV*
- $\uparrow V_D{:}V_T, \downarrow$ FRC
- $\uparrow$ spread $V/\dot{Q}$ ratios, $\uparrow$ venous admixture
- Increased pulmonary vascular resistance due to compression and stretching of vessels
- Impaired venous return.

*Large tidal volume ($V_T$)*
- Compensates for $\uparrow$ dead space that occurs with IPPV.
- Reduces basal atelectasis.
- Better tolerated by conscious patients.

Therefore, in the absence of lung pathology, use 12–15 ml/kg at 10–12 breaths/min.

### IMV, SIMV and MMV

*Intermittent mandatory ventilation (IMV).* Patient able to breathe spontaneously on CPAP between mandatory tidal volumes.

*Synchronized intermittent mandatory ventilation (SIMV).* As above, but synchronized with patient's respiratory efforts.

*Mandatory minute ventilation (MMV).* Spontaneous ventilation but if minute ventilation falls below set level, IPPV takes over.

### Advantages of IMV, SIMV and MMV
- Lowers mean airway pressure (improves myocardial and renal blood flow)
- More physiological gas distribution
- Reduces sedation requirements
- Avoids hyperventilation causing respiratory alkalosis
- Easier and earlier weaning, exercises respiratory muscles

### Disadvantages of IMV, SIMV and MMV
- Increases work of breathing if resistance is present in spontaneous breathing circuits
- Respiratory muscle fatigue
- Prolongs weaning if decrease in IMV is too slow
- Hypoventilation may cause respiratory acidosis
- Added dead space.

## High-frequency ventilation

*High-frequency positive pressure ventilation (HFPPV)* (1–2 Hz). Jet injector delivers gas into normal ventilator tubing. Low-velocity wavefront acts as a piston within the tracheal tube. Expiration is passive.

*High-frequency jet ventilation (HFJV)* (2–6 Hz). High-pressure (5 bar) pulses of gas delivered into tracheal tube, entraining air in the flow. Expiration is passive.

*High-frequency oscillatory ventilation (HFOV)* (3–20 Hz). Loudspeaker cone used to produce a sinusoidal pattern of gas flow superimposed on a continuous oxygen flow. Expiration is also active. Not shown to be of any benefit for preterm infants where the mortality and incidence of chronic lung disease are not improved in comparison with conventional ventilation. Associated with higher incidence of intraventricular haemorrhage (possibly from interference with cerebral vascular autoregulation) and inotropic support (possibly from interference with baroreflex).

### Advantages
- ↓ mean airway pressure, thereby reducing pulmonary barotrauma
- Provides PEEP (↑ as frequency increases)
- Less depression of cardiac output
- Reduction in pulmonary shunting
- Allows patient to breathe spontaneously
- Reduced sedation requirements
- Reduced air leak with pneumothorax.

### Disadvantages
- Humidification difficult

- Atelectasis in dependent areas of lung
- Inefficient $CO_2$ removal at > 3 Hz
- Difficult to monitor lung volumes and pressures.

Oxygenation of alveoli occurs by several proposed mechanisms:

- Direct alveolar ventilation of proximal alveoli
- Central core of oxygen
- Convective streaming – peripheral flow to alveoli
- Turbulent dispersion
- Resonance enhances spread of oxygen
- Pendelluft – exchange of gas between alveoli with different time constants at end of inspiration.

## Continuous positive airway pressure (CPAP)

### Advantages
- Increased airway pressure
- Increased FRC
- Recruitment of collapsed alveoli
- Decreased airway resistance
- Reduced $\dot{V}/\dot{Q}$ mismatch
- Improved distribution of inspired gas
- Reduced work of breathing.

### Disadvantages
- Impaired $CO_2$ elimination
- Reduced cardiac output
- Reduced GFR.

## Positive end expiratory pressure (PEEP)

### Effects of PEEP
- $\uparrow$ pulmonary vascular resistance. $\downarrow$ flow in West's zone 1 causes increased dead space
- $\uparrow$ work of breathing if patient breathing spontaneously because patient must generate a negative inspiratory pressure greater than the PEEP pressure to inspire
- $\uparrow P_aO_2$ due to $\uparrow$ FRC > CC
- Prevents surfactant aggregation, reducing alveolar collapse
- Worsens right-to-left shunt and may worsen shunt if applied just to lower lung in one-lung ventilation.

### Optimum PEEP/CPAP is that which:
- Reduces physiological shunt to < 15%
- Restores FRC to normal

- Corresponds to optimal compliance
- Minimizes work of breathing.

CPAP may be uncomfortable for the awake patient and cause gastric distension. Therefore, patient must be cooperative, able to protect the airway, cough and have the energy to breathe spontaneously.

## OTHER VENTILATORY MODES

### Pressure support ventilation

Ventilator senses inspiratory flow and then increases airway pressure to a set level. This inspiratory pressure is then maintained until expiration is triggered by low inspiratory gas flow or increasing airway pressure. Limits peak airway pressure and may improve distribution of alveolar gas in poorly compliant lungs.

### Airway pressure release ventilation (APRV)

A continuous flow system in which airway pressure is alternately switched between a high pressure and a lower expiratory pressure. Tidal volume is determined by the difference between the two pressures. Improves alveolar ventilation, decreases peak airway pressure but has little effect on oxygenation.

### BiPAP – Biphasic Positive Airway Pressure

Similar to APRV except that inspiration:expiration ratios are normal, not inversed, and it is partially synchronized with the patient's ventilation.

### Inverse ratio ventilation

Allows reduction in airway pressures and may improve expansion and thus gas exchange across slow alveolar units. Causes an abnormal breathing pattern and discomfort, requiring patient sedation.

*Permissive hypoxaemia.* A $P_aO_2$ of 8 kPa is not thought to be detrimental in critically ill patients if it allows avoidance of high PEEP, high airway pressures or $F_iO_2 > 0.6$.

*Permissive hypercapnia.* In diseased lungs, the large minute volume needed to achieve normocapnia may cause overdistension of the lungs and further alveolar damage. $P_aCO_2 > 6.7$ kPa is acceptable if pH > 7.25 with adequate cardiovascular function.

## WEANING FROM VENTILATION

The following criteria must first be met:

- Adequate oxygenation ($P_aO_2 > 8$ kPa with $F_iO_2 < 0.6$)
- Adequate $CO_2$ clearance
- Able to protect airway
- Control of pain, agitation and depression
- Control of precipitating illness, fever and infection
- Optimization of electrolytes and haemoglobin
- Optimization of nutritional state.

### Prognostic variables for failure to wean

- Tidal volume < 5 ml/kg
- Vital capacity < 10 ml/kg
- Minute volume < 10 l/min
- Max. inspiratory pressure < −20 cmH$_2$O
- A–aO$_2$ difference > 300 mmHg
- Dead space/tidal volume > 0.6
- Respiratory rate:tidal volume > 100.

### CROP index

Calculated from:

- thoracic compliance ($C_{dyn}$)
- respiratory rate
- arterial oxygenation – $P_aO_2 > 8.0$ kPa on $F_iO_2 < 0.35$
- maximum inspiratory pressure ($P_i$max) > −30 cmH$_2$O is a good predictor.

$$\text{CROP} = C_{dyn} \times P_i\text{max} \times [P_aO_2/P_AO_2]/\text{rate}$$

The threshold value predicting successful weaning was 13 ml/breath per min, giving a sensitivity of 0.81 and a specificity of 0.57.

All variables are of limited value in predicting the success of weaning because it generally requires maximum effort from the patient and there are difficulties in obtaining accurate measurements.

Other factors to be considered are:

- Cuff deflation improves laryngeal and pharyngeal muscle function and coordination pre-extubation.
- Normalizing arterial $P_aCO_2$ pre-extubation increases the ventilatory response to hypercapnia.
- Respiratory muscle strength, endurance and coordination are maximized by ventilation strategies that increase respiratory muscle work during weaning.
- Psychological state is difficult to measure quantitatively but is a major factor in success of weaning.

Overlooked factors contributing to failure to wean include:

- acute left ventricular failure
- sleep deprivation
- excessive $CO_2$ production from overfeeding.

## References

Hawker F F 1996 PEEP and CPAP. Current Anaesthesia and Critical Care 7: 236–242

Hayes B 1994 Ventilators: a current assessment. In: Atkinson R S, Adams A P (eds) Recent advances in anaesthesia and analgesia 18. Churchill Livingstone, Edinburgh p 83–102

Keogh B F 1996 New modes of ventilatory support. Current Anaesthesia and Critical Care 7: 228–235

Krishna G, Raffin T A 1999 Terminal weaning from mechanical ventilation. Critical Care Medicine 27: 9

MacIntyre N R 1998 High-frequency ventilation. Critical Care Medicine 26: 1955–1956

Pinsky M R 1994 Cardiovascular effects of ventilatory support and withdrawal. Anesthesia and Analgesia 79: 567–576

Shelly M P, Nightingale P 1999 ABC of intensive care: respiratory support. British Medical Journal 318: 1674–1677

Shneerson J M 1997 Are there new solutions to old problems with weaning? British Journal of Anaesthesia 78: 238–240

Silver M R 1998 BIPAP: useful new modality or confusing acronym? Critical Care Medicine 26: 1473–1475

Sydow M, Burchardi H 1997 Inverse ratio ventilation and airway pressure release ventilation. Current Opinion in Anaesthesiology 9: 523–528

# 3. Neurology

## EPILEPSY

Affects 1/200 of the general population. Continue anticonvulsants peri-operatively.

### Anaesthetic problems

- *Enzyme induction*. Chronic medication induces hepatic enzymes with resistance to i.v. induction agents and volatiles.
- *Risk of seizures*. Particularly with enflurane in hypocapnic patient, methohexitone, ketamine and etomidate. Although propofol has not been demonstrated to cause significant EEG changes, excitatory phenomena are more common. Because patients risk losing their driving licence after an epileptiform event, it is recommended to avoid propofol in patients who are driving. Several case reports document successful use of propofol for the treatment of status epilepticus.
- *Underlying pathology causing epilepsy.*

## CEREBROVASCULAR DISEASE

A cerebrovascular accident (CVA) is defined as a rapidly evolving episode of loss of cerebral function with symptoms lasting more than 24 h (< 24h = transient ischaemic attack) or leading to death. Annual incidence is 1–2 per 1000 in the UK, with a mortality of 15–30%.

Risk of perioperative stroke following general surgery is 0.2–0.7% in patients without a history of cerebrovascular disease. Most CVAs occur 2–10 days postoperatively with an average of 7 days and have an associated mortality of 26%. In those with a history of cerebrovascular disease, the risk is 2.9% with a mortality of 60%.

Risk factors include age, systolic hypertension, atrial fibrillation (AF), peripheral vascular disease and diabetes. Hyperextension of the patient's neck during head surgery may reduce flow in vertebral and internal carotid arteries.

**Preventative measures**

*Preoperative measures* include treating risk factors and anticoagulation for patients in AF. The European Carotid Surgery Trial (ECST) and the North American Symptomatic Carotid Endarterectomy Trial (NACEST) suggest that carotid endarterectomy would benefit symptomatic patients with > 70% carotid stenosis. Surgery should be deferred for 4–6 weeks after an acute event.

*Intraoperative measures.* Avoid hypocapnia (steal syndrome) or hypercapnia (inverse steal syndrome), avoid hypo- or hyperglycaemia, and avoid extreme cervical spine rotation or extension. Maintain BP within normal range.

*Postoperative measures.* Avoid hypotension, dehydration and hypoxia.

## PARKINSON'S DISEASE

Disorder of the extrapyramidal system with degeneration of the substantia nigra, giving rise to intention tremor, 'cogwheel' rigidity, akinesia and postural changes.

Patients are already confused in a strange environment, which is worsened by GA. Regional anaesthesia is well tolerated. Patients are often difficult to assess preoperatively. There is reduced pulmonary function, upper airway obstruction, weakness and incoordination of inspiratory and expiratory muscles. If patient is well controlled on L-DOPA, a GA is usually well tolerated. Autonomic neuropathy. Most antiemetics aggravate symptoms through dopamine antagonism.

Continue anti-Parkinsonian medication immediately postoperatively, via nasogastric (NG) tube if necessary. Delayed mobilization postoperatively increases risk of respiratory complications and deep vein thrombosis (DVT).

## MULTIPLE SCLEROSIS (MS)

Chronic progressive demyelinating disease characterized by repeated exacerbations and partial remissions. Affects 1:2000; equal incidence in both sexes. Upper motor neurone lesions, cerebellar lesions and sensory deficits are common.

*General anaesthesia* does not exacerbate MS. Use normal doses of muscle relaxants.

*Regional blockade.* New lesions may develop coincidentally at the time of regional blockade and subsequent symptoms may be difficult to differentiate from nerve injury or may be blamed on the block. Therefore regional blockade is relatively contraindicated.

## MOTOR NEURONE DISEASE

Progressive degeneration of motor function with sparing of higher mental function and sensory function. Involves both upper and lower motor neurones. Progressive muscle atrophy, spasticity, pseudobulbar palsy. Affects smooth, striated and cardiac muscle.

*General anaesthesia.* Risk of aspiration from delayed gastric emptying and bulbar weakness. Weak respiratory muscles. Suxamethonium may cause hyperkalaemia. Increased sensitivity to non-depolarizing relaxants and induction agents.

*Regional anaesthesia.* Avoid impairment of respiratory muscles but otherwise safe.

## AUTOIMMUNE DISEASE

### Myasthenia gravis

Affects 1:20 000. A result of autoantibodies directed against the neuromuscular junction.

*Preoperative.* Continue anticholinesterases and steroids. Intubate if vital capacity falls below 1000 ml. Consider β-blockers and atropine to stabilize the autonomic nervous system.

*GA.* Greatly increased sensitivity to non-depolarizers; decreased sensitivity to depolarizing blockers. Give conventional anticholinesterase dose at end of surgery and then restart anticholinesterases at a decreased dose. Extubate when inspiratory pressure $> -30$ cmH$_2$O or FVC $> 15$ ml/kg.

*Postoperative.* Risk factors for postoperative ventilation are:

- disease for 6 years
- chronic respiratory disease
- pyridostigmine $> 750$ mg/day
- FVC $< 2.9$ l.

### Eaton–Lambert syndrome

Severe muscle weakness found in association with 1% of patients with bronchial carcinoma, thyroid disease and connective tissue disorders (systemic lupus erythematosus, polyarteritis nodosa). Unlike myasthenia gravis, causes proximal rather than bulbar weakness, muscle power increases with exercise and no fade occurs on tetanic stimulation.

Increased sensitivity to both non-depolarizing and depolarizing blockers.

Associated with ↑ ACTH (hypertension, diabetes) and ↑ PTH (↑ Ca$^{2+}$, dehydration).

## MYOTONIA

### Myotonic dystrophy

Affects 1:25 000. Autosomal dominant. Myotonia with difficulty releasing hand grip, muscle weakness, cataracts, 'inverted smile', bilateral ptosis, frontal balding, masseter and sternomastoid wasting, and bulbar weakness (aspiration and chest infections); also cardiac conduction defects, cardiomyopathy, valve defects, obstructive sleep apnoea, dysphagia and reduced gastric emptying.

Sensitivity to sedatives, induction agents (barbiturates, propofol), opioids and non-depolarizing neuromuscular blockers. Anticholinesterases, cold and shivering may worsen myotonia. Suxamethonium may produce a generalized myotonic response. Non-depolarizing relaxants are safe. Myotonic contraction with surgical diathermy may be a major problem. Postoperative complications are usually related to cardiac pathology or muscle weakness leading to aspiration. Postoperative shivering may induce a myotonic crisis.

Pregnancy may exacerbate myotonia and muscle weakness.

### Myotonia congenita (Thomsen's disease)

Affects 1:25 000. Autosomal dominant. Generalized muscular hypertrophy, stiffness on initiating movement, relieved by exercise. Myotonia may be severe but no muscle weakness. Anaesthetic problems are as for myotonic dystrophy. Association with malignant hyperthermia.

## FAMILIAL PERIODIC PARALYSIS

### Hyperkalaemic periodic paralysis

Episodes of flaccid paralysis associated with hyperkalaemia. Paralysis may occur with potassium levels no greater than 4.0 mmol, possibly due to a defect in the sarcolemma causing spontaneous depolarization. Triggered by stress, cold, hunger and exercise. Vital to avoid hyperkalaemia perioperatively, using insulin/dextrose and loop diuretics. Suxamethonium may cause sufficient hyperkalaemia to precipitate an attack.

### Hypokalaemic periodic paralysis

Unrelated to hyperkalaemic periodic paralysis. Asymmetric paralysis involving arms, legs, trunk and neck. Usually spares diaphragm and facial muscles. Associated with reduced cell membrane potential, making muscle more excitable. Precipitated by heavy carbohydrate meals, diuretics, alkalosis and hypothermia. The effect of muscle relaxants may be clinically similar to the paralysis itself.

### References

Berrouschot J, Baumann I, Kalischewski P et al 1997 Therapy of myasthenic crisis. Critical Care Medicine 25: 1228–1235

Eriksson L I 1995 Neuromuscular disorders and anaesthesia. Current Opinion in Anaesthesiology 8: 275–281

Kam P C A, Calcroft R M 1997 Perioperative stroke in general surgical patients. Anaesthesia 52: 879–883

Le Corre F, Plaud B 1998 Neuromuscular disorders. Current Opinion in
   Anaesthesiology 11: 333–337
Russell S H, Hirsch N P 1994 Anaesthesia and myotonia. British Journal of
   Anaesthesia 72: 210–216
Sneyd J R 1999 Propofol and epilepsy. British Journal of Anaesthesia 82: 168–169

## NEUROANAESTHESIA

## PHYSIOLOGY

### Cerebrospinal fluid (CSF)

Secreted by the choroid plexus in the lateral, III and IV ventricles. Flows
through foramen of Magendie and Lushka and is absorbed by arachnoid
villi: 720 ml/day. Contents are:

- pH 7.3
- CSF > plasma: $Na^+$, $Cl^-$, $Mg^{2+}$
- CSF < plasma: $K^+$, $HCO_3^-$, glucose, protein.

### Intracranial pressure (ICP)

Munro–Kelly hypothesis (1852) stated that the contents of cranium are not
compressible (60% water, 40% solid). Therefore, increasing the volume within
the cranium causes a rapid increase in pressure (Fig. 3.1).

However, compression of veins and communication of CSF with spinal
column result in a small range of compensation before pressure increases
(Fig. 3.2).

Normal CSF pressure is 0–10 mmHg. Neurosurgical patients often have
raised ICP and so are already on the steep part of curve. Active treatment is
needed above 25–30 mmHg. CSF pressure oscillates with arterial pulse and
swings with respiration.

*Cushing reflex.* Increased ICP causes hypertension and bradycardia.

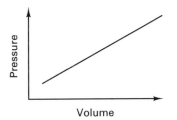

**Fig. 3.1** Theoretical intracranial pressure–volume relationship.

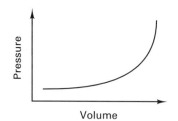

**Fig. 3.2** Actual intracranial pressure–volume relationship.

## Coning

All coning causes an autonomic storm. High pulmonary artery pressures may then result in neurogenic pulmonary oedema. ECG changes are now thought to be indicative of myocardial ischaemia. Reduced ADH secretion causes diabetes insipidus. Metabolic response is similar to that of the stress response following surgery.

- *Temporal (tentorial) coning.* Ipsilateral III nerve palsy, ↓ consciousness, Cushing reflex, decerebrate rigidity.
- *Cerebellar (medullary) coning.* Cheyne–Stokes breathing, sudden apnoea, neck stiffness.

## Pressure waves in CSF (described by Lundberg in 1960)

- *A-waves* – large amplitude waves lasting 5–20 min. Indicate failure of vasomotor compensation for raised ICP
- *B-waves* – 1/min. Associated with brainstem disorders
- *C-waves* – 6/min. Indicative of cerebral disorders.

## Cerebral circulation

$$CPP = MAP - (ICP + CVP)$$

where CPP = cerebral perfusion pressure, MAP = mean arterial pressure, ICP = intracranial pressure, CVP = central venous pressure at jugular bulb (usually zero).

Raised intrathoracic pressure increases CVP and reduces CPP further.

- *Normal flow* = 50 ml/100 g per min ≡ 15–20% of cardiac output.
- *Critical flow* occurs if MAP < 50 mmHg, i.e. < 20 ml/100 g per min.

Local metabolites are the main regulator of cerebral blood flow (CBF) by effects on extracellular $H^+$ concentration. Lactic acid metabolites maximally vasodilate diseased tissues, e.g. infarct, tumour, head injury, subarachnoid haemorrhage. Subsequently, any cerebral vasodilator will increase flow to normal tissue and may reduce flow in diseased tissue. Known as 'reverse steal'.

Normal brain autoregulates over a range of 50–130 mmHg (Fig. 3.3).

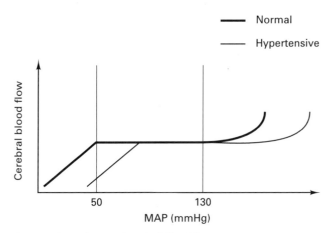

**Fig. 3.3** Autoregulatory limits of cerebral blood flow.

Hypertension shifts the curve to the right. Autoregulation is lost with volatile anaesthetic agents, tumour, trauma, infarction, intracranial bleed, hypoxia, hypercarbia, seizure disorders, hypotension and hypertension. In these conditions, CBF $\propto$ MAP.

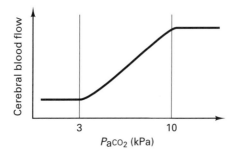

**Fig. 3.4** Effect of $P_a\text{CO}_2$ on cerebral blood flow.

## CO$_2$

Affects CBF through vasodilation by changing the pH of extracellular fluid (ECF) (Fig. 3.4).

Aim for a $P_a\text{CO}_2$ of 3.5 kPa to lower ICP without excessive vasoconstriction and prevent 'reverse steal'. Volatile agents increase effects of $CO_2$ on vasodilation. A 3% change in CBF occurs for each 0.1 kPa change in $P_a\text{CO}_2$.

Acute changes of hyperventilation return to normal values after 48 h due to normalization of CSF pH and a compensatory increase in CSF volume.

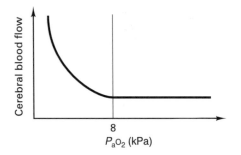

**Fig. 3.5** Effect of $P_aO_2$ on cerebral blood flow.

## $O_2$

Has less influence on CBF until $P_aO_2 < 8$ kPa (Fig. 3.5). Hyperoxia causes mild cerebral vasoconstriction of 5–10% at 60 kPa.

## MONITORING

**Table 3.1** Glasgow Coma Scale

| Eye opening | | Motor response | | Verbal response | |
|---|---|---|---|---|---|
| Spontaneous | 4 | Obeys commands | 6 | Orientated | 5 |
| To speech | 3 | Localizes pain | 5 | Confused | 4 |
| To pain | 2 | Normal flexion | 4 | Inappropriate words | 3 |
| Nil | 1 | Abnormal flexion | 3 | Sounds | 2 |
| | | Extension | 2 | Nil | 1 |
| | | Nil | 1 | | |

### EEG

- Unmodified EEG
- Cerebral function monitor – EEG filtered to derive mean amplitude
- Fourier analysis – displays frequency versus amplitude.

    *Waves*
- alpha (α):    8–13 Hz; awake, eyes closed
- beta (β):    > 13 Hz; alert, eyes open
- theta (θ):    4–7 Hz; abnormal in elderly patients
- delta (δ):    0.5–1 Hz; abnormal in all patients.

    Sudden reduction in CBF reduces amplitude of all waves and increases β and δ activity.

### Evoked potentials

Measure latency and amplitude.

- *Somatosensory* – e.g. median or posterior tibial nerve. Record over sensory cortex. Used for spinal cord and posterior fossa surgery.
- *Auditory* – auditory clicks. Record over mastoid to assess brainstem function, e.g. acoustic neuroma surgery.
- *Visual* – flashes of light over eyes. Record over visual cortex, e.g. for pituitary surgery.

### Measurement of intracranial pressure

- *Intraventricular catheter* – attached to transducer. Most accurate but risk of infection
- *Subdural bolt* – tends to under read at high pressures
- *Subdural catheter*
- *Extradural catheter* – either pressure transducer at tip of catheter or fibreoptic light shining onto mirror at tip which is displaced as ICP increases and alters amount of light reflected back onto the catheter.

## ANAESTHETIC DRUGS

Alter CBF by effects on vascular smooth muscle, cerebral metabolism and alveolar ventilation ($P_a\text{CO}_2$).

### Volatile agents

All volatiles reduce cerebral metabolism and oxygen demand. Effect is most marked with isoflurane. All increase ICP and abolish autoregulation in sufficient doses.

Halothane causes most cerebral vasodilation (Fig. 3.6). Enflurane may

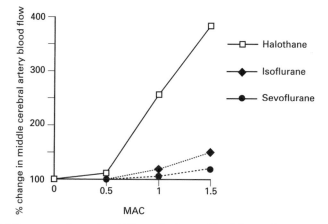

**Fig. 3.6** Percentage change in middle cerebral artery blood flow with increasing MAC.

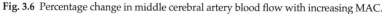

cause seizures, particularly at low $P_a\text{co}_2$. At 1 MAC (minimum alveolar concentration), isoflurane has the smallest effect on ICP, autoregulation or EEG depression. At 2.5 MAC, the EEG becomes isoelectric. Isoflurane reduces cerebral $O_2$ demand more than any other volatile and reduces cerebral blood flow without evidence of ischaemia.

Sevoflurane and desflurane appear similar to isoflurane in their CNS and CVS effects. $N_2O$ is a weak vasodilator causing moderate increases in CBF and cerebral metabolic rate (CMR). Changes in CBF are variable and may be more related to changes in $F_iO_2$.

### Intravenous agents

All i.v. induction agents decrease ICP except ketamine, and all have little effect on autoregulation. Both thiopentone and propofol cause dose-related decreases in CBF (Fig. 3.7) and $O_2$ demand and both are good attenuators of increased ICP during intubation. Propofol has nine Committee on Safety of Medicines reports (August 1987) warning of grand mal seizures.

Ketamine increases CBF, ICP and $O_2$ demand. Avoid in neuroanaesthesia.

Suxamethonium causes a transient rise in ICP through muscle fasciculations, increasing venous pressure and muscle spindle efferents activated by fasciculations.

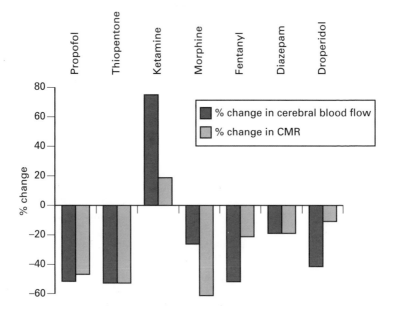

**Fig. 3.7** Effect of i.v. anaesthetics on cerebral blood flow (CBF) and cerebral metabolic rate (CMR).

## ANAESTHESIA FOR NEUROSURGERY

### Aims

- Maintain safe airway
- Maximize $O_2$ delivery
- Minimize $O_2$ demand
- Avoid sudden hypertensive insults
- Maintain CPP ($\rightarrow$ MAP, $\downarrow$ ICP, $\downarrow$ CVP)
- Use agents allowing rapid postoperative recovery.

### Preoperative

Assess gag reflex (?aspiration), $\downarrow$ cough reflex (?sputum retention), drowsiness (?drug-induced or CNS pathology), nausea and vomiting causing electrolyte disturbance and dehydration. Assess signs of raised ICP (headache, nausea and vomiting, Cushing reflex, downward gaze of eyes). Assess drug treatment: steroids decrease ICP, anticonvulsants induce liver enzymes, cimetidine inhibits liver enzymes. Assess pituitary dysfunction.

### Premedication

Avoid drugs causing neurological or respiratory depression. Prescribe midazolam and glycopyrrolate if necessary.

### Monitoring

Arterial line, CVP via long line (neck lines impair venous drainage of head), ECG, temperature, end-tidal $CO_2$, $S_aO_2$, neuromuscular stimulator, regular blood gases and electrolytes.

### Positioning

Avoid obstructing venous drainage of head. 15° head up. Protect eyes.

### Induction

Thiopentone is the drug of choice because of its anticonvulsant properties. Give slowly to avoid a decrease in BP reducing CPP. Consider additional agent to attenuate pressor response to intubation, e.g. lignocaine, high-dose opioids, β-blockers, hydralazine. Topical anaesthesia to larynx. Etomidate causes coughing, hiccoughs and vomiting which raises ICP. Propofol causes epileptiform EEG.

Suxamethonium causes hyperkalaemia in the presence of spastic paraplegia. Wait for full paralysis before intubation to avoid coughing and straining on endotracheal tube (ETT). Use armoured ETT to prevent kinking. Tape ETT, because a tie may cause venous obstruction of head and neck, increasing ICP. Consider NG tube.

### Maintenance

Use a balanced technique with fentanyl in combination with $O_2$ and $N_2O$/air and muscle relaxants, which produces good cardiovascular stability. Isoflurane is the volatile of choice. If greatly increased ICP, avoid volatiles until dura has been opened. Vecuronium is the relaxant of choice – use high dose to avoid coughing or straining. Ventilate to maintain $P_aCO_2$ at 3.5 kPa.

### Reversal

Avoid coughing. Early extubation allows CNS monitoring for signs of deterioration. Avoid sudden hypertension which causes cerebral oedema through loss of autoregulation.

### Fluids

Maintain plasma osmolality at the upper end of normal. Avoid fluids with low osmolality which increase free brain water (Table 3.2). Avoid glucose-containing solutions which accelerate anaerobic metabolism and may worsen neurological morbidity.

**Table 3.2** Osmolality of intravenous fluids

| Solution | Osmolality (mOsm/l) |
| --- | --- |
| Normal saline | 310 |
| Mannitol | 300 |
| Hartmann's solution | 272 |
| Dextrose saline | 262 |
| 5% dextrose | 250 |

### Postoperative

Any change in Glasgow Coma Scale can be assumed to be due to surgical complications. Aim for a similar BP as the preoperative value. Codeine phosphate is usually sufficient for analgesia. Start anticonvulsants. Watch for diabetes insipidus, tension pneumocephalus and cranial nerve injury.

## ANAESTHESIA FOR INTRACRANIAL ANEURYSM

Nimodipine reduces the risk of rebleeding in patients following a subarachnoid haemorrhage and may reduce the severity of vasospasm. Vasospasm is maximal between days 3 and 10. Generally aim for early surgery (within 48 h) if no severe neurological deficit, or late surgery if patient is comatose (to assess potential degree of recovery over about 10 days). Hyperventilation may worsen vasospasm.

Opening the dura reduces ICP, resulting in increased transmural pressure across the aneurysm wall. Therefore, may need perioperative hypotensive anaesthesia. Vasodilation with sodium nitroprusside causes increased ICP unless dura is opened. Trimetaphan can be used with the dura closed but is of slower onset, causes dilated pupils (ganglion blockade), making CNS assessment difficult, and triggers histamine release. Both drugs may cause rebound hypertension on cessation.

If aneurysm ruptures, press on ipsilateral carotid artery, give 100% $O_2$ and consider transient hypotension with sodium nitroprusside.

## ANAESTHESIA FOR POSTERIOR FOSSA SURGERY

The posterior fossa comprises midbrain, pons, medulla, cerebellum and cranial nerves V–XII. Patient position to be either:

- sitting – reduces blood loss but high risk of air embolus and hypotension
- park bench position – greatly reduces the risk of air embolus.

### Complications of surgery

*Air embolus.* Usually gradual leak rather than sudden bolus. Occurs due to veins being prevented from collapsing by tethering to dura (dural sinuses) or periosteum (emissary sinuses). Reduce incidence with 10 cm PEEP, neck tourniquet and G-suit.

Spontaneous respiration provides further indicators of brainstem function but increased risk of air embolus (negative intrathoracic pressure) and hypercapnia.

*Sensitivity of detection.* Precordial Doppler > $P_aO_2$ > $P_{ET}CO_2$ > PAP > $P_aCO_2$ > CVP > CO > BP > ECG> 'mill-wheel' murmur using stethoscope.

*Treatment.* Occlude wound with wet swab, 100% $O_2$, raise CVP by levelling table and neck compression, aspirate CVP line (tip should be placed in RA preoperatively), position patient in left lateral position with head down if possible.

### Other complications
- Stimulation of posterior fossa causing the Cushing reflex
- Vagal stimulation causes bradycardia
- Stimulation of V (trigeminal) cranial nerve causes hypertension
- Damage to dorsal group neurones causes postoperative apnoea
- Bulbar palsy
- Increased sensitivity to respiratory depressants.

### Postoperative

Loss of gag (glossopharyngeal [IX] damage) increases risk of aspiration following extubation. Therefore assess prior to extubation. Watch for respiratory failure and hydrocephalus.

## TREATMENT OF RAISED ICP

- 15° head-up tilt. Ensure good venous drainage of head and neck
- Avoid hypoxia. Keep $P_aCO_2$ lower limit of normal. No PEEP
- Keep CVP low
- Avoid cerebral vasodilating drugs
- Adequate muscle relaxation
- Osmotic/loop diuretics (Mannitol 1 g/kg; effect prolonged by frusemide)
- Consider CSF drainage.

---

**RECOMMENDATIONS FOR THE TRANSFER OF PATIENTS WITH ACUTE HEAD INJURIES TO NEUROSURGICAL UNITS**
Neuroanaesthesia Society of Great Britain and Ireland and the Association of Anaesthetists of Great Britain and Ireland 1996

1. There should be a designated consultant in the referring hospital with overall responsibility for the transfer of patients with head injuries to the neurosurgical unit and one at the neurosurgical unit with overall responsibility for receiving the transfers.
2. Local guidelines on the transfer of patients with head injury should be drawn up between the referring unit trusts and neurosurgical unit.
3. Thorough resuscitation and stabilization of the patient must be completed before transfer to avoid complications during the journey. A patient persistently hypotensive, despite resuscitation, must not be transported until all possible causes of the hypotension have been identified and the patient stabilized.
4. Only in exceptional circumstances should a patient with a significantly altered conscious level not be intubated for transfer.
5. Patients with head injuries should be accompanied by a doctor with at least 2 years' experience in an appropriate speciality (ideally anaesthesia). They should be familiar with the pathophysiology of head injury, the drugs and equipment they will use, working in the confines of an ambulance, and should have received supervised training in the transfer of patients with head injuries. They must have an appropriately trained assistant, have appropriate clothing, medical indemnity and personal insurance.

---

### References

Andrews P J D 1998 Head injury: complications and management. Current Opinion in Anaesthesiology 11: 473–477

Bullock R, Chesnut R, Clifton G et al 1996 Guidelines for the management of severe head injury. European Journal of Emergency Medicine 3: 109–127

Chesnut R M 1997 Hyperventilation in traumatic brain injury: friend or foe? Critical Care Medicine 25: 1275–1278

Chesnut R M 1998 Hyperventilation versus cerebral perfusion pressure management: time to change the question. Critical Care Medicine 26: 210–212

Fitch W 1998 Neuroanaesthesia. Current Opinion in Anaesthesiology 11: 457–458

Neuroanaesthesia Society of Great Britain and Ireland and Association of Anaesthetists of Great Britain and Ireland 1996 Recommendations for the transfer of patients with acute head injuries to neurosurgical units. NSGBI / AAGBI, London

Reinstrup P, Uski T K 1994 Inhalational anaesthetics in neurosurgery. Current Opinion in Anaesthesiology 7: 421–425

Werner C, Kochs E 1998 Monitoring of the central nervous system. Current Opinion in Anaesthesiology 11: 459–465

## AUTONOMIC NERVOUS SYSTEM

### SYMPATHETIC NERVOUS SYSTEM (Fig. 3.8)

Centres in brainstem give rise to descending tracts which innervate SNS preganglionic neurones in intermediolateral columns in the spinal cord.

**SNS**

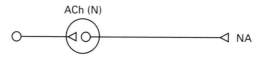

**Sweat-glands**

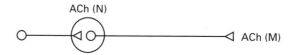

**Adrenal medulla**

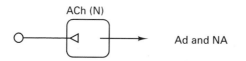

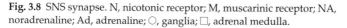

**Fig. 3.8** SNS synapse. N, nicotonic receptor; M, muscarinic receptor; NA, noradrenaline; Ad, adrenaline; ○, ganglia; □, adrenal medulla.

They emerge at $T_1$–$L_2$, then either synapse in SNS chain or synapse at a distance, e.g. coeliac plexus (splanchnic) or hypogastric plexus (bladder). SNS fibres for skin and vessels re-enter the cord to re-emerge with skeletal nerves.

## PARASYMPATHETIC NERVOUS SYSTEM

Parasympathetic nerve fibres run in cranial nerves II, V, VII, IX, X, $S_2$–$S_4$. 75% of PNS fibres run in the vagus to supply heart, lungs, upper GI tract and liver. Preganglionic fibres terminate in the end organ and postganglionic fibres are very short.

**PNS**

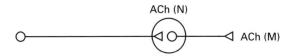

**Fig. 3.9** PNS synapse.

## VALSALVA MANOEUVRE

- *Phase I*
    — forced expiration against resistance (or a closed glottis) to a pressure of 40 mmHg for 10 s
    — raised intrathoracic pressure transmitted to arteries causing initial hypertension and compensatory bradycardia
- *Phase II*
    — reduced venous return causes hypotension with compensatory tachycardia
- *Phase III*
    — release of Valsalva
    — reduced intrathoracic pressure causes hypotension and compensatory tachycardia
- *Phase IV*
    — hypertension due to vasoconstriction as venous return and thus cardiac output increases, causing a reflex bradycardia.

## AUTONOMIC NEUROPATHY

**Causes**

- Elderly
- Diabetes (IDDM > NIDDM)
- CVA
- Guillain–Barré syndrome

- Parkinson's disease
- Shy–Drager syndrome
- AIDS.

## Symptoms and signs

- Loss of diurnal BP variation
- Fixed heart rate (tachycardia) and loss of R–R' variation
- Orthostatic hypotension
- Painless MI
- Failure of kidneys to concentrate urine at night, causing nocturia
- Increased gastric emptying time.

## Assessment

Abnormal response to Valsalva manoeuvre with BP continuing to fall during phase II. No overshoot of BP on release of Valsalva. No tachy- or bradycardia.

- *SNS*
  - degree of postural hypotension (decrease systolic > 30 mmHg)
  - thermoregulatory sweating test
- *PNS*
  - degree of bradycardia with Valsalva manoeuvre (< 5 beats/min is abnormal)
  - degree of sinus arrhythmia during deep breathing (difference between maximum and minimum HR < 15 beats/min is abnormal).

## Anaesthetic problems

- Blood pressure dependent upon ECF volume with subsequent hypotension on induction
- Arrhythmias common
- Reduced sensitivity to hypoxia and hypercapnia
- Ventilation not associated with the usual Valsalva-type response
- Reduced response to indirect-acting catecholamines (e.g. ephedrine) but exaggerated response to direct catecholamines (e.g. adrenaline) due to a denervation hypersensitivity.

### References

Foëx P 1994 The heart and autonomic nervous system. In: Nimmo W S, Rowbotham D J, Smith G (eds) Anaesthesia, 2nd edn. Blackwell Scientific Publications, Oxford, p 195–242
Keyl C, Lemberger P, Palitzsch K D, Hochmuth K et al 1999 Cardiovascular

autonomic dysfunction and haemodynamic response to anesthetic induction in patients with coronary artery disease and diabetes mellitus. Anesthesia and Analgesia 88: 985–991

Tusiewicz K 1988 The autonomic nervous system. In: Kaufman L (ed) Anaesthesia Review 5. Churchill Livingstone, Edinburgh, p 54–66

# 4. Other systems

First dental GA was given by Cotton & Wells in 1844. Currently, 300 000 dental GAs are given per annum (70% children) and, until recently, numbers have been declining owing to less tooth decay.

Mortality is 1:150 000 (2 deaths/year), compared with 1:250 000 non-dental day-case GAs, and is usually due to respiratory difficulties or sudden cardiovascular collapse.

Recent deaths in the dental chair have prompted moves to stop dental anaesthesia being carried out in dental surgeries.

**POSWILLO REPORT** Department of Health 1990

This report discusses general anaesthesia, sedation and resuscitation in dental surgeries. Its main recommendations are:

- Same standards required for GA in dental surgeries as in hospitals.
- Minimum monitoring standards.
- Dental surgeries to be inspected and registered.
- Accredited anaesthetists only.

**STANDARDS AND GUIDELINES FOR GENERAL ANAESTHESIA FOR DENTISTRY** The Royal College of Anaesthetists 1999

**Introduction**
- There are concerns over a recent increase in the number of dental anaesthetics administered in the community.
- Deaths (usually young, healthy patients) continue to occur. Criticism of anaesthetic standards has led to increase in public concern.
- The Royal College of Anaesthetists expects the same standards in dental anaesthesia as are widely accepted for anaesthesia in other clinical settings in the UK.

**Background**
- GAs are often used inappropriately as a method of anxiety control rather than pain relief.
- Risks of community GAs are often not appreciated, with frequent failings in standards of patient care, monitoring and resuscitation skills. Compromise in standards is almost inevitable because of economic pressure.
- The Poswillo report and guidelines from the General Dental Council have not improved standards as intended.

**Recommended standards**
General anaesthesia should be limited to:

1. control of pain that cannot be achieved with local anaesthesia ± sedation
2. patients with problems related to age/maturity or physical/mental disability
3. patients in whom dental phobia will be induced or prolonged.

*Patient assessment*
The final decision as to the benefit:risk of a dental GA can only be made after consultation between the patient, anaesthetist and dentist.

*Clinical setting*
Risks of death are greater should a complication occur. There must be written protocols for the management of patients requiring resuscitation or transfer.

*Equipment and drugs*
Equipment should be appropriate to the dental setting and anaesthetic technique. Routine maintenance must be performed and checks of equipment must be made before use. Back-up equipment and resuscitation drugs must be available.

*Staffing standards*
Dental anaesthesia should only be administered by:

1. anaesthetists on the Specialist Register
2. trainees working under supervision
3. non-consultant-grade anaesthetists working under the supervision of a named consultant.

Trained assistance must be provided by an operating department practitioner or dental nurse. Patients must be supervised in recovery until fully awake.

*Aftercare*
Patients must be discharged home according to the same criteria as day-case surgery.

*Audit*
This should examine all aspects of practice.

*The way forward*
- Greater patient education in non-GA techniques that are available
- Better anaesthetic training in control of pain and anxiety
- Centralization of GA services in centres with adequate facilities.

## MAIN ANAESTHETIC PROBLEMS

- Shared airway
- Day-case anaesthesia
- Paediatrics
- Mentally handicapped patients from institutions are at higher risk of hepatitis B.
- Lack of premedication causing ↑ anxiety, ↑ arrhythmias and difficult i.v. access.

## TECHNIQUES

### Local anaesthetic

### Sedation

A state of CNS depression during which *verbal contact with the patient is maintained*. Achieved with Entonox, oral/i.v. benzodiazepines, i.v. methohexitone.

### General anaesthetic

*Intubation.* Avoid suxamethonium which has high morbidity. High-dose alfentanyl (30 $\mu$g/kg) together with propofol enables intubation without relaxant.

Indicated for mental handicap, prolonged or painful surgery, and nasal airway obstruction. Use nasopharyngeal pack.

*Cardiovascular side effects*

*Dysrhythmias.* These are common due to sympathetic and parasympathetic activity, high levels of endogenous catecholamines, halothane and airway obstruction with hypoxia and hypercarbia:

- nodal rhythms   – 25%
- multifocal PVCs – 8%

They mostly occur during surgery and are worse during trigeminal nerve stimulation. Atropine increases the incidence of dysrhythmias.

Less common with i.v. induction than with gaseous induction. Less common with volatile agents other than halothane.

More common following recent Coxsackie B infection due to (?) viral myocarditis.

Arrhythmias may be the primary cause of high mortality seen with dental GAs .

*Fainting.* Only in conscious patients! May need large doses of atropine. Abandon procedure because CVS instability persists for up to 90 min.

High mortality in erect patients was attributed to unrecognized fainting, but mortality is the same in supine patients. Supine position is associated with more pharyngeal soiling. It is now recommended that all surgery should be performed in the supine position which gives better CVS stability.

### References

Cartwright D P 1999 Death in the dental chair. Anaesthesia 54: 105–107

Department of Health 1990 General anaesthesia, sedation and resuscitation in dentistry (Poswillo report). HMSO, London

Reilly C S 1992 Anaesthesia in the dental chair. Current Anaesthesia and Critical Care 3: 6–10

Royal College of Anaesthetists 1999 Standards and guidelines for general anaesthesia and dentistry. RCA, London

Worthington L M, Flynn P J, Strunin L 1998 Death in the dental chair: an avoidable catastrophe? British Journal of Anaesthesia 80: 131–132

## ANAESTHESIA FOR EAR, NOSE AND THROAT SURGERY

### GENERAL ANAESTHETIC PROBLEMS

- Competition with the surgeon for airway, loss of access to the airway and airway compromise with packs, blood, pus or tissue.
- Spontaneous ventilation has the advantage that the reservoir bag provides a good monitor of respiration and any disconnection hidden by the drapes is immediately obvious.
- Avoid halothane if repeated anaesthetics or if the surgeon is planning to use adrenaline.
- Extubate in a head-down, left lateral position to prevent aspiration of blood and debris and to protect the airway in the immediate postoperative period.

### EAR SURGERY

#### Myringotomy

This is a short, relatively painless operation. Premedication is not usually necessary.

Chronic otitis media is often associated with upper respiratory tract infection. Morbidity not increased with uncomplicated URTI if mask rather than intubation used. Need postoperative $O_2$ if oxygen saturation < 93% on room air.

### Middle ear surgery

Careful positioning is required to avoid obstruction of venous drainage of the head. Tympanoplasty and mastoidectomy usually require identification of facial nerve. Therefore, avoid long-acting neuromuscular blocking drugs.

Use hypotensive anaesthesia to minimize bleeding. Maximum recommended safe dose of adrenaline = 0.1 mg / 10 min.

Avoid $N_2O$ which diffuses into the middle ear to cause expansion, or on cessation diffuses out of the middle ear to cause negative pressure and disruption of ossicles.

Consider prophylactic antiemetics.

## NASAL SURGERY

### Anaesthesia of the nasal cavities

*Moffatt's solution*
- 2 ml 8% cocaine
- 2 ml 1% bicarbonate
- 1 ml 1:1000 adrenaline.

Give with head extended over trolley, with half into each nostril.

*Sluder's technique.* Four applicators are dipped into adrenaline and cocaine solution, and placed on middle turbinates under anterior and posterior ends.

*Packing of nasal cavities.* Spray nasal cavities with 4–10% cocaine and then pack with gauze soaked in 4–5% cocaine solution.

Gauze must contact area behind middle meatus (greater and lesser palatine nerves) and ethmoidal plate (anterior ethmoidal nerve).

## THROAT SURGERY

### Tonsillectomy

Avoid premedication if tonsils are large or there is a history of sleep apnoea.

Use gas or i.v. induction. Either deep gaseous intubation (patient more drowsy postoperatively) or suxamethonium. Use throat pack and endotracheal tube.

Spontaneous respiration tends to hypoventilation with risk of arrhythmias, especially with halothane.

Extubate awake (protective reflexes), with head down in left lateral position.

*Postoperative haemorrhage.* Affects 0.5%; 75% of postoperative haemorrhages occur within 6 h of surgery. Main problems are:

- hypovolaemia
- full stomach
- residual effects of earlier GA
- upper airway oedema from previous surgery and intubation
- anxious child and parents.

Assessing the patient can be difficult. Tachycardia due to hypovolaemia may also be due to anxiety or pain. Blood loss is usually underestimated as most is swallowed. Establish i.v. access, check BP sitting and lying (postural hypotension with hypovolaemia), check haematocrit and cross-match blood.

There are two approaches to induction:

- *Gas induction*. Head down, left lateral position, head-down tilt. If cords are visualized once lightly anaesthetized, give suxamethonium and intubate. Deep gaseous intubation worsens hypotension if hypovolaemic.
- *Rapid sequence induction*. Head down, left lateral position for intubation if practised in this technique.

Both approaches need a selection of laryngoscope blades, stylettes, range of ETTs, two suction units (one may become blocked with clot), emergency tracheostomy kit and tipping trolley.

Pass NG tube and aspirate stomach prior to extubation.

### Adenoidectomy

Usually performed in conjunction with tonsillectomy. Not as painful. May cause nasopharyngeal obstruction and obligate mouth breathing.

### Obstructive sleep apnoea

Grossly hypertrophied tonsils can cause partial upper airway obstruction when awake and complete obstruction during sleep. Associated with obesity, micrognathia (e.g. Pierre–Robin syndrome) and neuromuscular disorders (e.g. cerebral palsy). May present as failure to thrive, snoring, daytime somnolence, developmental delay, recurrent chest infections and, if severe, cor pulmonale. Airway obstruction may persist post-tonsillectomy.

### Peritonsillar abscess (quinsy)

The infected tonsil forms an abscess in the lateral pharyngeal wall with associated trismus and difficulty in swallowing. The abscess does not usually interfere with the airway, but there is a risk of rupture and aspiration of contents. Drainage under LA, otherwise treat as for epiglottitis. Consider tracheostomy under LA if abscess is likely to rupture on intubation.

**References**

Chambers W A 1994 ENT anaesthesia. In: Nimmo W S, Rowbotham D J, Smith G
(eds) Anaesthesia. Blackwell Scientific Publications, London, p 806–822

## ANAESTHESIA AND LIVER DISEASE

### NORMAL PHYSIOLOGY

The liver receives 25% of cardiac output. Portal venous blood contributes
70% of total flow and 50–60% of oxygen. The portal venous system has little
smooth muscle and is not as responsive to sympathetic tone as the hepatic
artery. When portal flow decreases, hepatic artery flow increases.
Autoregulation at a microvascular level is poorly developed in the liver but
hepatocytes can extract more oxygen from the blood than can any other
tissue.

Total hepatic blood flow is reduced by IPPV, PEEP, hypovolaemia,
hypocarbia, general anaesthesia and epidurals.

### PHYSIOLOGICAL CHANGES IN LIVER DISEASE

*CVS.* Hyperdynamic circulation, ↓ systemic vascular resistance, portal
hypertension, due to activation of renin–angiotensin system and intravascular
and interstitial fluid accumulation. Alcoholic cardiomyopathy.

*Respiratory.* Restrictive lung disease, pleural effusions. Impaired hypoxic
pulmonary vasoconstriction causing ↑$\dot{V}/\dot{Q}$ scatter and ↑ shunting, together
with impaired respiration from ascites, causing hypoxia.

*Haematology.* Anaemia, thrombocytopenia, coagulopathy.

*Renal.* Hepatorenal syndrome (especially with sepsis and ↑ bilirubin).
Prerenal failure causes acute tubular necrosis.

*GI.* Oesophageal varices, delayed gastric emptying. Increased gastric
volume and acidity.

*CNS.* Encephalopathy, cerebral oedema.

*Metabolic.* Metabolic and respiratory alkalosis, hyper- or hypoglycaemia.
Hyponatraemia (usually dilutional).

### PHARMACOKINETIC AND PHARMACODYNAMIC
### CHANGES

- Early alcoholic liver disease induces liver enzymes, causing drug
  resistance. In late stages, impaired function causes drug sensitivity.
  Phase I metabolism is reduced more than phase II metabolism.
- Sodium and water retention and ascites increase $V_D$ of water-soluble
  drugs.

- Hypoalbuminaemia increases free drug concentrations, e.g. barbiturates, propanolol, benzodiazepines etc.
- Increased CNS sensitivity to depressants due to increased blood–brain barrier permeability and altered CNS receptor kinetics.
- Decreased first pass of drugs due to shunting of portal blood flow into the systemic circulation, bypassing liver parenchyma.

## ASSESSMENT OF SURGICAL RISK

Child's (1963) classification assessed risk using albumin and bilirubin. Modified by Pugh et al (1973) (see Table 4.1).

Table 4.1 Pugh's (1973) modification of Child's (1963) classification of surgical risk in patients with liver disease

| | | | |
|---|---|---|---|
| Serum bilirubin (mg/dl) | < 2.3 | 2.3–3.0 | > 3.0 |
| Serum albumin | > 3.5 | 3.0–3.5 | < 3.0 |
| Ascites | None | Controlled | Decompensated |
| Neurological disorder | None | Minimal | Advanced |
| Nutritional status | Excellent | Moderate | Poor |
| Prothrombin ratio | 1–4 | 4–6 | > 6 |
| Surgical risk | Good | Moderate | Poor |
| Mortality rate | < 5% | 25% | > 50% |

## SPECIFIC DRUGS

*Anticholinergics.* Little change in pharmacokinetics. Use normal doses.

*Barbiturates.* Increased sensitivity and prolonged excretion of thiopentone. Use < 3–4 mg/kg.

*Benzodiazepines.* Lorazepam and oxazepam are metabolized by glucuronidation, which is minimally affected: therefore they are safe. Increased sensitivity to diazepam and midazolam due to impaired phase I reactions.

*Propofol.* Increased sensitivity. Use 2mg/kg for induction.

*Opioids.* Increased sensitivity and prolonged half-life of morphine, diamorphine and pethidine. No change in remifentanil pharmacokinetics.

*Muscle relaxants.* Suxamethonium has prolonged action due to reduced plasma cholinesterase. Resistance to tubocurarine and pancuronium due to increased $V_D$ of these drugs. Atracurium is probably the drug of choice due to spontaneous degradation and little change in pharmacokinetics. Action of vecuronium is prolonged even with mild liver disease.

*Anticholinesterases.* Normal doses of neostigmine may be used.

*Local anaesthetics.* Reduced metabolism of amides. Reduced plasma cholinesterase prolongs elimination of esters.

*Inhalational agents.* Halothane > enflurane > isoflurane decrease hepatic blood flow. Isoflurane vasodilates hepatic artery with only slight decrease in total flow. Overall $O_2$ delivery may be increased. Avoid halothane because of risks of hepatitis. Sympathomimetic effects of $N_2O$ may reduce hepatic blood flow.

*Other.* Adrenaline and ephedrine increase hepatic blood flow. Sodium nitroprusside and β-blockers decrease hepatic blood flow.

## ANAESTHETIC MANAGEMENT

### Preoperative

Assess cardiovascular and renal status. Optimize respiratory function with antibiotics, bronchodilators, physiotherapy and consider drainage of ascites. Correct coagulation with FFP, cryoprecipitate, vitamin K and platelets.

### Premedication

Avoid if possible.

### Monitoring

Routine monitoring, arterial line, CVP, urinary catheter, nerve stimulator, ± PCWP.

### Induction

Use small amounts of thiopentone or midazolam.

### Maintenance

Use isoflurane or enflurane in oxygen. High $F_iO_2$ needed because of pulmonary shunting. Avoid hyperventilation which increases mean intrathoracic pressure, thus reducing hepatic blood flow, accelerates formation of ammonia, causing hepatic encephalopathy, and increases urinary potassium loss through respiratory alkalosis.

Hepatic blood flow is proportional to mean arterial pressure.

Neuromuscular blockade with atracurium or pancuronium. Reversal with normal doses of anticholinesterases.

Maintain high urine output to protect against renal failure. Avoid excess sodium load in i.v. fluids to prevent dilutional hyponatraemia. Recheck clotting if surgery prolonged.

### Postoperative

IPPV may be necessary until patient is rewarmed and stabilized. Remove lines as soon as possible to reduce risk of infection. Analgesia with small doses of opioids. Regional block may reduce requirements, provided clotting is normal.

**References**

Brown B R 1994 Anaesthesia and liver disease. In: Nimmo W S, Rowbotham D J, Smith G (eds) Anaesthesia. Blackwell Scientific Publications, London, p 1264–1276

Childs C G 1963 The liver and portal hypertension. In: Major problems in clinical surgery, vol. 1. WB Saunders, Philadelphia

Gimson A E S 1996 Fulminant and late onset hepatic failure. British Journal of Anaesthesia 77: 90–98

Hayes P C 1992 Editorial. Liver disease and drug disposition. British Journal of Anaesthesia 68: 459–461

Pugh R N H, Murray-Lyon I M, Dawson J L, Pietroni M C, Williams R 1973 Transection of the oesophagus for bleeding varices. British Journal of Surgery 60: 646–649

## ANAESTHESIA FOR OPHTHALMIC SURGERY

## PHYSIOLOGY

### Aqueous humour

Made by ciliary plexus and secreted into anterior chamber. Absorbed through trabecular meshwork into Canal of Schlem.

### Intraocular pressure (IOP)

Normal value 15–25 mmHg. Once the eye is opened, IOP is equal to atmospheric pressure. Hypoxia, hypercapnia, coughing and vomiting all increase IOP.

### Oculocardiac reflex

Reflex pathway runs from the long and short ciliary nerves via the ciliary ganglion to the ophthalmic division of the trigeminal nerve (V) and then to the Gasserian ganglion. From here, the pathway runs to the trigeminal sensory nucleus in the brainstem, to the motor nucleus of the vagus (X) in medulla, through the reticular formation and finally to the heart via the vagus nerve.

Causes bradycardia, asystole, PVCs, A-V block, VT and VF. It is more marked and frequent in children, particularly during squint surgery.

Reflex fatigues quickly with cessation of stimulus.

Prophylaxis with glycopyrrolate is as effective as atropine.

## EFFECTS OF ANAESTHETIC DRUGS ON INTRAOCULAR PRESSURE

All volatile agents cause a dose-related decrease in IOP due to decreased extraocular muscle tone and increased aqueous humour outflow.

Etomidate and propofol lower IOP, as do (to a lesser degree) thiopentone, benzodiazepines, morphine and fentanyl. Ketamine increases IOP and causes blepharospasm and nystagmus.

Suxamethonium increases IOP, possibly by orbital smooth muscle contraction. Peak increase is 10 mmHg at 4 min, returning to baseline value by 6 min. Precurarization has a minimal effect on IOP.

d-Tubocurarine, pancuronium, vecuronium and atracurium all lower IOP.

## EYE SURGERY

### Requirements

- No coughing, straining or vomiting
- Soft, akinetic eye in central position.

### Advantages of regional block over GA

- More suitable for day surgery
- Reduced anaesthetic morbidity (less nausea and sore throat)
- Safer for sick patients
- Better postoperative analgesia
- Faster patient turnover.

### GA

More suitable for painful procedures, anxious patients, chronic cough, penetrating eye injuries, deaf and mentally handicapped patients, children and long operations. Assess other pathology associated with the eye disease, e.g. trauma, diabetes, myotonic dystrophy. Patient is often elderly with associated pathology, e.g. hypertension (47%), ischaemic heart disease (38%), hypothyroidism (18%), diabetes (16%), new malignancy (3%).

### Premedication

- Opiates – respiratory depression increases IOP and causes nausea and vomiting
- Benzodiazepines – good
- Anticholinergics – do not ↑ IOP at premedication doses and are safe with narrow angle glaucoma.

### Monitoring

Often in dark room (to prevent glare interfering with surgical microscope) with minimal access to patient. Expose limb and illuminate a limb to allow access to a pulse and observe for cyanosis.

### Induction

Propofol decreases IOP more than thiopentone and causes less nausea and vomiting. Laryngeal mask airway (LMA) results in less rise in IOP compared with ETT and less postoperative coughing and sore throat. If patient is ventilated, ETT avoids risks of regurgitation, but spray cord with local anaesthetic to reduce coughing. Tape ETT in place because a tie causes venous obstruction to drainage of head, raising IOP.

Smooth extubation to avoid coughing by extubating deep, deflating cuff before reversal and using lignocaine 1.5 mg/kg pre-extubation.

Ecothiopate (organophosphate – no longer available) inhibited plasma cholinesterase and prolonged action of suxamethonium. Avoid suxamethonium with myotonic dystrophy.

Keep IOP low by:

- 10° head-up tilt
- adequate neuromuscular blockade, which ensures low peak airway pressure
- keeping end-tidal $CO_2$ at the lower limit of normal (if IPPV)
- avoiding mechanical pressure on eyeball, e.g. lid retractors
- i.v. mannitol
- choroidal autoregulation – lost with systolic < 90 mmHg.

*Nitrous oxide.* Intraocular bubbles of sulphur hexafluoride ($SF_6$) or perfluoropropane ($C_3F_8$) are used in surgery for detached retina to push the retina against the choroid. Nitrous oxide will cause rapid expansion of the bubble if used within 10 days.

## REGIONAL ANAESTHESIA

First local anaesthetic (LA) eye surgery using topical cocaine was performed by Koller in 1880. It is becoming more popular: 80% of all cataracts are now operated on under LA.

*Absolute contraindications*
- Changes in eye shape
- Orbital pathology
- Penetrating eye injury
- Previous retinal detachment surgery in that eye.

*Relative contraindications*
- Large eye (> 26 mm)
- Warfarin (check INR < 2.5).

### Local anaesthetic solution

Use:

- equal volumes of lignocaine 2% and bupivacaine 0.75%
- hyaluronidase 5 units/ml
- +/– adrenaline 1:200 000 (5 μg/ml) to prolong block.

Less painful injection if solution warmed to 35°C.

Retrobulbar and peribulbar blocks are equated with spinal and epidural blocks, respectively.

*Retrobulbar block.* First described by Atkinson in 1955. Patient looks straight ahead. Use a 25G 40 mm blunt needle.

1. Inject through inferior conjunctiva in vertical line through edge of lateral border of iris. Advance needle in posterior direction to 1 cm then superomedially 2–3 cm to enter muscle cone (max. depth 25 mm) when the eye will bob downwards. Inject 4 ml LA solution.

2. Superior rectus block through upper lid in midline to depth of 15 mm.

3. Facial nerve block – there are several techniques:
- Van Lint – along lateral upper and lower orbital rims
- Atkinson – over zygomatic arch
- O'Brien – over temporomandibular joint.

The popularity of retrobulbar block has declined due to a greater risk of neurovascular damage compared with peribulbar block.

*Peribulbar block.* First described by Davis & Mandel in 1986. Aim to keep the needle always at a tangent to the globe, advancing the tip no further than the equator of the globe, outside the muscle cone. Uses larger dose of LA and has a longer onset time. Use a 25 G 25 mm blunt needle.

1. Insert needle at fornix of conjunctiva at junction of lateral third and medial two-thirds, directed towards the floor of the orbit, and inject 4–10 ml LA.

2. Insert medial to the medial caruncle to a depth of 20 mm: inject 2–5 ml LA.

Compress eyeball for 10 min after injection to aid spread of LA using small pneumatic/lead balloon strapped over eye.

Block of facial nerve is not usually required.

### Complications of regional blocks

Of 60 000 annual LA operations, life-threatening complications occur in 1:750. There are fewer complications with peribulbar block, but less akinesia.

- *Injection into optic nerve sheath* – solution may spread via optic chiasm to CNS, causing drowsiness, convulsions, cardiorespiratory arrest and loss of consciousness
- *Muscle damage* – avoid inferior and lateral rectus muscles
- *Oculocardiac reflex*
- *Retrobulbar haemorrhage (arterial)* – avoid superior–medial quadrant. Avoid damaging arterial branches of ophthalmic artery on upper border of medial rectus muscle by directing needle 5° caudally
- *Venous haemorrhage* – reassure patient; generally not a problem
- *Chemosis* – worse with excessive LA volume. Massage orbit to reduce. May interfere with trabeculectomy surgery
- *Postoperative diplopia* – until LA worn off. Reassure patient
- *Respiratory deterioration* – patients with respiratory disease are prone to hypoxia and hypercarbia

- *Penetration of the eye*, causing:
  - — intraocular haemorrhage
  - — immediate / delayed retinal detachment
  - — intraocular toxicity of local anaesthetic drugs
    and the following symptoms:
  - — movement of the eye with the needle
  - — acute pain
  - — sudden loss of vision
  - — loss of ocular tone.

## OPEN EYE INJURY AND FULL STOMACH

There is a conflict between protection of the airway and prevention of increased IOP. Discuss with surgeons. Can surgery be delayed until stomach is empty?

A study of rapid sequence induction using suxamethonium in 228 patients failed to show any loss of vitreous through the penetrating wound (Libonati et al 1985).

Three approaches to rapid sequence induction:

1. Suxamethonium preceded by lignocaine 1.5 mg / kg and a small dose of non-depolarizing drug
2. High-dose non-depolarizing muscle relaxant, e.g. vecuronium 0.2 mg / kg. Give anti-aspiration medication preoperatively ($H_2$ antagonist and metoclopramide) together with cricoid pressure
3. Awake intubation using topical anaesthesia.

---

**REPORT OF THE JOINT WORKING PARTY ON ANÄESTHESIA IN OPHTHALMIC SURGERY** Royal College of Anaesthetists and College of Ophthalmologists 1993

- If GA planned, the anaesthetist is responsible for assessing the patient's fitness for anaesthesia and perioperative supervision of the patient.
- Special investigations: ECG if > 60 years or evidence of CVS disease. CXR if chronic lung disease, evidence of malignancy or pulmonary TB. Urea, creatinine and electrolytes if > 60 years or evidence of renal impairment. Blood sugar in all diabetics. Hb in all women and men > 60 years.
- If LA, monitor verbally, pulse oximeter, ECG, non-invasive BP. Intravenous access is mandatory. Anaesthetist to administer regional block and remain present in case resuscitation is required.
- No need for antibiotic prophylaxis for patients with valvular heart disease undergoing intraocular surgery.

## References

Barker J P, Vafidis G C, Hall G M 1996 Postoperative morbidity following cataract surgery. A comparison of local and general anaesthesia. Anaesthesia 51: 435–437

Hamilton R C 1995 Techniques of orbital regional anaesthesia. British Journal of Anaesthesia 75: 88–92

Johnson R W 1995 Anatomy for ophthalmic anaesthesia. British Journal of Anaesthesia 75: 80–87

Libonati M M, Leahy J J, Ellison N 1985 The use of succinylcholine in open eye surgery. Anesthesiology 62: 637–640

Royal College of Anaesthetists and College of Ophthalmologists 1993 Report of the Joint Working Party on Anaesthesia in Ophthalmic Surgery. Royal College of Anaesthetists and College of Ophthalmologists, London

Rubin A P 1995 Complications of local anaesthesia for ophthalmic surgery. British Journal of Anaesthesia 75: 93–96

# ANAESTHESIA FOR ORTHOPAEDIC SURGERY

## EPIDEMIOLOGY

Two main age groups:

- young males, due to trauma
- elderly females, due to osteoporosis and osteoarthritis. Increasing numbers as the elderly population increases.

## ANAESTHETIC MANAGEMENT

### Preoperative

Most elderly patients have coexisting diseases. Carry out cardiovascular and respiratory assessment. Treat other pathology as necessary, e.g. dehydration, diabetes, renal failure, infection. Osteoarthritis and joint immobility are common.

Excessive delays awaiting surgery cause pressure sores, increase the risk of DVT and pulmonary embolus (PE), increase the risk of pneumonia and thus increase overall mortality. Therefore, do not prolong patient optimization longer than necessary.

### Anaesthetic technique

Most studies comparing regional and general anaesthetic techniques have not shown any difference in mortality between them. Postoperatively, no significant CVS differences have been shown. However, regional techniques may have several advantages, including:

- better, earlier postoperative gas exchange (no difference by 24 h)
- reduced blood transfusion requirements

- reduced bleeding from bone, which may be of importance in preventing excess blood compromising bone cement fixation
- improved cardiovascular stability
- improved postoperative mental function
- good postoperative analgesia
- reduced incidence of DVT.

Preoperative autologous blood donation, cell salvaging and mild deliberate hypotension reduce transfusion requirements. Mild hypothermia (35.0 vs 36.6°C) has been shown to increase blood loss during hip arthroplasty.

### Bone cement

Hypotension and cardiac arrest were initially attributed to free methyl-methacrylate monomer forced into circulation during insertion of cement. However, they are now thought to be due to fat, air, platelet and marrow embolization with $\dot{V}/\dot{Q}$ mismatching and release of vasoactive substances from the lungs. Severe pain during intramedullary nailing may also contribute.

Hypotension during cement insertion is more common with increasing age, uraemia and pre-existing hypertension. Incidence is reduced if normovolaemia maintained during cement insertion.

### Fat embolism syndrome (FES)

Fat is released into the circulation in most patients from long bones at the time of fracture or during intramedullary nailing to cause asymptomatic embolization. However, in 2% of patients following femoral fractures, 0.1% after hip/knee replacements, and as many as 90% of multiple trauma patients, the degree of embolization may be sufficient to cause a triad of symptoms:

1. respiratory insufficiency
2. cerebral decompensation
3. skin petechiae.

Severe FES may cause cardiovascular collapse, multiorgan failure and death. Pathophysiological changes occur in three steps, as illustrated in Figure 4.1.

*Prophylaxis.* Surgical measures to minimize intramedullary pressure. Ensure adequate hydration. Consider delaying medullary reaming in major trauma patients.

*Treatment.* Early recognition is vital (desaturation, petechiae, confusion, hypotension). Consider bronchoalveolar lavage for diagnostic cytology. Oxygen, fluid management, anticoagulation. Steroids are unproven.

### Postoperative hyponatraemia

Iatrogenic hyponatraemia is particularly common following orthopaedic surgery due to fluid overload from 5% dextrose which after metabolism of dextrose leaves free water. Compounded by:

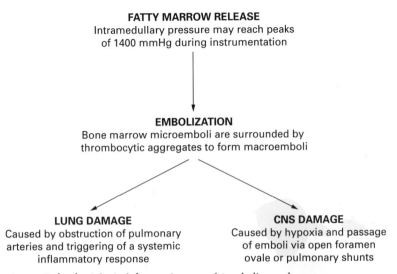

**Fig. 4.1** Pathophysiological changes in severe fat embolism sydnrome.

- thiazide diuretics – commonly used in the elderly to control hypertension, causing mild preoperative hyponatraemia
- surgical stress – causing a syndrome of inappropriate ADH secretion resulting in fluid retention and mild hyponatraemia for several days postoperatively
- impaired fluid homeostasis in elderly.

20% of patients with symptomatic hyponatraemia die or suffer serious brain damage. Brain damage reported with sodium as high as 128 mmol/l. Postmenopausal women are usually not symptomatic until sodium < 120 mmol/l.

*Early symptoms.* Weakness, nausea, vomiting and headache.

*Late symptoms.* Encephalopathy, convulsions, respiratory arrest, brain damage. Aim to raise serum sodium 1–2 mmol/l per hour until symptoms resolve. Risk of treatment is far less than risk of osmotic demyelination from treatment. Consider fluid restriction or hypertonic saline. Loop diuretics (e.g. frusemide) enhance free water excretion.

---

**ANTIBIOTIC PROPHYLAXIS FOR PROSTHETIC JOINT IMPLANTS**
Recommendations of a Working Party of the British Society for Antimicrobial Chemotherapy 1997. From the British National Formulary

Patients with prosthetic joint implants (including total hip replacements) do not require antibiotic prophylaxis for dental treatment. The Working Party considers that it is unacceptable to expose patients to the adverse effects of antibiotics when there is no evidence that such prophylaxis is of any benefit.

### References

Hofmann S, Huemer G, Salzer M 1998 Pathophysiology and management of the fat embolism syndrome. Anaesthesia 53(suppl. 2): 35–37

Lane N, Allen K 1999 Hyponatraemia after orthopaedic surgery. British Medical Journal 318: 1363–1364

Winkler M, Marker E, Hetz H 1998 The perioperative management of major orthopaedic procedures. Anaesthesia 53(suppl. 2): 37–41

## ANAESTHESIA AND RENAL FAILURE

### ACUTE RENAL FAILURE

**Table 4.2** Diagnosis of acute renal failure

|  | Prerenal | Renal |
|---|---|---|
| Urine:plasma (U:P) osmolality | > 2:1 | < 1:2 |
| U:P urea | > 20 | < 10 |
| U:P creatinine | > 40 | < 10 |
| Urine Na$^+$ (mEq/l) | < 20 | > 60 |

### CHRONIC RENAL FAILURE

Plot of 1/creatinine against time gives an approximation of rate of deterioration of renal function and an estimate of time before renal support is necessary (Fig. 4.2).

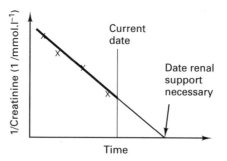

**Fig. 4.2** Progression of chronic renal failure with time.

#### Common indications for renal transplantation

- Diabetes
- Hypertensive nephropathy

- Polycystic disease
- Chronic glomerulonephritis
- Interstitial nephritis.

## Pharmacokinetic and pharmacodynamic changes

- Decreased active tubular excretion and decreased GFR
- Decreased protein binding secondary to hypoalbuminaemia
- Phase I hepatic metabolism (reduction, hydrolysis etc) reduced by uraemia. Phase II metabolism (conjugation) reduced by accumulating drug metabolites
- Competition for protein binding by accumulation of endogenous substances and drug metabolites
- Impaired salt and water excretion.

These changes result in hypertension, water retention, peripheral oedema and hyperdynamic circulation; also accumulation of ionized, water-soluble compounds, e.g. non-depolarizing neuromuscular blockers, digoxin, atropine, neostigmine, water-soluble β-blockers, e.g. atenolol.

## Common conditions associated with chronic renal failure

*CVS.* Hypertension, LVF exacerbated by A-V fistula, accelerated atherosclerosis causing ischaemic heart disease and peripheral vascular disease. Pericardial effusion and cardiomyopathy secondary to uraemia and dialysis.

*Respiratory.* Peritoneal dialysis causes diaphragmatic splinting, atelectasis and shunting. Respiratory infection is common. Fluid overload between periods of dialysis, causing pulmonary congestion.

*GI.* Delayed gastric emptying and increased gastric acid secretion. High risk of aspiration. GI bleeding. Deranged liver function secondary to transfusion-related hepatitis.

*Neurological.* Peripheral and autonomic neuropathy. Mild uraemic encephalopathy.

*Haematology.* Normochromic normocytic anaemia due to decreased erythropoietin, bone marrow depression from anaemia, iron, folate and $B_{12}$ deficiency and increased red cell fragility. Decreased $O_2$ delivery compensated for by $\uparrow$ CO, metabolic acidosis and $\uparrow$ 2,3-DPG, shifting $O_2$ dissociation curve to the right. Defective platelet function, increased factor VIII and fibrinogen, and decreased antithrombin III result in hypercoagulable state despite increased bleeding time.

*Post-dialysis.* Residual heparinization for 10 h post-dialysis. Large fluid shifts may cause hypotension, nausea and vomiting.

*Other.* Metabolic acidosis, hyperkalaemia, hypomagnesaemia, hypo-calcaemia, hyperphosphataemia, bone decalcification and carbohydrate intolerance.

## Specific Drugs

1. *Anticholinergics.* Atropine and glycopyrrolate are both water-soluble and therefore accumulate. Hyoscine has minimal renal excretion.

2. *Barbiturates.* Decreased dose requirements of thiopentone due to decreased protein binding and increased blood–brain barrier permeability.

3. *Ketamine.* Increases renal blood flow through altered autoregulation but reduces urine output. May worsen hypertension.

4. *Benzodiazepines.* Slight decrease in dose requirement due to reduced protein binding; more marked with those that are more highly protein-bound, e.g. diazepam.

5. *Etomidate.* Decreased dose requirement due to reduced protein binding.

6. *Propofol.* Little change in pharmacokinetics.

7. *Opioids. Morphine* effect is prolonged due to accumulation of renally excreted metabolite morphine-6-glucuronide. *Pethidine* causes excitation due to accumulation of renally excreted metabolite norpethidine.
*Fentanyl* and *alfentanyl* have relatively unaltered pharmacokinetics.

8. *Muscle relaxants*
*Suxamethonium.* Prolonged action due to plasma cholinesterase depletion with dialysis. Also increases $K^+$ by 0.5 mmol/l (same degree as healthy adults) which may be dangerous in the presence of hyperkalaemia.
Clearance of non-depolarizing drugs depends upon degree of renal excretion:
> 70% – gallamine, pancuronium, pipercuronium
< 25% – vecuronium, atracurium, mivacurium.
*Atracurium.* Little change in pharmacokinetics. Considered by many to be the muscle relaxant of choice. Accumulation of laudanosine to levels > 17 µg/ml causes fits in dogs but the highest level recorded in a patient is 8.65 µg/ml.
*Vecuronium.* Accumulates with repeated doses.
*Mivacurium, doxacurium, pipercuronium.* All are renally excreted and therefore action is prolonged.
*Rocuronium* is a medium-duration steroid mostly excreted by the liver. Does not appear to have prolonged action in renal failure. May be a useful alternative to atracurium.

9. *Anticholinesterases.* Impaired renal excretion results in significant prolongation of action of anticholinesterases, outlasting non-depolarizing neuromuscular blockers. Neuromuscular blockers may also be prolonged with acidosis and hypokalaemia.

10. *Local anaesthetics.* Reduced protein binding increases risk of toxicity.

11. *Inhalational agents*
*Indirect effects.* Decreased myocardial function, reducing GFR.
*Direct effects.* Renal toxicity of fluoride ion (methoxyflurane, enflurane)

causes high-output renal failure. Minimum toxic level is 50 $\mu$mol/l. Enflurane in renal failure may reach 40 $\mu$mol/l.

## ANAESTHETIC MANAGEMENT FOR CHRONIC RENAL FAILURE PATIENTS

### Preoperative

Measure baseline creatinine clearance. Preoperative haemodialysis to correct fluid and electrolytes, avoid cannulae in limbs (in case they are needed for fistula formation), correct hypertension and dehydration, control diabetes, administer anti-aspiration premedication.

### Monitoring

ECG (CM5), invasive BP, pulse oximetry, CVP, urinary catheter, ± PCWP. Regular blood glucose.

### Induction

Hypertension is common during induction. Thiopentone, etomidate or propofol is suitable. Suxamethonium (if $K^+ < 5.0$), atracurium and fentanyl/alfentanyl.

### Maintenance

Patients with CRF are acidotic so avoid spontaneous respiration. Isoflurane has least metabolism to $F^-$ and minimal nephrotoxicity. $N_2O$ is safe. Effective antihypertensive drugs are GTN or trimetaphan. Sodium nitroprusside in end-stage renal failure (ESRF) may cause cyanide toxicity.

Keep well hydrated. Replace fluid loss with salt-containing solutions (avoid Hartmann's as this contains $K^+$). Low threshold for blood transfusion since patient is already anaemic.

### Regional anaesthesia

Spinal and epidural anaesthesia can maintain renal blood flow if hypotension is avoided. Bladder innervation via SNS from $T_{12}$–$L_3$ and PNS from $S_2$–$S_4$. Therefore, aim for regional anaesthesia extending $T_{10}$–$S_4$.

### Other

Aminoglycoside antibiotics increase frusemide nephrotoxicity and potentiate non-depolarizing neuromuscular blockers.

NSAIDs impair production of prostaglandins ($PGE_1$) and prostacyclins ($PGI_2$), which modulate the vasoconstrictor effects of angiotensin II, noradrenaline and vasopressin. In the presence of renal disease or hypovolaemia, NSAIDs reduce renal blood flow and thus glomerular filtration rate. May worsen renal function or cause acute renal failure. May also cause oedema, heart failure and hypertension secondary to sodium retention.

## Postoperative

Patient is usually extubated immediately postoperatively. Monitor CVP and renal function closely.

### References

Amoroso P, Lanigan C 1995 Renal dysfunction and anaesthesia. Current Opinion in Anaesthesiology 8: 267–270
Cottam S, Eason J 1991 Anaesthesia for renal transplantation. In: Kaufman L (ed) Anaesthesia Review 8. Churchill Livingstone, London
Lote C J, Harper L, Savage C O S 1996 Mechanisms of acute renal failure. British Journal of Anaesthesia 77: 82–89
Pollard B J 1992 Editorial. Neuromuscular blocking drugs and renal failure. British Journal of Anaesthesia 68: 545–546
Short A, Cumming A 1999 ABC of intensive care. Renal support. British Medical Journal 319: 41–44

# ANAESTHESIA FOR UROLOGICAL SURGERY

## TRANSURETHRAL RESECTION OF THE PROSTATE

### Specific problems

- Increased age-related pathology
- Pharmacokinetic and pharmacodynamic changes related to age
- Risks from diathermy to pacemakers
- Lithotomy position
- Risk of hypothermia
- Fluid overload and hyperglycinaemia following bladder irrigation
- Haemorrhage from surgery and release of urokinase
- Bacteraemia.

### Anaesthetic techniques

Both GA and spinal anaesthesia cause decreased BP and cardiac output after induction, with changes more marked with GA. The resection period is not associated with significant haemodynamic changes in either group (Dobson et al 1994).

*General anaesthesia.* Fit elderly patients can be managed with a laryngeal mask and spontaneous ventilation, but those with significant respiratory or cardiovascular disease are best managed by intubation and IPPV.

*Regional anaesthesia*
- Need sensory block from $T_{10}$ to $S_4$
- Not suitable if patient unable to lie still or has cough

- Allows early warning of TURP syndrome
- Increased intravascular space may reduce risk of TURP syndrome
- Reduced blood loss. Reduced incidence of DVT
- Incidence of postdural puncture headache (PDPH) is low in the elderly
- Crystalloid preloading has no effect on the incidence of hypotension. More effective to use vasopressors to maintain blood pressure.

### Lithotomy position

Lithotomy position may result in hypoventilation and hypoxaemia due to a fall in FRC with age and supine position, and compression of lungs by abdominal contents. Thus, awake surgery may not be tolerated by all patients.

Lithotomy position increases the risk of gastric aspiration, particularly in obese patients and those with hiatus hernia. There is a further risk in the elderly due to impaired protective upper airway reflexes.

Increased CVP in the lithotomy position may cause angina or precipitate heart failure.

### Bladder irrigation

Glycine 1.5% is slightly hypotonic (osmolality = 220 mOsm/l). It is used because it is non-conductive, thus preventing dispersion of the diathermy current. Fluid absorbed through open venous sinuses in the prostate causes the TURP syndrome, characterized by:

- *Fluid overload.* Proportional to height of irrigation fluid. Absorption may be as rapid as 30 ml/min. Limit height of irrigation fluid to 60 cm with irrigation time no more than 1 h. Spiking irrigation fluid with ethanol and measuring expired ethanol concentration has been used to measure the degree of fluid absorption. The amount of fluid absorbed correlates well with hyponatraemia.

  Spinal anaesthesia can increase speed and volume of irrigation fluid absorbed compared with general anaesthesia. Probably due to lowered hydrostatic pressure in the prostatic veins.

  Symptoms due to fluid overload and dilutional hyponatraemia include bradycardia, hypertension progressing to hypotension, heart failure, headache, mental confusion and convulsions.

  Treat with fluid restriction and hypertonic saline. Rapid correction of $Na^+$ may cause central pontine myelinosis. Correction of no more than 12 mmol/day is suggested as safe.
- *Hyperglycinaemia.* Glycine is an inhibitory neurotransmitter in the brain and spinal cord. Temporary blindness may be due to inhibition of retinal transmission. Metabolism of glycine to ammonia may contribute to neurological symptoms. Glycine is also cardiotoxic. Addition of ethanol to irrigation fluid and measurement of expired ethanol have also been used to assess degree of glycine absorption.

- *Haemolysis.* Now distilled water has been replaced by glycine, this is no longer a problem.

### Haemorrhage

Assess blood loss by measuring Hb in irrigation fluid collected from washout. Average blood loss is 500 ml.

Release of prostatic urokinase triggers conversion of plasminogen to plasmin with resulting fibrinolysis. This phenomenon may account for persistent bleeding in some patients. Plasminogen activators may be of benefit in extreme cases.

### Bacteraemia

Urinary outflow obstruction predisposes to urinary tract infection. Prophylactic antibiotics are necessary if infection is present or if there is a risk of endocarditis.

### References

Dobson P M, Caldicott L D, Gervish S P, Cole J R, Channer K S 1994 Changes in haemodynamic variables during transurethral resection of the prostate: comparison of general and spinal anaesthesia. British Journal of Anaesthesia 72: 267–271

Gehring H, Nahm W, Baerwald J, Fornara P et al 1999 Irrigating fluid absorption during percutaneous nephrolithotripsy. Acta Anaesthesiologica Scandinavica 43: 458–463

Ryall D M, Dodds C 1992  Anaesthesia for urological surgery in the elderly. Current Anaesthesia and Critical Care 3: 200–206

# 5. Metabolism

## DIABETES

*CVS.* Results in micro- and macrovascular disease, accelerated atherosclerosis and cardiomyopathy. There is a reduced VF threshold and increased autonomic neuropathy, causing increased HR and BP during induction of anaesthesia. Increased need for inotropic support following CABG. Increased platelet aggregation.

*Respiratory.* Reduced $FEV_1$ and FVC. Reduced sensitivity to hypoxia and hypercapnia. Increased risk of chest infections, decreased pulmonary diffusing capacity, central and peripheral obstructive sleep apnoea, aspiration pneumonia.

*CNS.* Neuropathy impairs neuromuscular transmission. Decreased response to tetanic stimulation.

*Renal.* Chronic failure is common, heralded by onset of microalbuminuria. Progress of chronic renal failure can be limited with good diabetic control.

*GI.* Delayed gastric emptying and gastroparesis are secondary to autonomic neuropathy.

*Other.* Poor wound healing, increased risk of infection. Juvenile-onset diabetics may have reduced atlanto-occipital movement, making intubation difficult.

### Drugs

*Sulfonylureas,* e.g. glibenclamide and tolbutamide, stimulate release of insulin by increasing β-cell sensitivity to glucose.

*Biguanides,* e.g. metformin and phenformin, reduce basal glucose production. Phenformin has been withdrawn because of a high incidence of lactic acidosis.

### Perioperative management

If possible, avoid drugs that may interfere with glycaemic control. Ketamine causes hyperglycaemia, β-blockers result in a slower recovery from hyperglycaemia and ganglion-blocking drugs reduce sympathetic-mediated gluconeogenesis.

Sympathomimetics and diuretics antagonize insulin. β-blockers, clonidine, monoamine oxidase inhibitors (MAOIs) and salicylates potentiate insulin.

Epidurals/spinals have minimal effect on glucose.

Check anion gap (= $[Na^+ + K^+] - [HCO_3^- + Cl^-]$) in ketoacidotic patients. Above 16 mEq/l is due to ketone bodies in ketoacidosis, lactic acid in lactic acidosis, increased organic acids from renal failure or a combination of these.

Avoid lactate-containing solutions, e.g. Hartmann's.

Assess degree of stability by:

- frequency of hypoglycaemic attacks
- variations in insulin dosage
- glycosylated Hb < 10%.

### Control regimes

There are several different regimes. Omission of insulin avoids hypoglycaemia but risks severe hyperglycaemia and catabolism. Insulin infusion produces more stable blood glucose levels than bolus administration and is more physiological. Tight control of perioperative blood glucose may improve wound healing and reduce the risk of infection.

*Non-tight regime*
- Nil by mouth from midnight
- Commence 5% dextrose i.v. at 125 ml/h at 06.00 on morning of surgery
- Give half the morning insulin dose s.c.
- Continue 5% dextrose perioperatively
- Check BM stix 2–4 hourly and adjust blood glucose according to sliding scale.

*Alberti regime* (Alberti & Thomas 1979)
- 500 ml 10% glucose
- 10 mmol KCl
- 10 U soluble insulin (e.g. Actrapid)
- Give over 4 h with 2-hourly BM stix.
  If glucose is:
  - < 5 mmol, use 5 U/bag
  - 5–10 mmol, as above
  - > 10 mmol, use 15 U/bag
  - > 20 mmol, use 20 U/bag.

*Infusion regime.* Provides the tightest control of all regimes and is now becoming the method of choice for insulin-dependent diabetic patients.

**GUIDELINES FOR THE MANAGEMENT OF DIABETIC PATIENTS UNDERGOING SURGERY** *British National Formulary* 37 (section 6.1.1)

When an insulin-dependent patient requires surgery that is likely to require an i.v. infusion for > 12 h, the following regimen provides for i.v. administration of insulin (for an indefinite period):

- Give an injection of the patient's usual insulin on the night before the operation
- Early on the day of the operation, start an i.v. infusion of 5% glucose containing 10 mmol/l KCl (providing that the patient is not hyperkalaemic) and run at a constant rate appropriate to the patient's fluid requirements (usually 125 ml/h); make up a solution of soluble insulin 1 unit/ml in sodium chloride 0.9% and infuse i.v. using a syringe pump piggy-backed to the i.v. infusion
- The rate of the insulin infusion should normally be:
  — blood glucose < 4 mmol/l, give 0.5 units/h
  — blood glucose < 4–15 mmol/l, give 2 units/h
  — blood glucose < 15-20 mmol/l, give 4 units/h
  — blood glucose > 20 mmol/l, review.

In resistant cases (such as those who are shocked or severely ill or those receiving corticosteroids or sympathomimetics) 2–4 times these rates or even more may be needed.

The rate of i.v. infusion depends on the volume depletion, cardiac function, age and other factors. Blood glucose concentration should be measured preoperatively and then every 2 hours. The duration of action of i.v. insulin is only a few minutes and the infusion must not be stopped unless the patient becomes frankly hypoglycaemic (blood glucose < 3 mmol/l) in which case it should be stopped for up to 30 min. The amount of KCl required in the infusion needs to be assessed by regular measurement of plasma electrolytes. Sodium chloride 0.9% infusion should replace glucose 5% if the blood glucose is persistently above 15 mmol/l.

## INSULINOMA

Small β-islet cell tumours of the pancreas producing marked hypoglycaemia from insulin release. May be precipitated by food or starvation.

Diagnose by Whipple's triad:

1. Plasma glucose < 45 g/dl
2. Symptoms and signs of hypoglycaemia with fasting or exercise
3. Symptoms relieved by glucose.

Diazoxide may suppress insulin release. Discontinue preoperatively and initiate glucose infusion with BM stix every 15 min and every 5 min during tumour manipulation. Hyperglycaemic rebound may occur after tumour removal.

Suppressed islet cells take several days to recover, so monitor glucose for this period.

## CUSHING'S SYNDROME

Caused by excess cortisol from steroid therapy, adrenal hyperplasia, adrenal carcinoma or ectopic ACTH. Cushing's disease is due to an ACTH-secreting pituitary tumour.

*Symptoms and signs.* Moon face, 'buffalo hump', thin skin, hirsutism, easy bruising, hypertension (60%), diabetes (10%), osteoporosis (50%), pancreatitis (2%), muscle weakness, poor wound healing.

*Perioperative problems.* Hypertension, congestive cardiac failure, hyperglycaemia, careful positioning due to osteoporosis and fragile skin.

## ADDISON'S DISEASE

Adrenocortical insufficiency due to autoimmune disease, TB, adrenal infiltration with amyloid, tumour, leukaemia, pituitary failure or surgical adrenalectomy.

*Symptoms and signs.* Tiredness, lethargy, weight loss, nausea, hyperpigmentation, muscle weakness, hypotension, hyponatraemia, hyperkalaemia and hypoglycaemia.

*Perioperative problems.* Hypotension, low intravascular volume and small heart causing heart failure with minor fluid overload. Hyperkalaemia (care with suxamethonium) and hypoglycaemia. Remember steroid replacement.

## ACROMEGALY

This is characterized by excess growth hormone secretion resulting in soft tissue overgrowth.

*Anatomical.* Visual field defects, epiglottis and tongue overgrowth, recurrent laryngeal nerve palsy, headaches, rhinorrhoea.

*Endocrine.* Causes diabetes and hypertension, osteoarthritis and osteoporosis, muscle weakness, peripheral neuropathy.

*Surgery.* Via transfrontal craniotomy or transethmoidal approach.

*Postoperative.* Addison's disease, hypothalamic damage, CSF leak, diabetes insipidus.

## THYROID DISEASE

### Hyperthyroidism

*Symptoms.* Excitability, tremor, sweating, weight loss, palpitations, exophthalmos.

*Signs.* Tachycardia, atrial fibrillation (AF), heart failure, sweating, neuropathy, proximal myopathy and autoimmune diseases.

*Diagnosis.* Thyroid-stimulating hormone (TSH), free $T_3/T_4$, resin uptake, thoracic inlet X-ray/CT.

### Hypothyroidism

*Symptoms.* Tiredness, lethargy, cold sensitivity, obesity, dry skin, constipation.

*Signs.* Bradycardia, pericardial effusion, hypothermia, polyneuropathy and hyponatraemia.

*Diagnosis.* TSH, free $T_3/T_4$, autoantibodies.

### Anaesthetic management of thyroid disease

Aim for euthyroid patient, but risk of thyroid storm still remains in treated hyperthyroid patients. Antithyroid drugs may depress immune function. Check cord movement preoperatively. Assess tracheal compression and deviation by X-ray of thoracic inlet and CT scan. Thyroid hypertrophy may cause superior vena cava (SVC) obstruction and, if malignant, may invade surrounding structures. Exclude other autoimmune diseases.

Check that the patient can be manually ventilated before administration of a neuromuscular blocker. Enlarged tongue may make intubation difficult. Use armoured tube. Avoid atropine if hyperthyroid. Halothane increases risk of arrhythmias. Isoflurane causes least increase in $T_4$ of any volatile agent. CVS and respiratory depressant effects of drugs are magnified in hypothyroidism.

Thyroid replacement therapy may precipitate myocardial ischaemia. Take care with fluid overload. There is a tendency to hypothermia with hypothyroidism. Provide eye care.

Extubate light, following direct inspection of the vocal cords. Damage to both nerves results in cords fixed in adduction. Postoperative airway obstruction may occur due to peritracheal haematoma or tracheal oedema. There is a risk of hypoparathyroidism or hypothyroidism following thyroid resection.

## HYPOPARATHYROIDISM

Usually occurs following thyroidectomy. Symptoms include paraesthesia, muscle cramps, tetany, laryngeal stridor, CNS irritability and convulsions. Similar symptoms arise with metabolic/respiratory alkalosis.

Severe hypocalcaemia indicated by:

*Trousseau's sign.* Tourniquet inflated above arterial pressure causes carpopedal spasm.

*Chvostek's sign.* Percussion of the facial nerve produces facial muscle contraction.

Treat with 10–20 ml 10% calcium chloride.

## HYPERPARATHYROIDISM

Symptoms and signs are due to hypercalcaemia: renal stones (50%), polyuria and renal calculi; bone pain (10%), osteoporosis and fractures; abdominal pain (5%), vomiting, pancreatitis and ulcers; psychoses.

## PHAEOCHROMOCYTOMA

### Pathology

Arises from chromaffin cells which secrete noradrenaline >> adrenaline. May be part of multiple endocrine neoplasia (MEN) syndrome. 10% are extra-adrenal.

### Symptoms

Continuous or paroxysmal hypertension, headache, sweating, palpitations. Dilated and hypertrophic cardiomyopathies.

Noradrenaline causes systolic and diastolic hypertension with reflex bradycardia; adrenaline causes systolic hypertension, diastolic hypotension and tachycardia. Intraoperative cardiovascular instability is related to preoperative catecholamine levels.

### Diagnosis

Diagnose by urine vanillyl mandelic acid (VMA) and metaiodobenzyl-guanidine (MIBG) scan.

### Preoperative

Aim to:

- lower BP and prevent paroxysmal hypertensive crises
- increase intravascular volume
- decrease myocardial dysfunction.

Block catecholamine synthesis with $\alpha$-methyltyrosine. Preoperative $\alpha$- and then $\beta$-blockade, e.g. phenoxybenzamine ($\alpha_1 > \alpha_2$ blockade) followed by $\beta$-blocker if tachycardia persists. Consider ACE inhibitors and calcium-channel blockers.

### Monitoring

Arterial line, CVP ± PCWP, glucose and temperature.

### Induction and maintenance

Minimize sympathetic response to intubation. Suxamethonium causes abdominal muscle contraction, compressing tumour and releasing catecholamines. Induction with etomidate or propofol. Maintenance with isoflurane or enflurane with $O_2/N_2O$ and fentanyl/alfentanyl.

Avoid atropine, halothane and histamine-releasing drugs. Droperidol causes hypertension. Draw up antihypertensive drugs for immediate administration, e.g. nitroprusside, phentolamine.

Sudden decrease in catecholamines following ligation of the tumour causes severe hypotension, corrected with fluid loading ± noradrenaline infusion. Decrease in catecholamines also causes hypoglycaemia, so check plasma glucose frequently.

### Postoperative

50% remain hypertensive for several days postoperatively, as catecholamine levels do not return to normal for 7–10 days.

## CARCINOID TUMOUR

### Pathology

Vasoactive amines are released from enterochromaffin cells of neural crest. Asymptomatic if tumour lies proximal to liver portal flow where amines are deactivated. Secondaries in liver secrete amines (5HT, bradykinin, prostaglandins, histamine, substance P, neurotensin, neuropeptide K, pancreatic polypeptide), which escape into venous blood to cause hypertension (5HT), hypotension (bradykinin), flushing, wheezing, pulmonary stenosis, tricuspid regurgitation and diarrhoea.

### Diagnosis

Measure 24-h urine 5-hydroxyindoleacetic acid (5-HIAA) levels.

### Preoperative

Block amine production preoperatively with α-methyldopa. Preoperative octreotide also reduces amine secretion. Correct fluid and electrolyte balance. Give antibiotic prophylaxis for endocarditis if there is heart valve involvement.

### Monitoring

Potential for wide swings in BP. Therefore, carry out invasive BP and CVP monitoring. Consider pulmonary artery pressure measurement if there are cardiac complications.

### General anaesthesia

Avoid histamine-releasing drugs, which may cause cardiovascular instability and worsen wheeze. Benzodiazepine premedication and benzodiazepine + fentanyl induction provide good cardiovascular stability. Etomidate and propofol are also suitable.

Suxamethonium causes 5HT and histamine release. Vecuronium or pancuronium are the most suitable neuromuscular blocking drugs. Isoflurane produces good cardiovascular control and is rapidly eliminated postoperatively.

If regional techniques are used, avoid hypotension, which causes histamine release.

Use amine antagonists to control BP perioperatively:

- ketanserin or methysergide antagonize 5HT
- aprotinin antagonizes bradykinin production (but more effective to use preoperative octreotide and steroids)
- chlorpheniramine antagonizes histamine
- give boluses of octreotide if patient is hypotensive during surgery.

Perioperative hyperglycaemia may occur.

Use of catecholamines to treat perioperative cardiovascular collapse may precipitate peptide release and impair resuscitation efforts.

### Postoperative

Hypotension may occur up to 3 days postoperatively and usually responds to octreotide. Good analgesia with continuous epidural infusion or fentanyl patient-controlled analgesia (PCA).

## ATRIAL NATURIETIC PEPTIDE

This is released in response to atrial distension, e.g. CCF. Promotes diuresis with loss of sodium and inhibition of renin–angiotensin system and aldosterone. Acts as a vasodilator. Decreases mean arterial pressure via (?) centrally acting opioids.

## PERIOPERATIVE STEROID SUPPLEMENTATION

Normal steroid response to surgery is dependent upon the magnitude and duration of the operation. Plasma cortisol increases rapidly, reaching a peak at 4–6 h and declining over a 48–72 h period. Major surgery is associated with as much as 100 mg endogenous cortisol release.

Therapy with glucocorticoids results in suppression of the hypothalamic–pituitary–adrenal (HPA) axis. Failure of cortisol secretion is due primarily to inhibition of synthesis of corticotrophin (ACTH). The HPA axis can be assessed preoperatively by the following:

1. *random cortisol*
2. *short synacthen test* – plasma cortisol is measured 0, 30 and 60 min after

an injection of synthetic ACTH. Normal function results in cortisol levels > 500 nmol/l

3. *insulin tolerance test* – 0.1 U/kg insulin injected into fasting patient. Resulting hypoglycaemia (< 2.2 mmol/l) causes release of ACTH from the pituitary. Normal function results in cortisol levels > 500 nmol/l.

## Anaesthetic implications

There is no evidence that aiming for cortisol levels higher than normal baseline values is of any benefit in patients with suppressed HPA function (i.e. those on steroid therapy). The current recommendations are summarized in Table 5.1.

**Table 5.1** Recommendations for perioperative steroid supplementation

|  | Preoperative | | Additional steroid cover |
|---|---|---|---|
| **Patients currently taking steroids** | < 10 mg/day | Assume normal HPA function | Additional steroid cover not required |
|  | > 10 mg/day | Minor surgery | 25 mg hydrocortisone on induction |
|  |  | Moderate surgery | Usual preoperative steroids + 25 mg hydrocortisone on induction + 100 mg/day for 24 h |
|  |  | Major surgery | Usual preoperative steroids + 25 mg hydrocortisone on induction + 100 mg/day for 48–72 h |
| **Patients stopped taking steroids** | < 3 months | | Treat as if on steroids |
|  | > 3 months | | No perioperative steroids necessary |

## Equivalent steroid doses

- Hydrocortisone        20 mg
- Prednisolone          5 mg
- Methylprednisolone    4 mg
- Betamethasone         0.75 mg
- Dexamethasone         0.75 mg

### References

Alberti K G M M, Thomas D J B 1979 The management of diabetes during surgery. British Journal of Anaesthesia 51: 693–703

Eldridge A J, Sear J W 1996 Perioperative management of diabetic patients. Any changes for the better since 1985? Anaesthesia 51: 45–51

Hall G M 1994 Insulin administration in diabetic patients – return of the bolus? Editorial. British Journal of Anaesthesia 72: 1–2

Hull C J 1986 Phaeochromocytoma. Diagnosis, preoperative preparation and anaesthetic management. British Journal of Anaesthesia 58: 1453–1468

Nicholson G, Burrin J M, Hall G M 1998 Peri-operative steroid supplementation. Anaesthesia 53: 1091–1104

Pullerits J, Ein S, Balfe J W 1988 Continuing medical education article: anaesthesia for phaeochromocytoma. Canadian Journal of Anaesthesia 35: 526–534

Roizen M F, Stevens A, Lampe G H 1989 Perioperative management of patients with endocrine disease. In: Nunn J F, Utting J E, Brown B R Jr (eds) General anaesthesia. Butterworths, London, p 731–738

Russell W J, Metcalfe I R, Tonkin A L, Frewin D B 1998 The preoperative management of phaeochromocytoma. Anaesthesia and Intensive Care 26: 196–200

Veall G R Q, Peacock J E, Bax N D S, Reilly C 1994 Review of the anaesthetic management of 21 patients undergoing laparotomy for carcinoid syndrome. British Journal of Anaesthesia 72: 335–341

## MALIGNANT HYPERTHERMIA

Malignant hyperthermia (MH) is defined as a fulminant hypermetabolic state of skeletal muscle. The UK incidence is 1:200 000 in adults and 1:15 000 in children. Inheritance is autosomal dominant. There is a mortality of about 10% (has improved from 24% in 1970s).

The first description was published in the *Lancet* by Denbrough (Australia) in 1960. Animal model in Landrace pigs.

### Signs

*Early.* Tachypnoea, rise in end-tidal $CO_2$, tachycardia, hypoxaemia, fever ($> 2°C/h$).

*Late.* Generalized muscle rigidity ($> 75\%$ cases), metabolic and respiratory acidosis, hyperkalaemia, increased muscle enzymes (CPK, LDH, SGOT) and myoglobinaemia.

### Disease associations

ENT and trauma surgery (?because triggering agents used more often). Possibly myopathies and periodic paralysis. Kyphoscoliosis, pes cavus, squint and inguinal hernia are not now thought to be associated.

### Triggering factors

- *Definite* – suxamethonium (may accelerate the onset of MH when using

volatiles), all volatile agents (including desflurane – a weak trigger – and sevoflurane)
- *Possible* – atropine (may make attack more fulminant); phenothiazines (?neuroleptic malignant syndrome mistaken for MH)
- *Unsure* – stress, exercise.

### Safe drugs

Opioids, all local anaesthetics, nitrous oxide, non-depolarizing relaxants, benzodiazepines, propofol, thiopentone (delays onset of MH in animals), etomidate, ketamine, droperidol and metoclopramide.

### Pathophysiology

Muscle contraction results from flooding of the cytoplasm by $Ca^{2+}$ entering across the plasma membrane through voltage-gated $Ca^{2+}$ channels and released from the sarcoplasmic reticulum (SR) through ryanodine-sensitive $Ca^{2+}$ channels (Fig. 5.1). These channels occur in pairs where folds in the SR meet the sarcolemma of the t-tubule. The ryanodine ($Ry_1$) receptor is a large protein molecule comprising four identical monomers that sits between the two $Ca^{2+}$ channels. Depolarization results in charge movement in the voltage-operated $Ca^{2+}$ channels which activates the $Ry_1$ receptor to open and $Ca^{2+}$ is released into the myoplasm. Volatile anaesthetic agents may increase the leak of $Ca^{2+}$ through the $Ry_1$ protein, which does not cause clinical symptoms. In myopathic muscle, this leak may be sufficient to trigger a final common pathway with activation of contractile elements, ATP hydrolysis,

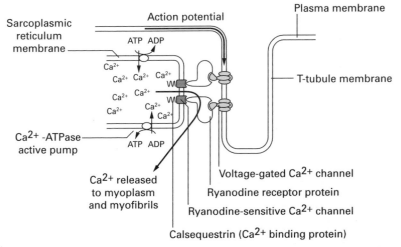

**Fig. 5.1** Mechanism of excitation–contraction coupling and calcium release in skeletal muscle.

$O_2$ consumption, $CO_2$ production, lactate and heat generation, uncoupling of oxidative phosphorylation, and cell breakdown with loss of myoglobin, CPK and $K^+$ to cause the clinical picture of MH.

All Landrace pigs have a defective ryanodine receptor, resulting from an arginine to cysteine mutation. Similar mutations have been found in about 5% of human MH cases, and glycine to arginine mutations have also been documented. The defective gene for mutations of the ryanodine receptor is located on or near the long arm of chromosome 19 (19q13.1 region). However, a number of MH families are not linked to this chromosome. There is evidence that mutations in other cytoplasmic proteins that contribute to the functioning of the Ry protein may also cause defective $Ca^{2+}$ homeostasis (e.g. calsequestrin). Mutation of the $\alpha_2\delta$ subunit of voltage-gated $Ca^{2+}$ channels has also been documented in some patients with MH. In many cases, no genetic defects have been identified.

Dantrolene may bind to multiple sites other than the Ry protein. There is evidence that it may actually increase $Ca^{2+}$ release, explaining why patients with MH treated with dantrolene may undergo a recrudescence of hypermetabolism.

---

**GUIDELINES FOR THE MANAGEMENT OF A MALIGNANT HYPERTHERMIA CRISIS** Association of Anaesthetists of Great Britain and Ireland 1998

**Diagnosis**
Consider MH if:
- masseter muscle spasm after suxamethonium
- unexplained, unexpected tachycardia, together with
- unexplained, unexpected increase in end-tidal $CO_2$

**Early management**
1. Withdraw all trigger agents (i.e. all anaesthetic vapours)
2. Install clean anaesthetic breathing system and hyperventilate
3. Abandon surgery if feasible
4. Give dantrolene i.v. 1 mg/kg initially and repeat p.r.n up to 10 mg/kg
5. Measure ABGs, $K^+$ and CPK
6. Measure core temperature
7. Surface cooling, avoiding vasoconstriction

**Intermediate management**
1. Control serious arrhythmias with β-blockers etc.
2. Control hyperkalaemia and metabolic acidosis

**Later management**
1. Clotting screen to detect DIC
2. Take first voided urine sample for myoglobin estimation
3. Observe urine output for developing renal failure

4. Promote diuresis with fluids/mannitol (20 mg dantrolene contains 3 mg mannitol)
5. Repeat CPK at 24 h.

**Late management**
1. Consider other diagnoses and do appropriate investigations, e.g. VMA, thyroid function test, WCC, CXR
2. Consider possibility of myopathy, neurological opinion, EMG
3. Consider possibility of recreational drug ingestion (ecstasy)
4. Consider possibility of neuroleptic malignant syndrome
5. Counsel patient and/or the family regarding implications of MH
6. Refer patient to MH unit.

## Treatment

Admit patient to ITU. Do not stop treatment until symptoms have completely resolved, otherwise MH may recur (morbidity $\propto$ duration of symptoms). Continue dantrolene 1 mg/kg i.v. q.d.s. for up to 48 h (same dose can be given p.o. after 24 h).

*Dantrolene.* Each vial contains 20 mg orange dantrolene crystals and 3 g mannitol to aid solubility. Made up with 60 ml water to pH 9.5. Side-effects include phlebitis, nausea and vomiting, muscle weakness, uterine atony, placental transfer with fetal weakness, potentiation of non-depolarizing neuromuscular blockers, hyperkalaemia and CVS collapse.

## Screening

MH is autosomal dominant, so all parents, siblings and children should be screened. Muscle biopsy taken for in vitro halothane and caffeine contracture tests. The latter has been shown to have 97% sensitivity (3% false negatives) and 78% specificity (22% false positives).

## Differential diagnosis

Overheating (blankets, heating mattress etc.), infection, thyrotoxicosis, phaeochromocytoma, transfusion reaction, CNS trauma, neuroleptic malignant syndrome, MAOIs, cocaine, tricyclics, atropine, glycopyrrolate, droperidol, ketamine, alcohol withdrawal and ecstasy.

## Perioperative management of patients with known MH

*Elective surgery.* Run $O_2$ at 8 l/min through machine for at least 12 h preoperatively. Fit with new breathing circuit. Avoid triggering agents. Regional/local blocks are safe. Only use dantrolene prophylaxis (2.5 mg/kg i.v. preoperatively) if there is a risk of stress-induced MH or hypermetabolic state (e.g. thyrotoxicosis) because of dantrolene side-effects.

*Dental patient.* Any major surgery must be performed in hospital.

*Obstetric patient.* Stress of labour and delivery may increase susceptibility but dantrolene prophylaxis causes both increased blood loss due to uterine atony and fetal weakness. Best managed with early epidural. Rapid sequence induction must avoid suxamethonium (e.g. vecuronium 0.25 mg/kg). Obstetric drugs (terbutaline, oxytocin etc.) not shown to trigger MH.

## Masseter muscle rigidity

There are three groups of patients:

1. *normal jaw stiffness*
2. *jaw tightness interfering with intubation* – change to safe drugs, carefully monitor and continue
3. *true masseter muscle rigidity* – jaw not able to be opened; 50% of children and 25% of adults are subsequently found to be MH-susceptible. Therefore, stop anaesthetic immediately and monitor closely for 24 h. Postoperative CPK > 20 000 is highly suggestive of MH.

### References

Association of Anaesthetists of Great Britain and Ireland 1998 Guidelines for the management of a malignant hyperthermia crisis. AAGBI, London

Halsall P J, Ellis F R 1996 Malignant hyperthermia. Current Anaesthesia and Critical Care 7: 158–166

Islander G, Twetman E R 1999 Comparison between the European and North American protocols for diagnosis of malignant hyperthermia susceptibility in humans. Anesthesia and Analgesia 88: 1155–1160

Mickelson J R, Louis C F 1996 Malignant hyperthermia – excitation-contraction coupling, $Ca^{2+}$ release channel, and $Ca^{2+}$ regulation defects. Physiological Reviews 76: 537–592

Pessah I N 1996 Complex pharmacology of malignant hyperthermia. Anesthesiology 84: 1275–1279

## ANAESTHESIA FOR THE MORBIDLY OBESE PATIENT

### DEFINITION

Body mass index (BMI) = weight (kg)/height (m)$^2$. Normal = 22–28 kg/m$^2$.

- *Obesity* = BMI > 30. Affects ≈ 33% of the population.
- *Morbid obesity* (MO) = BMI > 35, or weight > ideal body weight (IBW) + 45 kg. Affects 1% of the population.

## PATHOPHYSIOLOGY

*CVS.* Increased blood volume, increased cardiac output by increased stroke volume, left ventricular hypertrophy; hypertension; increased $O_2$ consumption; cardiac autonomic dysfunction increasing risk of sudden death; fatty infiltration causing conduction blocks and arrhythmias.

*Airway.* Large tongue, high and anterior larynx, multiple chin skin folds and large breasts limit neck and head flexion/extension; fatty pharyngeal tissue narrows the airway.

*Respiratory.* Increased work of breathing, decreased compliance, decreased FRC < CC causes V/Q̇ mismatch and hypoxia, obstructive sleep apnoea syndrome progressing to Pickwickian syndrome (cor pulmonale, hypoxia, hypercapnia, polycythaemia). Increased $O_2$ consumption and low FRC cause faster desaturation.

*GI.* Increased gastric acidity and volume (90% of MO patients have gastric pH < 2.5 and volume > 25 ml). Incompetent lower oesophageal sphincter and hiatus hernia are common. Impaired liver function is common.

*Other.* Glucose intolerance, hyperlipidaemia and malignancies.

## PHARMACOKINETIC AND PHARMACODYNAMIC CHANGES

- Water-soluble drugs have similar $V_D$, clearance and half-life.
- Fat-soluble drugs, e.g. thiopentone, benzodiazepines and lignocaine, have ↑ $V_D$, ↑ half-life but normal clearance. Prolonged recovery does not occur with fat-soluble anaesthetic agents.
- Plasma protein levels and plasma protein binding are not changed significantly by obesity.
- Impaired hepatic and renal function may alter drug metabolism and elimination. Increased GFR increases clearance of drugs not biotransformed before renal excretion.
- High plasma cholinesterase levels, so use suxamethonium 1.5 mg/kg lean weight.
- Vecuronium dose should be based on lean body weight for normal recovery times.
- Atracurium dose should be based on absolute weight for normal recovery times.

### Drug doses

Some drug dosages may need to be altered for morbidly obese patients (see Table 5.2).

## PERIOPERATIVE MANAGEMENT

### OR preparation

Equipment must be able to cope with weight. Positioning and padding of the patient should be done with care. Excessive extension of head and limbs as they hang off the obese trunk may cause nerve injury. Lumbar support reduces backache. Powerful ventilators may be needed.

**Table 5.2** Changes in drug doses for morbidly obese patients

| Unchanged dose per total weight | Unchanged dose per lean weight | Larger absolute dose but smaller dose per total weight |
| --- | --- | --- |
| Midazolam | Vecuronium | Thiopentone |
| Diazepam | Propofol | |
| Suxamethonium | Remifentanil | |
| Pancuronium | | |
| Atracurium | | |
| Fentanyl | | |
| Alfentanyl | | |
| Lignocaine | | |

### Premedication

Avoid intramuscular route. Give antacid, $H_2$ antagonists and metoclopramide. Give anticholinergic if awake intubation is planned.

### Monitoring

ECG should include $V_5$. Use arterial line in all but the shortest cases. Capnograph, pulse oximeter, temperature, peripheral nerve stimulator (may need percutaneous electrodes). Consider pulmonary artery catheter if there is cardiorespiratory disease.

### Airway management

Endotracheal intubation is necessary because maintaining an airway with a face mask is difficult. There is a need for IPPV due to hypoventilation and risk of aspiration. 13% of MO patients are difficult intubations. Consider topically anaesthetizing upper airway and larynx in an attempt to visualize cords prior to induction. Awake intubation is recommended if > 1.75 of IBW.

### General anaesthesia

Rapid sequence induction with cricoid pressure. Larger induction doses needed, e.g. thiopentone 7 mg/kg, but exercise caution if there is CVS disease. Fastest recovery achieved with propofol. Balanced anaesthesia is recommended, using volatiles, opioids, non-depolarizing neuromuscular blockers ± extradural anaesthesia. Rapid metabolism of volatile agents causes higher than usual levels of fluoride ions. Therefore, consider avoiding halothane and enflurane. Volatiles do not cause prolonged postoperative recovery. $N_2O$ has low fat solubility and minimal metabolism, but its use limits $F_iO_2$.

Lithotomy, head-down and subdiaphragmatic packs may further impair respiration. IPPV is usually necessary. Use large tidal volumes based on IBW at 8–10 breaths/min. $P_aCO_2 < 4$ kPa increases shunt fraction. PEEP may improve oxygenation but lowers cardiac output and may reduce $O_2$ delivery.

### Reversal

Neuromuscular block must be fully reversed and patient awake with protective upper airway reflexes before extubation.

### Postoperative

Consider elective admission to ITU because of high risk of cardiorespiratory complications. Postoperative hypoxaemia may last for 6 days after intra-abdominal surgery so consider supplemental $O_2$ therapy on ward. Nurse at 30° head-up to reduce pressure of gut on diaphragm. High incidence of DVT so use prophylactic measures. Increased dose of anaesthetic drugs increases risk of renal and hepatic side-effects.

*Postoperative analgesia.* There is perhaps a lesser need for opioid analgesics. Intramuscular injections are likely to be intrafat. Most reliable route is i.v., e.g. PCA. Epidural local anaesthetic or epidural opioid is associated with fewer postoperative respiratory complications and faster discharge home compared with i.v. opioids. Obstructive sleep apnoea syndrome is worse with opioids.

## REGIONAL/LOCAL ANAESTHESIA

Local blocks may be difficult because of hidden anatomical landmarks. Use nerve stimulator. Epidural and subarachnoid blocks may not be as difficult as anticipated because there is less fat in the midline over the spine. Doses reduced by 20–25%, except normal doses for obstetric epidurals. Blocks above $T_5$ may cause respiratory compromise. Give supplemental $O_2$.

Never perform regional/local block unless able and ready to convert to a GA.

### References

Buckley F P 1997 Anesthetic risks related to obesity. Current Opinion in Anaesthesiology 10: 240–243

Shenkman Z, Shir Y, Brodsky J B 1993 Perioperative management of the obese patient. British Journal of Anaesthesia 70: 349–359

## METABOLIC RESPONSE TO STRESS

The stress response is an evolutionary response that has evolved to protect the body from injury and enhance chances of survival. There are cardiovascular, thermoregulatory and metabolic components. It was first described by Cuthbertson in 1929.

The **metabolic response** is initiated by:

- *afferent neuronal input* (somatic and autonomic) from operative site triggering neuroendocrine response
- *release of interleukins* and histamine from damaged tissue, triggering synthesis of acute-phase proteins (cytokines [IL-1β, IL-2, IL-6], tumour necrosis factor, C-reactive protein, fibrinogen, complement and interferons) involved in haemostasis, tissue repair and regeneration.

This **neurohumoral response** (Fig. 5.2) converges on the hypothalamus to trigger:

- *sympathetic response* (rapid) – release of adrenaline and noradrenaline
- *hormonal response* (slow)
    - increased catabolic hormones: ACTH, prolactin, glucagon, catecholamines, GH
    - decreased anabolic hormones: insulin, testosterone, $T_3$
- *metabolic response* – increased breakdown of carbohydrate, lipid and protein and reduced peripheral glucose utilization. Results in thermogenesis, hyperglycaemia, acute-phase protein synthesis, leucocytosis, salt and water retention, and mineral and electrolyte

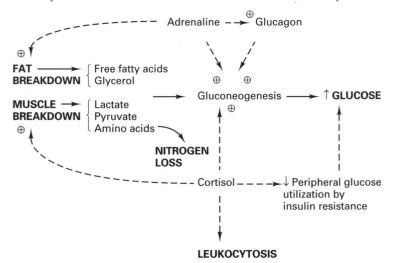

**Fig. 5.2** Metabolic changes triggered by the stress response.

imbalance. Decreased muscle protein, plasma divalent cations and zinc.

## EFFECTS OF SURGERY

The major circulating interleukin is IL-6. The magnitude and duration of IL-6 changes are proportional to tissue damage. Laparoscopy is associated with reduced IL-6 levels compared with open laparotomy, but adrenaline and noradrenaline release is the same in both groups, i.e. visceral afferent stimulus is the main factor triggering the neuroendocrine response and is only ablated by complete block of sensory fibres.

## EFFECTS OF ANAESTHESIA ON THE STRESS RESPONSE

### Opioids

Fentanyl < 15 $\mu$g/kg does not modify cytokine response to surgery. High-dose fentanyl (>50 $\mu$g/kg) inhibits cortisol and GH responses to pelvic surgery but > 100 $\mu$g/kg is required for upper abdominal surgery. High-dose opioids suppress most hormonal responses to surgery but not those triggered by cardiopulmonary bypass.

### Induction agents

Etomidate inhibits 11$\beta$-, 17$\alpha$- and 18$\beta$-hydroxylase and increases mortality in critically ill patients sedated with the drug. A single induction dose is not associated with adverse effects. Midazolam reduces adrenocortical response to major upper abdominal surgery.

### Volatiles

Less effective than narcotics in suppressing the stress response. May contribute to hyperglycaemia by inhibiting insulin release.

### Regional anaesthesia

Only affects those aspects of the stress response that are mediated by afferent neuronal stimulation. There is no evidence that neuronal blockade can decrease the inflammatory response to surgery. Complete afferent blockade (somatic and autonomic) is required to prevent the neuroendocrine response. Complete neuronal block can only be achieved for limbs, pelvic organs and the eye. Extradural for pelvic surgery does not affect IL-6 levels but prevents anterior pituitary hormone changes and blocks catecholamine-mediated metabolic changes. Less effective for upper abdominal and thoracic procedures, probably because of incomplete blockade of afferent fibres.

## BENEFITS OF MODIFYING THE STRESS RESPONSE

It is generally agreed that it is beneficial to decrease stress response in patients with cardiovascular disease. Neonates undergoing cardiac surgery showed decreased stress response when anaesthesia was supplemented with sufentanil and may suffer fewer postoperative complications.

There is no evidence that limiting the endocrine and metabolic responses to surgery is of benefit in all patients. However, regional anaesthesia may reduce complications in elderly high-risk patients (decreased CVS and respiratory complications, reduced hospital stay) but further studies are needed.

Patients on steroid therapy require supplementary doses perioperatively. However, excess may cause side-effects, particularly:

- impaired wound healing
- increased risk of infection
- hyperglycaemia
- stress ulcers
- fluid retention causing hypertension
- psychiatric disturbance.

### References

Desborough J P, Hall G 1993 Endocrine response to surgery. In: Kaufman L (ed) Anaesthesia review 10. Churchill Livingstone, London, p 131–148

Hall G M, Ali W 1998 The stress response and its modification by regional anaesthesia. Anaesthesia 53(suppl. 2): 10–12

Hall G M, Desborough J P 1996 Endocrine and metabolic responses to surgery and injury – effects of anaesthesia. In: Prys Roberts C, Brown B R (eds) International practice of anaesthesia. Butterworth-Heinemann, Oxford

## THERMOREGULATION

## PHYSIOLOGY

### Normal thermoregulation

- Closely controlled at $37 \pm 0.2°C$
- Small deviation causes large physiological impact.

### Afferent input

*Warm receptors*
- Quiescent at normothermia and increase rate of firing as temperature increases
- Unmyelinated C fibres.

### Cold receptors
- Fire continuously and increase rate of firing as temperature decreases
- Aδ nerve fibres.

Five main areas each supply approximately 20% of sensory thermal input (Fig. 5.3). Core structures comprise 80% of this input, whereas the periphery is only 20% of the total input.

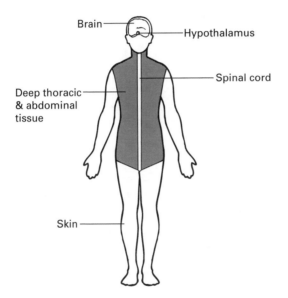

**Fig. 5.3** Sensory thermal input to the hypothalamus.

### Central control
- Integration of afferent input begins in the spinal cord
- Further integration in the pre-optic nuclei of the anterior hypothalamus
- Reflex spinal cord pathways may control some responses
- Impaired control in elderly, obese, malnourished and severely ill.

### Efferent mechanisms

#### Hypothermia
- *Cutaneous vasoconstriction*
  — reduces heat loss from radiation and convection
  — regulated by α-adrenergic action on arteriovenous shunts

- *Non-shivering thermogenesis*
  - doubles heat production in infants
  - probably of little significance in adults
- *Shivering*
  - doubles heat production in adults.

  **Hyperthermia**
- *Sweating*
  - mediated by postganglionic, cholinergic nerves
  - blocked by atropine or nerve blocks
  - non-athletes can sweat up to 1 l/h
- *Active vasodilation*
  - mediated by an unknown protein released from sweat glands
  - cutaneous blood flow can reach 7.5 l/min
  - less effective than sweating at heat loss.

## MEASUREMENT

Nasopharyngeal and tympanic membrane temperature are good indicators of brain temperature. Axillary temperature is a less accurate measure of core temperature. Changes in rectal temperature lag behind changes at other core sites. Also blood temperature (via pulmonary artery catheter), bladder temperature and oesophageal temperature. Skin temperature is dependent upon skin blood flow.

## PERIOPERATIVE HYPOTHERMIA

Perioperative hypothermia develops in three phases (see Figs 5.4 and 5.5):

1. *Change in temperature distribution.* GA causes peripheral vasodilation with ↑ peripheral temperature and ↓ core temperature, redistributing

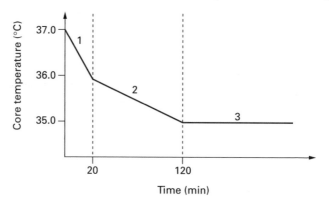

**Fig. 5.4** Development of perioperative hypothermia. 1, heat redistribution; 2, linear phase, 3, plateau phase.

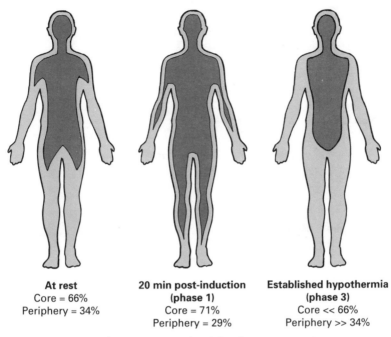

|  | | |
|---|---|---|
| **At rest**<br>Core = 66%<br>Periphery = 34% | **20 min post-induction<br>(phase 1)**<br>Core = 71%<br>Periphery = 29% | **Established hypothermia<br>(phase 3)**<br>Core << 66%<br>Periphery >> 34% |

**Fig. 5.5** Perioperative changes in core and peripheral compartment size.

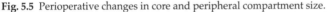

heat from core to periphery. Temperature (heat) *content* remains constant.

2. *Linear phase.* Slow decrease for 2–3 h as heat loss exceeds production. Heat is lost by radiation (40%), convection (30%), evaporation (20%) and respiration (10%). Heat loss is accelerated by naked patient in cold environment, cold skin preparation, cold i.v. fluids and cold gases from ventilator. GA decreases basal metabolic rate (BMR) with 15% less heat production and impairment of compensatory mechanisms. The greatest influence on heat loss is the operating room temperature.

3. *Plateau phase.* Temperature becomes constant as thermoregulatory vasoconstriction limits heat loss to a rate equal to heat production.

## EFFECTS OF GENERAL ANAESTHESIA

GA inhibits behavioural responses to hypothermia, decreases metabolic rate, inhibits hypothalamic function and attenuates homeostatic reflexes. The threshold at which compensatory mechanisms to hypothermia are activated is lowered by 2.5°C and the threshold for mechanisms protecting from hyperthermia is increased by 1.0°C, i.e. widening of thresholds with ↑ MAC (Fig. 5.6).

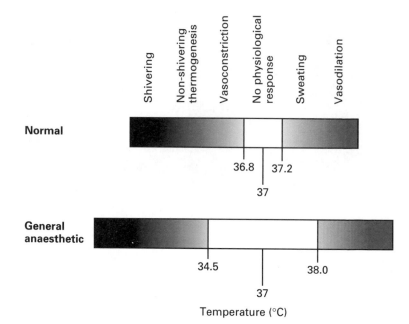

**Fig. 5.6** Changes in thermoregulatory thresholds.

Thermoregulatory thresholds vary depending upon the anaesthetic agents used:

- *Vasoconstriction threshold*
  - — all volatiles decrease threshold to 34.5°C
  - — propofol, fentanyl and nitrous oxide appear to have similar effects
  - — gain and maximum intensity are generally maintained.
- *Shivering threshold*
  - — rarely seen during general anaesthesia because shivering threshold is decreased to below that of core temperature.

## EFFECTS OF REGIONAL ANAESTHESIA

Similar three-phase pattern of hypothermia to that seen with GA. However, sympathetic inhibition below the level of the block prevents thermoregulatory vasoconstriction in the lower half of the body so the core temperature plateau (phase 3) may not be established because heat loss continues to exceed heat production.

Despite a marked core hypothermia, shivering is rarely seen, even in awake patients. This may be because the continuously firing cold receptors are blocked, fooling the hypothalamus into overestimating the peripheral temperature.

# EFFECTS OF HYPOTHERMIA

## CVS

- Decreased CO below 32°C, bradycardia and reduced MAP
- Vasoconstriction occurs below 32°C, increasing afterload and thus increasing myocardial work
- Increased PR interval, widening of QRS complex, prolonged QT interval. Risk of VF below 28°C. J waves on ECG
- Increased blood viscosity, increasing myocardial work.

## Respiratory

- Decreased $CO_2$ production
- Increased anatomical and physiological dead space
- Diaphragm fatigue
- Metabolic acidosis, causing pulmonary hypertension.

## GI

- Decreased hepatic and renal blood flow, prolonging action of anaesthetic drugs
- Decreased liver metabolism, prolonging action of anaesthetic drugs.

## Metabolism

- Decreased metabolic rate 8% per °C
- Shivering increases $O_2$ consumption by up to 800%. Resultant increased muscle blood flow may accelerate heat loss
- Hypothermia shifts $O_2$ dissociation curve to the left, reducing $O_2$ delivery
- Increased stress response and increased nitrogen loss postoperatively
- Hyperglycaemia secondary to increased glycogenolysis and reduced insulin production
- Reduced drug metabolism. Hypothermia increases neuromuscular resistance to non-depolarizing muscle relaxants, but increased sensitivity occurs as hypothermia progresses.

## CNS

- Decreased MAC
- CNS protection below 24°C
- Pupils become fixed and dilated < 30°C
- Risk of intraventricular haemorrhage in neonates.

## Other

- Shivering worsens postoperative pain and is unpleasant for the patient
- Poor wound healing and increased risk of infection

- Increased bleeding time of skin, increased prothrombin time (PT) and partial thromboplastin time (PTT)
- Decreased platelet count and white cell count
- Increased risk of DVT and PE
- Immunosuppression.

## SHIVERING FOLLOWING GENERAL ANAESTHESIA

Shivering during recovery from anaesthesia may be due to spinal reflex hyperactivity resulting from inhibition of descending cortical control by residual anaesthetic rather than being a thermoregulatory mechanism. In addition, pre-optic nuclei may become hypersensitive to local changes in temperature, causing an exaggerated shivering response.

Shivering is reduced with radiant heat, pethidine, tramadol and doxapram.

## TECHNIQUES TO AVOID HEAT LOSS

- Maintain ambient temperature > 24°C and ambient humidity > 50%
- Prevent draughts
- Prevent skin contact with cold surfaces
- Prevent exposure of patients by use of drapes, blankets and head covering
- Silver blankets reflect heat and may reduce heat loss
- Cover exposed bowel
- Use warm fluids for washout of body cavities
- Warm i.v. fluids
- Use low fresh gas flow (FGF) in circle system
- Use heat and moisture exchanger or warmed and humidified inspiratory gases
- Use warming mattress/blankets, forced-air convective warming (Bair Hugger)
- Use radiant heat.

### References

Carli F, MacDonald I A 1996 Perioperative inadvertent hypothermia: what do we need to prevent? British Journal of Anaesthesia 76: 601–603

Sessler D I 1997 Perioperative thermoregulation and heat balance. Annals of the New York Academy of Sciences 813: 757–777

Wood M L B, Carli F 1991 Inadvertent hypothermia in the operating theatre. Current Anaesthesia and Critical Care 2: 222–231

# 6. General

ASA status is a good risk predictor of perioperative death in patients aged over 80 years. Operations in this age group are more common as the numbers of elderly increase.

## PHYSIOLOGY

### CVS

- Reduced cardiac output and cardiac reserve, $\uparrow$ SVR, $\uparrow$ circulation time
- Reduced sympathetic and parasympathetic responses
- Loss of vascular compliance causes systolic > diastolic hypertension.

### Respiratory

- $\downarrow$ lung total surface area, $\downarrow$ compliance
- $\uparrow$ closing capacity, $\uparrow$ FRC, $\uparrow\uparrow$ RV, $\downarrow$ expiratory reserve volume (ERV), $\downarrow$ VC
- $\downarrow$ response to $CO_2$.

### Renal

- $\downarrow$ renal blood flow, GFR and concentrating ability
- $\downarrow$ active tubular excretion.

### GI

- GI tract – $\downarrow$ motility, $\downarrow$ gastric acidity, $\downarrow$ blood flow, $\downarrow$ mucosal surface area. However, little overall effect on oral drug absorption
- $\downarrow$ hepatic blood flow, $\downarrow$ hepatic metabolism ($\downarrow$ liver mass, not $\downarrow$ microsomal enzyme activity). $\downarrow$ plasma albumin, thus decreased plasma binding, e.g. benzodiazepines, barbiturates.

## CNS

- ↓ cerebral blood flow
- ↓ cognitive, motor and sensory function.

### Other

- Decreased bone mass and strength, periodontal disease, and reduced subcutaneous fat increasing the chance of peripheral nerve injury. Chronic and iron deficiency anaemia. Impaired temperature homeostasis. Decrease in basal metabolic rate decreases drug metabolism.
- Among the elderly, 47% are hypertensive, 31% have renal disease, and 22% have heart failure/cardiomegaly.

## PHARMACOKINETIC AND PHARMACODYNAMIC CHANGES

- ↓ lean body mass
- ↓ total body water
- ↑ total body fat
- ↓ blood volume.

Therefore, ↓ $V_D$ for water-soluble drugs, ↑ $V_D$ for fat-soluble drugs.

- ↓ protein binding but effect minimal (except pethidine)
- ↓ hepatic and renal clearance so reduced clearance of drugs excreted by these routes
- ↓ MAC
- ↓ blood:gas solubility (?changes in cholesterol, triglycerides and albumin)
- Faster inhalational induction with ↓ cardiac output and ↓ blood:gas solubility countered by ↑ intrapulmonary shunting and ↓ cerebral blood flow
- Prolonged recovery due to decreased tissue perfusion and higher proportion of body fat acting as drug reservoir
- Drug interactions more likely due to polypharmacy. One-third of patients > 75 years are taking ≥ 3 drugs/day.

## SPECIFIC DRUGS

*Anticholinergics.* Increased $V_D$ atropine with ↑ half-life. Causes central anticholinergic syndrome unlike glycopyrollate because of passage across blood–brain barrier.

*Barbiturates.* Larger $V_D$ with prolonged clearance; 30–40% ↓ dose requirement.

*Benzodiazepines* (Table 6.1). Increased CNS sensitivity. High protein binding of diazepam results in greater free drug in elderly in contrast to lesser change in dose requirements of midazolam. The latter may cause severe hypotension in the elderly (Committee on Safety of Medicines warning).

**Table 6.1** Half-life of benzodiazepines

|  | $t_{1/2}$ (hours) | |
| --- | --- | --- |
|  | **Young adult** | **Elderly** |
| Diazepam | 24 | 72 |
| Midazolam | 2.8 | 4.3 |

*Propofol.* 50% reduced dose requirement. More enhanced CVS depression and greater hypotensive effect (diastolic > systolic). Reduce hypotension on induction by slower rate of injection. Propofol reduces postoperative mental confusion compared with other induction agents.

*Volatiles.* MAC decreases linearly with age. Volatiles with rapid elimination, e.g. desflurane, may reduce postoperative mental confusion. Isoflurane, desflurane and sevoflurane have fewer cardiovascular side-effects than other volatiles.

*Opioids* (Table 6.2). Smaller $V_D$ with higher initial plasma concentrations. Increased elimination half-life ($\downarrow$ clearance greater than $\downarrow V_D$). Decreased protein binding of pethidine with increasing age.

**Table 6.2** Half-life of opioids

|  | $t_{1/2} \beta$ (min) | |
| --- | --- | --- |
|  | **Young adult** | **Elderly** |
| Alfentanyl | 90 | 130 |
| Fentanyl | 250 | 925 |

*Muscle relaxants.* Reduced plasma cholinesterase but minimal effect on hydrolysis. There are conflicting results for atracurium and vecuronium. Probably little change in initial dose requirements but prolonged elimination. No change in dose requirements or elimination of cisatracurium, but 30% increase in time to effective block. Pancuronium and gallamine cause tachycardia, worsening any myocardial ischaemia.

*Anticholinergics.* No change in dose but slower onset of action and prolonged muscarinic side-effects.

*Local anaesthetics.* Decreased elimination of lignocaine and bupivacaine with increased risk of toxicity.

## REGIONAL ANAESTHESIA

In the elderly, regional anaesthesia decreases postoperative mental confusion and allows immediate recognition of angina, TIAs and mental confusion during TURP. Although some studies show benefits from regional anaesthesia, e.g. decreased blood loss and less CNS and respiratory dysfunction, long-term studies show little difference in outcome between GA and regional techniques.

## CENTRAL ANTICHOLINERGIC SYNDROME

- Occurs with atropine, hyoscine and promethazine
- Causes confusion, amnesia, agitation, ataxia, hallucinations and coma
- Reverse with physostigmine 1 mg/kg i.v.

## GENERAL PRINCIPLES OF ANAESTHETIC MANAGEMENT

- Avoid premedication. Use temazepam if necessary.
- Take care with placement of i.v. cannulae
- Reduce all drug doses and allow time for induction agents to circulate
- Decrease % MAC of volatiles and increase $F_iO_2$
- Avoid fluid overload
- Take care with immobile joints (especially the neck) and bony prominences.

### References

Bittenbinder T M, McLeskey C H 1994 Geriatric anesthesiology. Current Opinion in Anaesthesiology 7: 481–482

Waldmann C 1992 Anaesthesia for the elderly. In: Kaufman L (ed) Anaesthesia review 9. Churchill Livingstone, London

## ANAPHYLACTIC REACTIONS

## HISTORY

- 2640 BC – Egyptian hieroglyphics describe the sudden death of a Pharaoh following a wasp sting
- 1902 – Richet and Porter describe the death of dogs following a second injection of sea anemone toxin.

## EPIDEMIOLOGY

Between 1991 and 1994, 90 (four were fatal) suspected anaphylactic reactions associated with anaesthesia were reported by British anaesthetists to the Medicines Control Agency (MCA) on yellow cards. It is estimated, however, that there may be as many as 175–1000 severe reactions in the UK each year (1:5000–25 000 anaesthetics), with an overall mortality of 3.4%.

90% occur within 10 min of drug administration. It is more common in females (5:1 neuromuscular blocking drugs; 3:1 thiopentone).

## TYPES OF ALLERGIC REACTION

### Anaphylactic reaction

An exaggerated response to a foreign protein, associated with the release of vasoactive substances, e.g. type I hypersensitivity reaction, histamine, serotonin or complement activation (classical pathway). Tends to be self-perpetuating and therefore more severe.

### Anaphylactoid reaction

Clinically identical to an anaphylactic reaction but is not mediated by sensitizing IgE antibody, e.g. direct stimulation of histamine release or complement activation (alternate pathway). May be equally as severe but tends to be short-lived.

## HYPERSENSITIVITY REACTIONS

- *Type I* – anaphylactic; previous sensitization. Mediated via mast cells and IgE
- *Type II* – cytotoxic; antibodies directed against the cell membrane
- *Type III* – immune complex
- *Type IV* – delayed-type hypersensitivity; T-cell mediated.

## MAST CELLS

Found in perivascular tissue, gut mucosa, lung and skin. Up to 10% of their total weight is histamine. Stimulation causes release of histamine, eosinophil and neutrophil chemotactic factors, leucotrienes, prostaglandins, platelet-activating factor and kinins.

## HYPERSENSITIVITY TO DRUGS (Fig. 6.1)

A previous history of specific drug exposure does not seem necessary, particularly for neuromuscular blocking drugs where there may be no history of previous exposure in as many as 80% of cases. Cross-reactivity may occur between drugs with similar structures, causing a type I

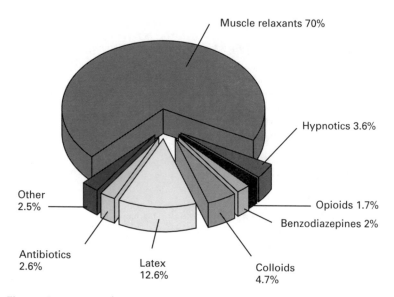

**Fig. 6.1** Causes of life-threatening allergic reactions during anaesthesia. (Data from Laxenaire 1993.)

hypersensitivity reaction to a drug to which the patient has not previously been exposed.

### Opioids

Usually cause anaphylactoid reactions. Mostly morphine. Reactions to synthetic opioids are rare.

### Induction agents

20% of reactions to thiopentone are anaphylactic; the remainder are anaphylactoid (90% direct histamine release, 10% complement activation) – methohexitone > thiopentone > propofol > etomidate.

### Muscle relaxants

Are the commonest cause of drug reactions. Steroid-based compounds (vecuronium, pancuronium) cause anaphylactic reactions, whereas benzyl-isoquinoliniums (doxacurim, mivacurium, atracurium) tend to cause anaphylactoid reactions. Of drug reactions caused by muscle relaxants, 43% are due to suxamethonium, 37% to vecuronium and 7% to atracurium. Least with pancuronium.

## Colloids

Fluids used for resuscitation following anaphylaxis may themselves cause histamine release and worsen any reaction.

### Volatile agents

No reports are known of anaphylactic reactions to volatile agents.

### Latex

Latex hypersensitivity is increasingly common, especially in gynaecological and abdominal surgery. High-risk groups include patients exposed to repeated bladder catheterizations, health care workers and patients with an occupational exposure to latex. Risk factors include male gender, non-Caucasian race, young age, atopy (asthma, allergic rhinitis, eczema and hay fever), spinal cord abnormality and food allergies (particularly banana or kiwi fruit; also chestnuts, potato, tomato and avocado). Unlike most other forms of anaphylaxis, the reaction is often delayed, beginning 30–60 min after the start of the procedure rather than at induction.

## CLINICAL SYMPTOMS (Fig. 6.2)

Awake patients may experience a metallic taste and a sense of impending doom. Commonest symptoms are hypotension (80%), rash/erythema (50%)

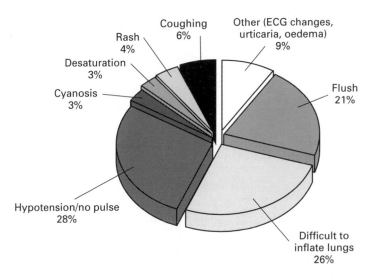

**Fig. 6.2** The first clinical feature of an anaphylactic reaction (Association of Anaesthetists 1995).

and bronchospasm (36%). Tachycardia due to chronotropic effects of histamine and secondary release of adrenaline and noradrenaline. SVR is decreased by as much as 80% due to direct effect of histamine.

Other symptoms include the following:

*CVS.* Arrhythmias, pulmonary hypertension.

*Respiratory.* Pharyngeal and laryngeal oedema (24%), rhinitis, pulmonary oedema.

*GI.* Nausea and vomiting, diarrhoea, abdominal colic.

*Other.* Generalized oedema (7%).

## TREATMENT

**ANAPHYLACTIC REACTIONS ASSOCIATED WITH ANAESTHESIA** Association of Anaesthetists of Great Britain and Ireland and the British Society of Allergy and Clinical Immunology, revised guidelines, 1995

Every anaesthetist should know and practise an anaphylaxis drill.

**Treatment**

*Initial therapy*

- Stop administration of drug(s) likely to have caused anaphylaxis
- Call for help
- Maintain airway: give 100% oxygen
- Lay patient flat with feet elevated
- Give adrenaline (epinephrine). This may be given i.m. in a dose of 0.5–1.0 mg and may be repeated every 10 minutes according to the arterial pressure and pulse until improvement occurs. Alternatively, 50–100 μg i.v. over 1 minute has been recommended for hypotension, with titration of further doses as required.

   In a patient with cardiovascular collapse, 0.5–1.0 mg may be required i.v., in divided doses by titration. This should be given at a rate of 0.1 mg/min, stopping when a response has been obtained
- Start intravascular volume expansion with suitable colloid or crystalloid

*Secondary therapy*

- Antihistamines – chlorpheniramine 10–20 mg by slow i.v. infusion; consider $H_2$ antagonists
- Corticosteroids – hydrocortisone 100–300 mg i.v.
- Catecholamine infusions (starting doses)
  — adrenaline: 0.05–0.1 μg/kg per min
  — noradrenaline: 0.05–0.1 μg/kg per min
- Perform arterial blood gas analysis; consider sodium bicarbonate (0.5–1.0 mmol/kg i.v.) for acidosis

- Airway evaluation (before extubation)
- Bronchodilators may be required for persistent bronchospasm

**Investigations**

Diagnosis is made on clinical grounds. Make a detailed written record of all events, including timing of administration of all drugs in relation to onset of reaction. There are no tests that are of use during anaphylaxis to identify the cause. Approximately 1 h after the beginning of the reaction, take 10 ml of venous blood into a plain glass tube. Separate serum and store at –20°C until the sample can be sent to a reference laboratory for estimation of serum tryptase concentration. Elevated levels occur in both anaphylactic and anaphylactoid reactions. A negative test does not exclude anaphylaxis.

**Tests to investigate the causative agent**

No test confidently identifies the causative agent.

Radioallergosorbent (RAST) tests are only available for suxamethonium and morphine (RAST test measures IgE). Cross-reactivity occurs with drugs of similar structure. The CAP system is an alternative to RAST. It is a fluoroimmunoassay for the measurement of antigen-specific antibodies and is usually more sensitive than RAST.

Skin prick test is a useful diagnostic test for drug allergy. Repeat with 1 in 10 dilution if test is initially positive to reduce chance of false-positive results. Cross-reactivity occurs with muscle relaxants. False positives are common with muscle relaxants and opioids but not with induction agents.

**Other tests**

*Mast cell tryptase* is the principal protein content of mast cell granules and is released, together with histamine and other amines, in anaphylactic and anaphylactoid reactions. Its concentration in the plasma or serum is raised between 1 and 6 h after reactions which involve mast cell degranulation. Thus postmortem analysis of plasma tryptase may yield meaningful results. The normal value of basal plasma tryptase is < 1 ng/ml. Plasma tryptase levels > 20 ng/ml may be seen after anaphylactic reactions.

In reactions to anaesthetic drugs, the analysis of mast cell tryptase appears to be a specific and sensitive diagnostic test for anaphylactic and anaphylactoid reactions. It is the most useful acute test available at present but requires further validation in mild/moderate reactions.

Some agents may release histamine without tryptase, e.g. agents acting through neuropeptide receptors.

*Methylhistamine* is the principal metabolite of histamine and is excreted in the urine. Raised urinary concentrations occur after reactions which involve systemic histamine release.

## PROPHYLAXIS

Prophylaxis with antihistamines ($H_1$ and $H_2$) does not reduce the incidence of allergic reactions, but reduces mortality if they occur.

## SCREENING

There is no method of predicting sensitivity to anaesthetic drugs. A history of previous exposure is not necessary for an anaphylactic reaction. The use of test doses of intravenous drugs is not an appropriate method of testing for anaphylaxis. Anaphylaxis has resulted from very small doses.

## ANAESTHESIA FOR THE ATOPIC PATIENT

There is some evidence that mast cells may degranulate more readily in atopic patients, but no evidence that atopic patients are any more susceptible to drug-mediated allergic reactions. Consider using drugs with low incidence of reaction, i.e. ketamine, etomidate and pancuronium.

### References

Association of Anaesthetists of Great Britain and Ireland / British Society of Allergy and Clinical Immunology 1995 Suspected anaphylactic reactions associated with anaesthesia (revised edition). AAGBI, London

Bouaziz H, Laxenaire M-C 1998 Anaesthesia for the allergic patient. Current Opinion in Anaesthesiology 11: 339–344

Dakin M J, Yentis S M 1998 Latex allergy: a strategy for management. Anaesthesia 53: 774–781

Hunter J M 1993 Histamine release and neuromuscular blocking drugs. Editorial. Anaesthesia 48: 561–563

Kam P C A, Lee M S M, Thompson J F 1997 Latex allergy: an emerging clinical and occupational health problem. Anaesthesia 52: 570–575

Laxenaire M C 1993 Drugs and other agents involved in anaphylactic shock occurring during anaesthesia. A French multicenter epidemiological inquiry. Annales Françaises d'Anesthésie et de Réanimation 12: 91–96

Watkins J 1987 Investigations of allergic and hypersensitivity reactions to anaesthetic agents. British Journal of Anaesthesia 59: 104–111

Wildsmith J A W, McKinnon R P 1995 Histaminoid reactions in anaesthesia. British Journal of Anaesthesia 74: 217–228

## BLOOD

## BLOOD DONORS

Seventeen million units of blood are donated in Europe each year. Each unit is screened for antibodies to:

- syphilis
- hepatitis B and C
- HIV 1 & 2
- +/− CMV.

## BLOOD GROUPS

The ABO blood groups are summarized in Table 6.3.

**Table 6.3** Summary of ABO blood groups

| Group | % | Erythrocyte antigens | Antibodies | |
|-------|-----|----------------------|-------------|---|
| O | 47 | Nil | Anti-A, anti-B | Universal donor |
| A | 42 | A | Anti-A | |
| B | 8 | B | Anti-A | |
| AB | 3 | AB | Nil | Universal recipient |

## PRODUCTS

### Whole blood

- 500 ml per bag with a haematocrit of 0.40
- No functioning platelets after 2–3 days; ↓ 2,3-DPG by 2 weeks
- Normal concentrations of albumin and clotting factors, except factors V and VIII, which are reduced to 10–20% of normal
- Not sterilized, so there is a risk of transmitted pathogens.

### Red cell concentrate (packed cells)

- 250 ml per bag with haematocrit of 0.60
- No functioning platelets; 2,3-DPG levels maintained for 14 days
- Storage is 35 days with SAGM (saline, adenine, glucose, mannitol); 42 days with A-CPD (adenine, citrate, phosphate, dextrose).

### Platelet concentrates

- Usually as a pool of 5–6 single unit donations; 4 units of platelets contain 1 unit FFP
- Small numbers of red cells and leucocytes
- Infection risk as for whole blood, but increased by multiple donors
- Use ABO-compatible platelets. Maximum storage is 5 days at 4°C.

### Fresh frozen plasma (FFP)

- Prepared from plasma from single donation; 150 ml per bag

- Contains all clotting factors, albumin and gammaglobulin
- Use immediately after thawing. Usually give at least 4 units
- Must be ABO-compatible and Rh(D)-negative if recipient is a Rh(D) fertile female
- Risk of anaphylactic reactions.

### Cryoprecipitate

- Precipitates from FFP when slowly thawed; supplied as 6–8 units
- High in factor VIII, fibrinogen and von Willebrand factor
- Indicated for DIC and von Willebrand's disease.

### Human albumin solution

Prepared by fractionation of multiple units of plasma giving 96% albumin and 4% globulin. Available as 4.5 or 20% (hyperoncotic) solution. Each 20 g of albumin requires 20 000 blood donations. Pasteurized at 60°C for 10 h to kill all microorganisms including viruses.

### Plasma protein fraction (PPF)

Prepared in a similar manner to albumin but contains more globulin (83% albumin, 17% globulin).

### Factor VIII concentrate

- Freeze-dried protein as 250 units
- Sterilized to inactivate viruses.

### Factor IX concentrate

- Freeze-dried protein as 250 units
- Sterilized to inactivate viruses
- Also contains factors II and X.

### Immunoglobulin products

- Fractionation of plasma to produce pool with > 90% IgG
- No risk of viral transmission
- Used for immune thrombocytopenia and immunodeficiency states.

## TRANSFUSION REACTIONS

### Acute

- *Haemolysis* – due to antibodies directed against red cells

- *Fever* – donor leucocytes attack host red cells
- *Anaphylaxis* – due to antibodies directed against recipient IgA
- *Transfusion-related acute lung injury* – due to donor antibodies directed against leucocytes. Clinically identical to ARDS
- *Hyperkalaemia* – 5–10 mmol $K^+$ in a unit of blood stored for 4–5 weeks. Effects of additional $K^+$ are exacerbated by acidosis and hypothermia. Hyperkalaemia is usually transient
- *Citrate toxicity* – citrate is added as a preservative to bind excess calcium and prevent clotting. Metabolized to bicarbonate. Excess causes metabolic alkalosis
- *Acid–base disturbance* – citrate from preservative and lactate from red cells
- *Hypocalcaemia* – citrate anticoagulant binds ionized calcium; ↓BP, ↓ pulse pressure. Give $CaCl_2$ only if there are symptoms/signs (not $Ca^{2+}$ gluconate, which must be metabolized to release free $Ca^{2+}$)
- *Febrile reaction* – due to bacterial contamination
- *Microemboli* – aggregates of all cellular components, increase with age of blood. Cause complement activation, haemolysis and thrombocytopenia. Removed by 170 $\mu$m filter; +/– 40 $\mu$m screen and depth filters
- *Hypothermia* – left shift of $O_2$ dissociation curve, platelet and clotting dysfunction
- *Air embolus*
- *Fluid overload.*

### Delayed

- *Haemolytic transfusion reaction* – from red cell antibodies
- *Graft-versus-host disease*
- *Alloimmunization* (reaction to minor foreign antigens) – 10% of all transfusion reactions:
  — red cell antibodies including anti-Rh(D)
  — leucocyte antibodies
  — platelet antibodies
- *Viral infection* – hepatitis B (1:20 000 units) and C (1:1000 units), HIV (1:400 000 units), cytomegalovirus, parvovirus (causes aplastic anaemia in sickle cell patients)
- *Other infections* – syphilis, malaria, trypanosomiasis
- *Tumour recurrence* – increased risk
- *Sensitization* – resulting in antibody formation and subsequent difficulties with cross-matching
- *Iron overload* – occurs with repeated transfusions.

## MASSIVE BLOOD TRANSFUSION

Defined as the acute administration of more than 1.5 times the patient's blood volume, or replacement of the patient's total blood volume within 24 h.
  Blood groups for urgent transfusion are:

- O Rh(D)-negative if patient not cross-matched
- uncross-matched blood (type-specific) if patient's blood group is known.

Blood transfusions can be avoided by:

- reducing blood loss – hypotensive anaesthesia, antifibrinolytic agents
- tolerating a lower haematocrit
- transfusing autologous blood – prior donation, use of cell saver
- artificial blood
- erythropoietin.

### Cell saver

Returned blood is warm, with normal levels of 2,3-DPG: Contraindicated with sepsis, contamination with intestinal contents or tumour cells.

---

**GUIDELINES FOR AUTOLOGOUS BLOOD TRANSFUSION** British Committee for Standards in Haematology Blood Transfusion Task Force 1997

The purpose of all forms of autologous transfusion (acute preoperative haemodilution and preoperative donation or intraoperative cell salvage) is to avoid the transfusion of allogeneic blood and the associated risks. Autologous transfusion procedures are not usually acceptable to Jehovah's Witnesses, although some accept intraoperative cell salvage.

**Intraoperative cell salvage**
*Indications.* Elective and emergency surgery with expected blood loss >20% total body volume.
*Contraindications.* Bacterial contamination of wound, malignant disease and sickle cell disease.

**Acute preoperative haemodilution and preoperative donation**
*Indications.* Elective surgery with expected blood loss > 20% total body volume.
*Contraindications.* Aortic stenosis, unstable angina, and moderate to severe left ventricular impairment.

---

### Antifibrinolytic agents

For example tranexamic acid and aprotinin. Bind to plasminogen and plasmin to interfere with their ability to split fibrinogen. Prostatic plasminogen activator is released during prostate surgery to cause bleeding, inactivated by antifibrinolytic agents. Antifibrinolytic agents may reduce bleeding in cardiac surgery following cardiopulmonary bypass.

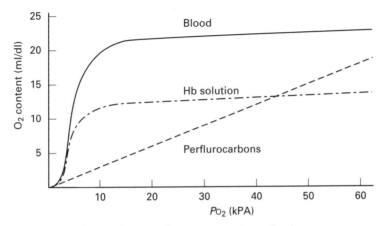

**Fig. 6.3** Oxygen dissociation curve for oxygen-carrying molecules.

## Artificial blood (Fig. 6.3)

*Perfluorocarbons.* Inert chemicals with oxygen solubility 20 times that of plasma. Difficulties with emulsification limit their development to 10% solution.

*Recombinant Hb (rHb1.1).* Modified human haemoglobin tetramer cross-linked with a glycine bridge between the alpha subunits. Produced from *E. coli* or yeast. Cross-linking prevents renal excretion. Cleared by the reticuloendothelial system within 24 h.

*Purified Hb.* From expired red cells, e.g. diaspirin cross-linked haemoglobin.

## Jehovah's Witnesses

'For the life of the flesh is in the blood: and I have given it to you upon the altar to make atonement for your souls: for it is the blood that maketh an atonement for the soul. Therefore I said unto the children of Israel, No soul of you shall eat blood, neither shall any stranger that sojourneth among you eat blood.' (Leviticus 17: 10–12; see also Genesis 9: 3–4 and Acts 15: 28–29).

There are an estimated 145 000 Jehovah's Witnesses in the UK. They refuse administration of all blood and usually all blood products. They will allow blood to be retransfused if it has not lost contact with the circulation, e.g. cardiopulmonary bypass. The Children and Young Persons Act 1933 states that parents have a duty of care to their children which is not fulfilled if permission for a life-saving blood transfusion is withheld. Doctors can apply to the courts for permission to give blood against the parents' wishes, but in an emergency, blood can be given to children without consulting the courts. Children under the age of 16 can consent to a blood transfusion if they understand the issues involved, but may not refuse blood.

Blood loss > 500 mL in adults is associated with increased mortality.

## MANAGEMENT OF ANAESTHESIA FOR JEHOVAH'S WITNESSES Association of Anaesthetists of Great Britain and Ireland, 1999

### Clinical management

Anaesthetists have the right to refuse to anaesthetize an elective case (when referral can be made to other colleagues) but must anaesthetize an emergency case if failure to do so would harm the patient. Ideally, consultant staff should be involved with patient care.

Preoperatively, patients must be seen alone to avoid undue influence from other family / church members. The patient must be made fully aware of the risks of refusal of blood products. It must be clarified which blood products and techniques (e.g. cell saver) are acceptable.

Preoperative assessment should take place as early as possible. Anaemia should be treated. Use of iron supplements and erythropoetin should be considered.

### Intraoperative management

Techniques to minimize blood loss include positioning to avoid venous congestion, hypotensive anaesthesia, use of tourniquets, meticulous haemostasis, use of vasoconstrictors, haemodilution and use of a cell saver.

Antifibrinolytics (e.g. tranexamic acid, aprotinin) may also reduce blood loss.

### Postoperative care

- Early detection and correction of postoperative oozing
- Consider elective ventilation to increase oxygen delivery
- Active cooling reduces oxygen demand and increases dissolved oxygen carriage
- Hyperbaric oxygen therapy may also be of benefit.

### References

Anon 1993 The risks and uses of donated blood. Drug and Therapeutics Bulletin 31: 89–92

Association of Anaesthetists of Great Britain and Ireland 1999 Management of anaesthesia for Jehovah's Witnesses. AAGBI, London

British Committee for Standards in Haematology Blood Transfusion Task Force: Autologous Transfusion Working Party (Napier J A, Bruce M, Chapman J et al) 1997 Guidelines for autologous transfusion. II. Perioperative haemodilution and cell salvage. British Journal of Anaesthesia 78: 768–771

Contreras M (ed) 1998 ABC of transfusion, 3rd edn. BMJ Publishing Group, London

Cox M, Lumley J 1995 No blood or blood products. Anaesthesia 50: 583–585

Donaldson M D J, Seaman M J, Park G R 1992 Massive blood transfusion. British Journal of Anaesthesia 69: 621–630

McClelland B 1996 Handbook of transfusion medicine, 2nd edn. HMSO, London

Van der Linden P, Vincent J-L 1997 Effects of blood transfusion on oxygen uptake: old concepts adapted to new therapeutic strategies? Critical Care Medicine 25: 723–724

Veeckman L 1997 Artificial blood substitutes. Current Opinion in Anaesthesiology 10: 280–283

## BURNS

### EPIDEMIOLOGY

There are 10 000 burns admissions per annum in the UK, of which 600 are fatal; 35% of burn injuries occur in children. Most burns are scalds, flame burns and flash burns; also electrical and chemical burns. Cold injury (frostbite) is rare in the UK.

### SYSTEMIC EFFECTS OF BURNS

Tissue damage is due to both direct thermal injury and secondary damage from inflammatory mediators.

*CVS.* Initial reduction in cardiac output due to hypovolaemia and myocardial depressant factor. Substantial amounts of water, sodium and protein are lost within 48 hours due to leakage from capillary beds. This increased capillary permeability may cause generalized oedema in large burns (> 30%). Hypermetabolic state leads to an increased cardiac output within a few days. Hypertension is common secondary to catecholamines and renin activation. Responds to ACE inhibitors.

*Respiratory.* Reduced chest wall compliance, reduced FRC, reduced pulmonary compliance. Mucosal damage from upper airway burn.

*Renal.* Renal failure due to reduced GFR (inadequate resuscitation), myoglobinuria, haemoglobinuria and sepsis.

*GI.* Impaired liver function due to hypovolaemia, hepatotoxins and hypoxia. Curling's ulcers form in the stomach.

*CNS.* Encephalopathy, seizures.

*Haematology.* Bone marrow suppression, anaemia, thrombocytopenia and coagulopathy.

*Skin.* Increased heat, fluid and electrolyte loss. Loss of protective antimicrobial barrier.

*Metabolism.* Full-thickness burn causes water loss of 200 ml/$m^2$ per hour; 500 calories are used to evaporate 1000 ml water. Therefore there is an increased energy demand.

Inhaled carbon monoxide and cyanide reduce tissue oxygen delivery.

Stress response causes a hypermetabolic state with accelerated nitrogen turnover, negative nitrogen balance, hyperinsulinaemia and insulin resistance. Large nutritional requirements necessitate early high-calorie feeding.

## PHARMACOKINETIC AND PHARMACODYNAMIC CHANGES

- Suxamethonium is contraindicated in burns because of the risk of hyperkalaemia. Probably due to the entire myocyte cell membrane acting as a receptor. There is resistance to non-depolarizing neuromuscular blockers due to increased $V_D$ and upregulation of ACh receptors. These changes are proportional to the size of burn and may persist for at least 2 years after the burn has healed.
- Renal and hepatic failure reduce drug clearance.
- There is increased tolerance to narcotics and sedatives despite decreased clearance.
- Hypocalcaemia is common.

## PATIENT ASSESSMENT

### Initial evaluation

Assess airway (A), breathing (B) and circulation (C). Establish venous access. Perform a secondary survey and exclude any other injuries. Assess neurological status (D) and expose the patient fully (E).

Wear protective clothing if there are chemical burns.

## TREATMENT OF BURN INJURY

### Airway

Direct thermal injury, toxic gases and smoke inhalation cause:

- upper airway oedema and obstruction
- lung parenchymal damage
- carbon monoxide poisoning
- cyanide poisoning (burning plastic).

### Breathing

Monitor respiratory function, especially if there is inhalational injury. Indicators of an upper airway burn include voice changes, CXR changes, carboxyhaemoglobinaemia > 15%, or compromised arterial blood gases.

Humidify inspired gases if there is upper airway burn. Intubate immediately if severe airway burn since facial oedema will develop rapidly over the initial 24 hours following a facial burn and may make intubation very difficult.

*Carbon monoxide poisoning.* The symptoms of CO poisoning are given in Table 6.4.

**Table 6.4** Symptoms of carbon monoxide poisoning

| %HbCO | Symptoms |
| --- | --- |
| 0–10 | None |
| 10–20 | Headache, malaise |
| 30–40 | Nausea and vomiting, slowing of mental activity |
| >60–70 | CVS collapse, death. Consider hyperbaric $O_2$ therapy |

The half-life of carbon monoxide (250 times the affinity of $O_2$ for Hb) is:

- room air – 5 h
- 100% $O_2$ – 1 h.

*Cyanide poisoning.* Causes metabolic acidosis, raised lactate, arterial hypoxaemia and increased anion gap. Consider treatment with cyanide-chelating agents (dicobalt edetate) or agents accelerating cyanide metabolism (sodium thiosulphate).

## Circulation

Risk of profound hypovolaemia with hypotension. Early fluid shifts result in loss of fluid from the plasma into the extracellular tissue around the burn. This fluid is similar in composition to plasma with equal electrolyte content but with slightly less protein. If crystalloid is used for resuscitation, larger volumes are necessary and may result in tissue oedema. Fluid loss is maximal in the first few hours and returns to basal levels by 36 h.

Blood loss during surgical debridement may be rapid and exceed 2 ml/kg per 1% of burn desloughed.

## Extent and depth of burn

*Burn size.* This is estimated using the 'Rule of Nines' (Fig. 6.4).
*Depth of burn*
*Superficial.* Damage to epidermis. Erythema but no blistering. Painful. Heals in 2–3 days.
*Partial thickness.* Destruction of epidermis and dermis with formation of blisters. If deep, may also include islets of fat. Painful. Heals within 10 days as fresh epidermis grows out from hair follicles but deep partial thickness burns may be slow to heal.
*Full thickness.* Complete loss of epidermis and dermis down to subcutaneous fat. Loss of pain receptors renders burn painless. The burn is either white or charred with eschar. Heals by wound contraction and thus if circumferential may require escharotomies in the acute stage.

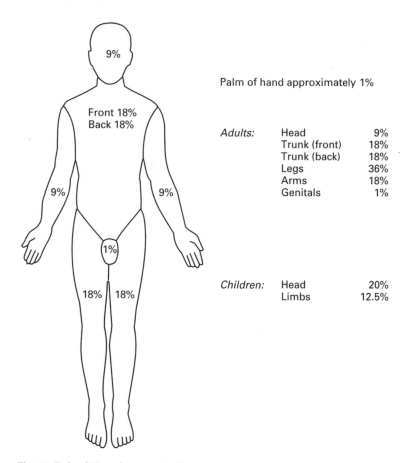

Palm of hand approximately 1%

| Adults: | Head | 9% |
|---|---|---|
| | Trunk (front) | 18% |
| | Trunk (back) | 18% |
| | Legs | 36% |
| | Arms | 18% |
| | Genitals | 1% |

| Children: | Head | 20% |
|---|---|---|
| | Limbs | 12.5% |

**Fig. 6.4** Rule of Nines for assessing burn area.

*Fluid replacement.* Formal fluid resuscitation is commenced in adults with > 15% burns or in children with >10% burns. Most UK centres use colloid-containing solutions, whilst crystalloid-based regimes are more popular elsewhere. Hypertonic saline may reduce fluid volumes and oedema, but some studies have shown that it causes hypernatraemia, renal failure and increased mortality.

These regimes are given in addition to the normal daily fluid requirements (usually given as 5% dextrose or dextrose saline). Volumes may need increasing if clinical indicators show inadequate resuscitation (mental status, vital signs, urine output, capillary refill, CVP etc.).

Check electrolytes, haematocrit and plasma and urine osmolality every 4 hours. Low volume urine with osmolality > 450 suggests continuing hypovolaemia. Transfuse blood if haematocrit < 0.3.

Common fluid replacement formulae:

- *Muir & Barclay (Mount Vernon formula)*
  0.5 ml/kg colloid (PPF/albumin) × % burn given over 4, 4, 4, 6 and 6 h.
- *Brook*
  0.5 ml/kg colloid and 1.5 ml/kg crystalloid × % burn
  ($\frac{1}{2}$ given over first 8 h, $\frac{1}{4}$ over next 8 h, $\frac{1}{4}$ over next 8 h)
- *Parkland*
  4 ml/kg crystalloid × % burn
  ($\frac{1}{2}$ given over first 8 h, $\frac{1}{4}$ over next 8 h, $\frac{1}{4}$ over next 8 h).

## Infection

May worsen depth of burn, risks spreading to become a systemic infection and may destroy any skin grafts. Patients at high risk both from loss of protective skin barrier and from generalized immunosuppression.

Nurse in as clean an area as possible because of high risk of infection. Take measures to avoid cross-infection. Use topical antimicrobial prophylaxis with silver sulphadiazine cream (Flamazine).

Antibiotic cover is necessary to cover dressing changes. Systemic antibiotics should not be given routinely.

## Hypothermia

Impaired homeostatic control and heat loss through burns result in rapid onset of hypothermia, accelerated by general anaesthesia and cold fluids. Keep room at 30°C to minimize energy requirements and ensure use of blood warmer and heated mattress.

## Multiple anaesthetics

Are required for dressing changes and skin grafting. Monitoring (e.g. ECG dot placement) may be difficult with extensive burns. Venous access may have to be gained through burnt tissue or by a cutdown.

## Nutrition and GI

Early feeding is vital because of high catabolic state. NG tube may be necessary for feeding and to prevent acute gastric dilatation. Gastric stasis is common, in which case a nasojejunal tube is necessary. Calculate amount of feed needed according to Sutherland or modified Curreri formula. Aim for a calorie:nitrogen ratio of 100:1. Give gastric stress ulcer prophylaxis. Monitor blood sugar closely.

## Analgesia

Any burns less than full thickness require large doses of opioid analgesia.

### Surgical management

*Superficial burns* usually heal spontaneously within 10 days and do not require surgery.

*Partial-thickness burns* require frequent debridement and may require grafting if unhealed by 3 weeks.

*Full-thickness burns* require early debridement and grafting. Although early debridement of a large area further traumatizes the patient and may result in loss of a large blood volume, a delay in debridement risks wound colonization and septic shock and prolongs the catabolic state following injury. If full-thickness burns are not grafted, they may never heal, or if they do they will result in contractures.

### References

Brazeal B A, Traber D L 1997 Pathophysiology of inhalation injury. Current Opinion in Anaesthesiology 10: 65–67

Carl P, Reich H 1998 Burns. Current Opinion in Anaesthesiology 11: 181–184

MacLennan N, Heimbach D M, Cullen B F 1998 Anesthesia for major thermal injury. Anesthesiology 89: 749–770

## DAY-CASE ANAESTHESIA

### ADVANTAGES

- More convenient for patient
- Reduced morbidity (pneumonia, DVT etc)
- Reduced risk of hospital-acquired infections
- Cost savings
- Increased hospital efficiency.

### PATIENT SELECTION

Generally limited to ASA I and II patients. Elderly and ASA III patients may be considered suitable if their systemic disease is well controlled preoperatively. Patients with morbid obesity are probably best treated as in-patients.

Healthy full-term infants < 6 months are suitable for day-case surgery. Infants < 50 weeks post-conceptual age are unsuitable because of risk of postoperative apnoea, poor gag reflex and poor temperature control. Admit overnight any patient with a history of near-miss sudden infant death syndrome (SIDS), or patients with a family history of SIDS.

Length of anaesthesia is directly related to postoperative morbidity.

## GENERAL ANAESTHESIA

### Requirements of a general anaesthetic

- Safe and effective anaesthesia
- Minimal side-effects
- Rapid recovery
- Good postoperative analgesia.

### Premedication

May impair coordination for 5–12 h postoperatively, therefore avoid if possible.
Use metoclopramide and ranitidine if there is an aspiration risk.

### Airway

Laryngeal mask airway (LMA) reduces the incidence of postoperative sore throat and avoids the need for intubation. Ventilation with LMA appears safe but does not protect against gastric aspiration. For patients at risk of aspiration, use cuffed endotracheal tube. Endotracheal intubation using propofol/alfentanyl may avoid the need for neuromuscular blockers.

### Induction agents

*Thiopentone* may impair motor skills for up to 8 h. Children induced with thiopentone are more sleepy for the first 30 min postoperatively compared with gas induction with halothane.

*Etomidate* is rapidly metabolized but is associated with a higher incidence of nausea and vomiting.

*Propofol* recovery is faster than thiopentone, methohexitone, etomidate, isoflurane, enflurane or halothane and causes less nausea and vomiting. More CVS depression than barbiturates. High incidence of pain on injection reduced with lignocaine or opioid and injection into a large vein. At 24 h, patients given propofol are more alert, less drowsy and less tired than those given thiopentone.

*Midazolam* is highly suitable for sedation during local procedures due to minimal cardiorespiratory depression and rapid clearance. However, CNS recovery is more rapid with propofol.

### Opioids

Short-acting opioids may reduce volatile requirements and actually decrease postoperative recovery time. Decrease pain on injection and movement with etomidate and methohexitone. Emergence is more rapid with alfentanyl than with fentanyl. Use with prophylactic antiemetics, although there is less nausea and vomiting if combined with propofol.

### Inhalational agents

*Desflurane* has the lowest blood:gas solubility of the current volatile agents (0.42) and therefore undergoes the fastest elimination with rapid recovery. Too irritant for gas induction.

*Sevoflurane* (blood:gas solubility = 0.6) is less pungent and can be used for gas induction with rapid elimination. Because both undergo rapid equilibration, a more rapid adjustment of anaesthetic depth is possible. Both allow more rapid recovery than a propofol infusion and cause less residual impairment of cognitive function. Neither causes nausea or vomiting. Both are more expensive than *isoflurane* and have not been shown to enable earlier discharge home.

### Muscle relaxants

Use of neuromuscular blockers may reduce recovery time by decreasing volatile requirements.

Suxamethonium can cause myalgia for up to 4 days.

Intubating dose of mivacurium (0.2 mg/kg) causes maximum blockade within 3 min and spontaneous recovery by 20–30 min. Mivacurium 0.08 mg/kg produces maximum blockade in 4 min and 95% recovery of twitch height within 25 min. It has the fastest recovery of any non-depolarizer, usually avoiding the use of reversal drugs.

Brief laparoscopic procedures may be possible with spontaneous ventilation and face mask.

Neostigmine and glycopyrrolate increase the incidence of postoperative nausea and vomiting.

### Recovery

Postoperative waking is faster with sevoflurane and desflurane.

Postoperative nausea, vomiting and headaches are associated with $N_2O$, etomidate, fentanyl and volatiles. Droperidol causes increased postoperative drowsiness.

## LOCAL/REGIONAL ANAESTHESIA

Avoids complications of GA, reduces aspiration risk and provides good postoperative analgesia. Cognitive defects are present at 3 days postoperatively in GA patients but are not present following local infiltration.

Day-case techniques include topical anaesthesia (including EMLA), Bier's block, field infiltration, peripheral nerve blocks, regional blocks.

Spinal headaches are more common in the young, especially with early ambulation. Use fine Sprotte or Whitacre needles (< 24 G). Discharge times using spinal for inguinal hernia are significantly longer than with field block.

## FLUID MANAGEMENT

Allow clear fluids up to 2 h preoperatively. This minimizes preoperative thirst and discomfort, avoids hypoglycaemia (particularly in children) and reduces hypotension on induction. Consider i.v. fluids if surgery is scheduled to last more than 30 min, blood loss > 300 ml or there is a risk of nausea and vomiting (e.g. squint surgery).

## ENT SURGERY

Day-case adenotonsillectomy for children is safe and cost-effective. Children undergoing tonsillectomy for airway obstruction are at continuing risk of obstruction in the postoperative period, so admit overnight.

## DISCHARGE CRITERIA

### General anaesthetic

- Awake, orientated and tolerating oral fluids
- Urine passed
- Stable observations for 60 min
- Responsible adult to accompany patient home.

### Regional anaesthetic

- As above, but also ensure regression of motor, sensory and sympathetic blockade
- Suitable criteria include normal perianal ($S_{4-5}$) sensation, plantar flexion of the foot and proprioception in the big toe.

## POSTOPERATIVE COMPLICATIONS

The 30-day postoperative mortality is 1:11 000. Incidence of stroke, MI and pulmonary embolus is extremely low, and less than would be expected in a similar population undergoing surgery involving a hospital stay.

Unanticipated postoperative admission rate is approximately 1%, mostly due to bleeding and inadequate pain relief; 3–12% patients discharged contact their GP/hospital due to bleeding, inadequate pain relief and headaches/dizziness.

---

**DAY CASE SURGERY** Association of Anaesthetists of Great Britain and Ireland 1994

**Patient selection**
- *Social* – responsible adult to care for the patient for 24 h postoperatively with easy access to a telephone. Suitable home situation

- *Medical factors* – patients should be fully fit or any illness should be well controlled. Obese patients are generally not suitable
- *Personnel factors* – good liaison between GP, hospital and community nurses.

**Anaesthetic management**
Use anaesthetic techniques minimizing morbidity and providing good analgesia. Recovery facilities should be of the same high standard as the main theatres.

**Discharge**
Local policy must be drawn up. If using spinal or epidural anaesthesia, ensure patient can pass urine and has return of sensation to $S_1$ (ability to walk). Must receive verbal and written instructions before discharge and be given a hospital contact phone number. Instruct to avoid drinking, driving and operating machinery for 24 h.

**Audit**
Must be developed by each unit.

**References**

Association of Anaesthetists of Great Britain and Ireland 1994 Day case surgery. AAGBI, London

Marshall S I, Chung F 1999 Discharge criteria and complications after ambulatory surgery. Anesthesia and Analgesia 88: 508–517

White P F 1998 Ambulatory anesthesia in the 21st century. Current Opinion in Anaesthesiology 11: 593–594

Wilkinson D J 1993 Modern day-surgery. In: Kaufman L (ed) Anaesthesia review 10. Churchill Livingstone, London, p 163–182

Wolverson A, Nathanson M H 1998 Volatile versus intravenous anaesthetic techniques for ambulatory anaesthesia. Current Opinion in Anaesthesiology 11: 595–600

# DEPTH OF ANAESTHESIA

## GUEDEL CLASSIFICATION

Described for spontaneous respiration with diethyl ether in 1937.

- **Stage 1: Analgesia** – beginning of induction to loss of consciousness
    Regular, small-volume respiration
    Pupils normal.
- **Stage 2: Excitement** – loss of consciousness to onset of automatic breathing

Irregular respiration
Divergent, dilated pupils
Active laryngeal/pharyngeal reflexes
Eyelash reflex abolished.

- **Stage 3: Surgical anaesthesia** – automatic respiration to respiratory paralysis:
  - *Plane 1:* Regular, large-volume respiration
    Central, pinpoint pupils. Cessation of eye movements
    Eyelid reflex abolished
  - *Plane 2:* Thoracic component of respiration decreased
    Loss of corneal reflex
  - *Plane 3:* Respiration becoming diaphragmatic. Small volume
    Laryngeal reflexes depressed
    Pupils normal
  - *Plane 4:* Irregular diaphragmatic, small-volume respiration
    Dilated pupils
    Carinal reflex depressed.
- **Stage 3:** More recent classification, replacing that of Guedel:
  - *Light anaesthesia:* until cessation of eyeball movement
  - *Medium anaesthesia:* increasing intercostal muscle paralysis
  - *Deep anaesthesia:* diaphragmatic respiration.
- **Stage 4: Coma**
    Apnoea, hypotension.

## MONITORING DEPTH OF ANAESTHESIA

*Autonomic responses.* BP, pulse, sweating, dilated pupils.

*Isolated forearm technique of Tunstall (1977).* Tighten tourniquet on upper arm above systolic pressure before injection of neuromuscular blocker.

*Spontaneous skeletal muscle activity.* Abolished with neuromuscular blockers.

*EEG.* Difficult to use and interpret because of specific effects of different anaesthetic agents. A drug-independent EEG parameter has not yet been identified. Fourier analysis (decomposes EEG into its component sine waves) correlates well with sedation but not depth of anaesthesia.

*Evoked potentials.* Auditory, visual and electrical. Measure change in latency and amplitude of EEG responses.

*Oesophageal smooth muscle provoked contraction.* Provoked with balloon dilation in lower third of oesophagus. Unaltered with neuromuscular blockers. Different volatiles affect the response in different ways.

## AWARENESS DURING ANAESTHESIA

Occurs in 0.1–1% of paralysed patients, and 0.3% of patients undergoing fast-track cardiac anaesthesia. Single case report of a patient aware during spontaneous respiration. Commonest during obstetric GA, often at intubation.

## Causes

- Use of minimal dose of induction agents and no opioids for lower segment caesarean section (LSCS) to avoid fetal depression
- Use of minimal drugs if patient seriously ill
- Prolonged attempts at intubation during which induction agent wears off and patient remains paralysed
- VOC with percentage of volatile within the circle lower than that set on the vaporizer
- Vaporizer exhausted of volatile
- Vaporizer not seated correctly on back bar, causing loss of volatile
- Leak within the breathing circuit
- Disconnection
- Total intravenous anaesthesia
  — infusion not commenced immediately after induction agent given
  — incorrect infusion rates, too low to be used without the addition of $N_2O$ and opioids
  — pump failure or occlusion of line
- Hypermetabolic states with increased volatile requirement, e.g. thyrotoxicosis.

### References

Aitkenhead A R 1994 The pattern of litigation against anaesthetists. British Journal of Anaesthesia 73: 10–21

Jessop J, Jones J G 1991 Conscious awareness during general anaesthesia – what are we attempting to monitor? British Journal of Anaesthesia 66: 635–637

Jones J G 1996 Depth of anaesthesia. Current Opinion in Anaesthesiology 9: 452–456

Rampil I J 1998 A primer for EEG signal processing in anesthesia. Anesthesiology 89: 1002

Tunstall M E 1977 Detecting wakefulness during general anaesthesia for caesarean section. British Medical Journal 1: 1321

## GENERAL TOPICS

## ASA GRADING (1963)

I   – Healthy. No systemic disease
II  – Mild/moderate systemic disease not limiting patient's activities
III – Severe systemic disease causing functional limitation
IV – Severe systemic disease which is a constant threat to life
V  – Moribund patient unlikely to survive > 24 h with/without surgery
E  – Additional coding for emergency surgery.

## CEPOD CLASSIFICATION OF DISEASES

- *Immediate* – resuscitation simultaneous with surgical treatment, e.g. ruptured aortic aneurysm
- *Urgent* – operation performed as soon as possible after resuscitation, e.g. congenital diaphragmatic hernia
- *Scheduled* – early operation but not immediately life-saving, e.g. cancer surgery
- *Elective* – operation at a time convenient to surgeon, anaesthetist and patient, e.g. plastic surgery.

## AIMS OF PREMEDICATION

- To reduce preoperative anxiety
- To reduce undesirable autonomic reflexes (salivation, bradycardia etc.)
- To assist in smooth induction and maintenance of anaesthesia
- To prevent and treat pain
- To prevent postoperative nausea and vomiting
- To reduce the risk from acid aspiration.

## CRICOID PRESSURE

First described by Sellick in 1961. Traditional teaching is that 44 N force is required to occlude the oesophagus. This is the equivalent of the force required to produce pain when 'cricoid pressure' is applied to the bridge of the nose.

More than 20 N cricoid pressure is uncomfortable and causes retching, risking pulmonary aspiration or oesophageal rupture. More than 40 N cricoid pressure applied after loss of consciousness can obstruct the airway, prevent ventilation and cause difficulty with intubation.

Although suxamethonium fasciculations can increase gastric pressure, peak intragastric pressure rarely exceeds 25 mmHg. In 10 cadavers, 30 N pressure prevented regurgitation of gastric contents at 40 mmHg in all cases. Additionally, reduction in upper oesophageal sphincter tone occurs before consciousness is lost.

Cricoid pressure should therefore be applied before loss of consciousness. Recent recommendations suggest 10 N (1 kg) pressure when the patient is awake, increasing to 30 N following loss of consciousness (Vanner & Asai 1999).

Cricoid pressure impairs insertion of the laryngeal mask airway.

Nasogastric tubes should be in position before induction of anaesthesia to empty gastric contents and the lumen then left open to vent gastric contents. Their presence does not reduce the efficiency of cricoid pressure.

## PROPHYLAXIS OF THROMBOEMBOLIC DISEASE

Recognized by CEPOD reports as a common cause of postoperative morbidity and mortality. Incidence of postoperative deep venous thrombosis (DVT) varies from 18% post-hysterectomy to 75% post-repair of femoral neck fracture.

Several studies have shown that regional techniques reduce the incidence of postoperative DVT and pulmonary embolism. However, there is less evidence that overall outcome is affected. Regional techniques only appear to be effective in reducing DVT risk if the block involves both legs. Thoracic epidurals for abdominal surgery do not reduce the incidence of DVTs. Mechanisms of action may include increased lower limb blood flow through vasodilation, reduced blood viscosity through vasodilation and fluid preload, and less suppression of fibrinolysis compared with GA.

Hormone replacement therapy and low-dose oestrogen/progesterone oral contraceptives do not appear to increase the risk of DVT.

Recent THRIFT (Thromboembolic Risk Factors Consensus) study and CEPOD reports recommend that prophylaxis is given to most surgical patients. Low dose heparin (5000 units b.d.) does not increase the risk of bleeding, and reduces the risk of DVT by 66% and the risk of PE by 50%.

Low-molecular-weight heparins have a greater anti-Xa activity, which makes them more effective at preventing thrombin formation. There may be an increased risk of spinal haematoma in patients with epidurals (see 'Epidural and spinal anaesthesia', p. 292).

### Risk factors for deep venous thrombosis

*Low-risk patients*
- < 40 years without additional risk factors
- Minor surgery (< 30 min)

*Moderate-risk patients*
- > 40 years
- Major surgery (> 30 min)
- Immobilized medical patients with active disease

*High-risk patients*
- Previous DVT/PE
- Major surgery for malignant disease
- Orthopaedic surgery to lower limbs
- Stroke, heart failure and acute MI.

## EYE INJURIES AFTER NON-OCULAR SURGERY

In a study of 60 965 patients (Roth et al 1996), eye injuries occurred in 0.06%. The commonest injury was corneal abrasion. This is usually due to the failure of the eyelids to close during anaesthesia with an associated reduction in tear production. Other common injuries include conjunctivitis, chemical injury and direct trauma. Risk factors are long surgical procedures, lateral positioning during surgery, operation to the head or neck and general anaesthesia.

# HUMAN IMMUNODEFICIENCY VIRUS

First reported in homosexual men in New York in 1981. The HIV virus was first identified as the causative agent in 1983. The virus is a retrovirus which targets the T-helper lymphocyte and impairs the immune response to antigens.

There were 15 712 cases reported in the UK by 1991, but the number now probably exceeds 50 000. About 10% of cases are thought to result from heterosexual transmission. HIV virus is present in all body fluids, but is particularly high in blood, semen, pericardial fluid, amniotic fluid and cerebrospinal fluid. Most transmission occurs through blood, sexual contact and vertically through placental transfer to the fetus.

The disease progresses through three stages:

- *Seroconversion illness.* Initial infection from the virus may result in a flu-like illness with fever, lymphadenopathy, arthralgia and sore throat. May not progress further for several years.
- *Persistent generalized lymphadenopathy.* Defined as enlarged nodes at least 1 cm in diameter in more than one extrainguinal site, persisting for at least 3 months in the absence of any other illness or cause.
- *Acquired immunodeficiency syndrome.* Characterized by tumours (Kaposi's sarcoma, non-Hodgkin's lymphoma, squamous cell carcinoma) and opportunistic infections (*Pneumocystis*, cytomegalovirus, herpes simplex, *Cryptococcus*).

Patients infected with the HIV virus present several anaesthetic problems:

- side-effects of drugs used in the treatment of AIDS
- patients presenting with respiratory failure
- risk of transmission of the HIV virus.

### Drug side-effects

#### Nucleoside analogues

*Zidovudine (AZT).* This drug acts as a false transmitter for reverse transcriptase, inhibiting the incorporation of HIV DNA into the host cell genome. It may delay progression of the disease. Inhibition of DNA polymerase results in a megaloblastic anaemia and neutropenia, made worse by $B_{12}$ or folate deficiency. Other side-effects of relevance to anaesthesia include convulsions, myopathy, impaired liver function and lactic acidosis.

*Didanosine (DDI).* Used as an alternative to AZT. May cause impaired liver function, diarrhoea, peripheral neuropathy and convulsions.

#### Protease inhibitors

*Ritonavir, Indinavir.* These drugs inhibit the cytochrome $P_{450}$ enzyme system. They increase plasma concentrations of benzodiazepines and cisapride. Ritonavir contains 43% alcohol, so its administration with disulfiram and metronidazole should be avoided.

### Antibiotics

*Co-trimoxazole (high dose).* A mixture of trimethoprim and sulphamethoxazole for the prophylaxis and treatment of *Pneumocystis carinii*. May cause megaloblastic anaemia, leucopenia, thrombocytopenia and impaired liver function.

### Antiviral agents

*Ganciclovir.* More active than acyclovir against cytomegalovirus. Causes anaemia, leucopenia and thrombocytopenia. Also arrhythmias, hypertension, hypotension and hypoglycaemia.

## Respiratory failure

AIDS often presents with opportunistic respiratory infections, usually due to *Pneumocystis carinii*. Respiratory failure is a common sequela of this infection and requires the decision as to the appropriateness of ventilatory support. Early studies showed that the outcome from mechanical ventilation was universally poor, with mortality rates approaching 100%. Recent studies, however, have shown survival rates following mechanical ventilation as high as 36–54% although the median survival of patients weaned from ventilation was less than 1 year. Recurrence of *Pneumocystis carinii* infection or symptoms for more than 4 weeks are particularly poor prognostic indicators.

## Anaesthetists infected with HIV

The General Medical Council (1988) advise that any anaesthetist who thinks that he or she may be infected with the HIV virus must seek appropriate counselling and treatment. Anaesthetists infected with HIV risk infecting patients following blood-to-blood contact. The Department of Health (1993) has defined procedures that place patients at risk as:

> surgical entry into tissues, cavities or organs, or repair of major traumatic injuries, cardiac catheterization and angiography, vaginal and Caesarian deliveries; the manipulation, cutting or removal of any oral or perioral tissues ... during which bleeding may occur.

Therefore an anaesthetist who is HIV-positive should not carry out procedures which involve opening the patient's skin or tissues.

Concern has been expressed by the Association of Anaesthetists (1988) that HIV encephalopathy may impair the physical and mental skills of an anaesthetist. However, encephalopathy usually presents late in the course of the illness, by which time the patient is too ill to work. Encephalopathy should be detected early if the patient is under regular medical care.

## Needlestick injury

- 0.3% risk of seroconversion if patient is HIV-positive

- 3% risk of seroconversion if patient is hepatitis C-positive
- 30% risk of seroconversion if patient is hepatitis B e antigen-positive.

*Protection*
- Avoid resheathing needles
- Use sharps bins
- Wear protective clothing
- Staff with open skin lesions should avoid patient contact
- Use of ventilation devices to avoid mouth-to-mouth ventilation
- Employers must have an exposure protection plan.

## GUIDELINES ON POST-EXPOSURE PROPHYLAXIS (PEP) FOR HEALTH CARE WORKERS OCCUPATIONALLY EXPOSED TO HIV
Department of Health 1997

The risk of acquiring HIV following needlestick injury is about 3 per 1000 injuries. Risk factors include deep injury, hollow bore needles, blood from terminally ill HIV patients, and needles that have been in arteries or veins. This risk can be reduced if zidovudine is taken prophylactically as soon as possible after exposure.

### Risk assessment
PEP should be considered whenever there has been exposure to material known to be infected with HIV. The three types of exposure in health care settings known to be associated with significant risk are:

- percutaneous injury (needles, instruments, bone fragments)
- exposure of broken skin (abrasions, cuts, eczema etc.)
- exposure of mucous membranes, including the eye.

### Choice of PEP drugs
The currently recommended drug regime is:
zidovudine 200 mg t.d.s. + lamivudine 150 mg b.d. + indinavir 800 mg t.d.s.

Any drug regime must take into account whether the health care worker is allergic to any of these drugs, is pregnant, whether there would be an interaction with any other medication, and whether the virus might be resistant to any of the medication. Expert advice must be sought.

### Making PEP available
PEP should be commenced as soon as possible after the incident, and ideally within the hour. Therefore, in a high-risk situation, it might be appropriate to give the initial doses immediately, pending full discussion and risk assessment later.

## HIV AND OTHER BLOOD BORNE VIRUSES Association of Anaesthetists of Great Britain and Ireland 1992

Risk of transmission of hepatitis B (HBV), human immunodeficiency virus (HIV) and HTLV-1 (causes T-cell leukaemia and adult tropical spastic paraparesis).

### Epidemiology

A total of 15 712 cases of HIV had been reported in the UK by June 1991, of which 1489 probably acquired the infection through heterosexual intercourse. The actual number of HIV-positive people is probably 50 000. There are 2000 clinical cases of HBV but many more have asymptomatic infections; 1:500 adults in the UK are HBV carriers.

### Transmission and occupational exposure

HIV is mostly transmitted by blood, sexual contacts and from mother to fetus (blood, vaginal delivery and breast milk).

- *High-risk fluids* – amniotic fluid, pericardial and pleural fluid, CSF, peritoneal fluid, semen and vaginal secretions
- *Low-risk fluids* – faeces, nasal secretions, sputum, saliva, sweat, urine and vomit.

HBV present in virtually all human fluids, particularly blood, semen and vaginal secretions.

Transmission of both HIV and HBV usually follows needlestick injury. HIV has been transmitted by infected blood on broken skin and mucous membranes. HBV transmission occurs more readily.

### Screening

Screening for HIV does not reduce the risks of occupational transmission. Window period of 3 months before antibodies appear. Patient consent must be obtained before HIV testing.

### Precautions against infection

Use mask, gloves and eye protection during invasive procedures. Needles must not be resheathed but placed into a sharps container. Cover all open skin lesions with waterproof plaster. Non-autoclavable equipment should be cleaned with 2% glutaraldehyde.

### Resuscitation and intensive care

No reports of HIV or HBV infection from basic life support but still a risk so use protective devices. Relatives of organ donors should be counselled about HIV testing.

### Protection against HBV

All anaesthetists should be immunized against HBV, with boosters at 3–5 years.

### Post-exposure management

Following inoculation injury, encourage wound to bleed and wash with soap and water. Irrigate splashes on mucous membranes with copious volumes of water. Designate a person to contact following exposure. Early treatment with HBV immunoglobulin, AZT, antibiotics or anti-tetanus immunization as deemed necessary.

### Anaesthetists with HIV infection
In 1988 the GMC set out the duties of doctors infected with HIV. Doctors must seek appropriate advice and modify their clinical practice accordingly. Similar guidelines apply for HBV-infected staff.

### BLOOD-BORNE VIRUSES AND ANAESTHESIA – AN UPDATE
Association of Anaesthetists of Great Britain and Ireland 1996

### Anaesthesia and exposure-prone procedures
Exposure-prone procedures (replacing the term 'invasive procedures') are:

> those procedures where there is a risk that injury to the health worker may result in the exposure of the patient's open tissues to the blood of the worker. These procedures include those where the worker's gloved hand may be in contact with sharp instruments, needle tips or sharp tissues (spicules of bone or teeth) inside a patient's open body cavity, wound or confined anatomical space where the finger tips may not be visible at all times.

The report recommended that:

- although anaesthetists put their fingers into patients' mouths, anaesthesia should not be regarded as an exposure-prone speciality
- it should be mandatory for anaesthetists to wear surgical gloves when carrying out procedures which involve putting their hands into patients' mouths.

### Transmission of hepatitis C virus (HCV) via the anaesthetic breathing system
A case report from Australia suggests that several patients may have become infected with HCV by cross-infection from a breathing system. The Council recommends that:

- either an appropriate filter should be placed between the patient and the breathing system, a new filter being used for each patient, or that a new breathing system be used for each patient
- where expired gas sampling is used, the sample should be taken from the breathing system side of the filter
- in paediatric practice where the use of a filter would increase dead space and/or resistance unacceptably, filters should not be used but the breathing system should be changed between patients.

## HEPATITIS C (HCV)

Discovered in 1989 as the causative agent of non-A, non-B hepatitis. Single strand RNA virus.

European prevalence is 0.3–1.2%; highest in Japan, Middle East and the Mediterranean. Most transmission is via i.v. drug abuse; also tattoos, sexual transmission and needlestick injury. Patient-to-patient transmission has been documented in chronic haemodialysis patients and via heat-and-moisture exchange filters.

Following acute HCV infection, a lag period of 2–3 months occurs before anti-HCV is detected in serum. Acute illness often progresses to chronic disease. Recombinant α-interferon normalizes liver function tests and renders serum free from HCV RNA in these patients.

### References

Anon. 1997 Major advances in the treatment of HIV-1 infection. Drug and Therapeutics Bulletin 35: 25–29

Association of Anaesthetists of Great Britain and Ireland 1988 AIDS and hepatitis B. Guidelines for Anaesthetists. AAGBI, London

Association of Anaesthetists of Great Britain and Ireland 1992 HIV and other blood borne viruses. Guidelines for Anaesthetists. AAGBI, London

Association of Anaesthetists of Great Britain and Ireland 1996 A report received by Council of the Association of Anaesthetists on blood borne viruses and anaesthesia – an update (January 1996). AAGBI, London

Department of Health 1993 AIDS-HIV infected health care workers. Occupational advice for health care workers, their physicians and employers. HMSO, London

Department of Health 1997 Guidelines on post-exposure prophylaxis for health care workers occupationally exposed to HIV (Professional Letter: PL/CO(97)1). Department of Health, Wetherby (West Yorkshire)

General Medical Council 1988 HIV infection and AIDS: the ethical considerations. GMC, London

Hopkins C C 1994 AIDS: universal precautions, transmission, and public health policies. Current Opinion in Anaesthesiology 7: 310–313

Liddle C 1996 Hepatitis C. Anaesthesia and Intensive Care 24: 180–183

Roth S, Thisted R A, Erickson J P, Black S, Screider B D 1996 Eye injuries after nonocular surgery. Anesthesiology 85: 1020–1027

Searle J F 1994 Human immunodeficiency and hepatitis viruses. In: Nimmo W S, Rowbotham D J, Smith G (eds) Anaesthesia, 2nd edn. Blackwell Scientific Publications, Oxford, p 1346–1354

Vanner R G, Asai T 1999 Safe use of cricoid pressure. Anaesthesia 54: 1–3

Wheatley T, Veitch P S 1997 Recent advances in prophylaxis against DVT. British Journal of Anaesthesia 78: 118–120

White E, Crosse M M 1998 The aetiology and prevention of perioperative corneal abrasions. Anaesthesia 53: 157–161

# DISEASES OF IMPORTANCE TO ANAESTHESIA

## CONGENITAL SYNDROMES

### Down's syndrome (trisomy 21)

Incidence of 1:700 live births, increasing with maternal age; 50% have congenital heart disease. Defects include (in order of decreasing frequency) complete AV canal, VSD, PDA and tetralogy of Fallot (VSD, overriding aorta, pulmonary stenosis, left ventricular hypertrophy). Down's is associated with large protruding tongue, small mandible, mental retardation, epilepsy, duodenal obstruction, hypothyroidism and impaired immune system. Institutionalized patients have a higher incidence of hepatitis B. About 20% have atlantoaxial instability (poor muscle tone, ligamentous laxity and abnormal odontoid peg). Obstructive sleep apnoea and respiratory complications are common.

Anaesthetic problems include difficult intubation, requirement for a smaller endotracheal tube size than expected, cervical spine instability and a higher incidence of postoperative atelectasis and pulmonary oedema.

### Pierre–Robin syndrome

Rare congenital syndrome with severe micrognathia and posterior prolapse of the tongue. Causes airway obstruction, which is worse in the supine position; improved by placing the child prone. If severe, may require tongue to be sutured to the lower gum. Can progress to cor pulmonale. There are also problems feeding, and a risk of aspiration. Difficult intubation.

### Marfan's syndrome

Autosomal dominant condition affecting connective tissue, causing ocular, skeletal and cardiac abnormalities. Premature death is common.

CVS lesions present in 50% by 22 years. Associated with ascending aortic aneurysm, aortic regurgitation, mitral regurgitation, myocardial infarction and myocardial fibrosis; also long thin extremities, high arched palate, upward lens displacement, spontaneous pneumothorax and scoliosis.

Anaesthetic problems include difficult intubation, cardiac and respiratory complications and joint dislocation.

## HAEMOGLOBINOPATHIES

### Sickle cell disease

Autosomal dominant inheritance. Affects people of African, Mediterranean,

Indian, Caribbean and Middle Eastern descent. Found in 10% of negroes in the UK.

The condition is due to substitution of glutamine by valine on position 6 of the β-chain of haemoglobin A to form HbS. Causes polymerization of deoxygenated haemoglobin at low $P_aO_2$ with alteration of the discoid cell to a rigid sickle shape. These abnormal cells increase blood viscosity and sludge in the microvascular circulation. Infarcts cause symptoms and signs of the disease. Sickling is precipitated by dehydration, acidosis, fever and hypoxia.

The *heterozygous form*, HbAS (sickle trait), has normal life expectancy with haemoglobin > 11 g/dl, no clinical symptoms or signs and sickling only if $P_aO_2$ < 2.5 kPa. Hb does not fall below 11.0.

The *homozygous form*, HbSS, usually presents by 6 months as HbF is replaced by HbS. Deoxygenation of HbS results in polymerization to form insoluble globin polymers. Associated with chronic anaemia, painful sickle crises, pulmonary thromboembolism, pulmonary, renal and bone infarcts, gallstones, priapism, TIAs and strokes. Splenic sequestration results in splenomegaly in infants, but multiple infarcts cause autosplenectomy by adulthood. Parvovirus causes aplastic crises. Target cells on blood film. HbSS sickles at $P_aO_2$ < 5.0 kPa.

Haemoglobin S may combine with other haemoglobins, e.g. HbC, to give HbSC or with β-thalassaemia haemoglobin.

***Diagnosis.*** Sickledex test causes sickling when affected erythrocytes are exposed to sodium metabisulphite. Unlike electrophoresis, it does not distinguish between homozygous and heterozygous conditions.

***Anaesthetic considerations.*** Consider exchange transfusion if HbA < 40%, aiming to reduce HbS to < 25%. Postoperative mortality is about 5%. Patients are not suitable for day-case surgery. Impaired renal concentrating ability.

Reduce risk of sickling by:

- keeping well oxygenated
- good analgesia
- avoiding tourniquets, which induce sickling
- keeping warm
- keeping well hydrated
- prophylactic antibiotics.

## Porphyria

Autosomal dominant metabolic disorder of porphyrin synthesis. Porphyrins are tetrapyrole rings involved in the synthesis of haemoglobin, myoglobin and cytochromes. There are two types of porphyria:

- erythropoietic – anaemia and liver disease only
- hepatic – potentially fatal.

Increased production of aminolaevulinic acid (ALA) and porphobilinogen (PBG), together with their reduced metabolism by porphobilinogen deaminase, causes symptoms:

$$\begin{array}{ccc} \uparrow \delta \text{ ALA synthetase} \\ \text{triggered by drugs} \end{array} \longrightarrow \begin{array}{c} \uparrow \text{ALA} \\ \uparrow \text{PBG} \end{array} \longrightarrow \begin{array}{c} \downarrow \text{activity of} \\ \text{porphobilinogen} \\ \text{deaminase} \end{array}$$

Acute intermittent porphyria (hepatic) is the commonest form, presenting as hypertension (36%), tachycardia (80%) and abdominal pain (95%) due to autonomic neuropathy; also peripheral neuropathy (30%), bulbar palsy (30%), convulsions (20%) and mental confusion (55%). Urine turns red after standing in sunlight. Underlying defect is decreased activity of porphobilinogen deaminase.

Acute episodes are precipitated by:

- infection, starvation and dehydration
- steroids, barbiturates, etomidate
- alcohol
- oral contraceptive pill
- cimetidine, erythromycin, sulphonamides
- prochlorperazine, metoclopramide.

*Safe drugs*
- Volatile agents and nitrous oxide
- Propofol, midazolam, diazepam
- Morphine, fentanyl
- Droperidol
- Lignocaine, bupivacaine
- All muscle relaxants
- Anticholinergics, anticholinesterases.

*Treatment.* Identify and remove cause if possible. Ensure adequate hydration and correct any electrolyte imbalance. Hypertension and tachycardia respond well to β-blockers. Treat generalized convulsions with diazepam. Ensure adequate analgesia with opioids. Specific treatment involves infusion of heme arginate, which directly increases negative feedback to ALA synthetase.

*General anaesthesia.* Best avoided by using regional techniques, although beware if there is any peripheral neuropathy. Postoperatively, good analgesia avoids the stress of pain triggering an acute attack. Monitor postoperatively for 5 days since onset may be delayed.


## Haemophilia

*Haemophilia A.* Sex-linked recessive inherited condition with reduced levels of factor VIII. Males are affected, females are carriers. Spontaneous bleeding, mostly into joints with ankylosis and permanent joint deformities.

Prolonged partial thromboplastin time (intrinsic pathway) with normal whole blood clotting time and normal bleeding time. Diagnose by factor VIII:C assay.

Haemophiliacs treated with factor VIII before it was available in its sterilized freeze-dried form may be carriers of hepatitis B or C and HIV. Avoid regional anaesthesia. Care is needed during laryngoscopy and intubation. Titrate factor VIII replacement against blood levels of factor VIII and nature of operation. Mild haemophiliacs may manage with an infusion of i.v. desmopressin. Avoid i.m. injections. NSAIDs may cause persistent bleeding.

*Haemophilia B (Christmas disease).* Sex-linked recessive inherited condition with reduced levels of factor IX. Coagulation tests are similar to those of haemophilia A with reduced factor IX assay. Treat with factor IX. Desmopressin is ineffective.

## OTHER CONDITIONS

### Ankylosing spondylitis

An inflammatory condition of unknown aetiology, characterized by high ESR, fever, weight loss and anaemia. Causes progressive fibrosis, ossification and ankylosis of sacroiliac joints and spine. 50% have extra-articular involvement.

Difficult intubation may occur as a result of limited cervical spine movement and ankylosis of temporomandibular joint, limiting mouth opening in > 10% patients. Cricoarytenoid arthritis presents as dyspnoea and hoarseness. Cardiovascular complications include aortic incompetence, mitral valve disease and conduction defects. Thoracic spine involvement limits chest expansion and is associated with pulmonary fibrosis.

### Rheumatoid arthritis

An autoimmune disease of unknown aetiology. Affects females much more than males. Primarily affects joints but 50% have extra-articular involvement.

Cervical instability (atlantoaxial and subaxial subluxation) presenting as sensory symptoms, weakness, flexor spasms and urinary incontinence; 25% of patients are asymptomatic. Cricoarytenoid involvement may result in upper airway obstruction. Assess cervical spine with lateral X-rays in flexion and extension. Distance > 3 mm between odontoid peg and posterior border of the anterior arch of the atlas suggests subluxation. Subluxation may necessitate awake fibreoptic intubation. Temporomandibular joint involvement may limit mouth opening.

Lung involvement includes generalized fibrosis with a restrictive defect, rheumatoid nodules and pleural effusions. Perform preoperative pulmonary function tests and arterial blood gases if necessary.

Cardiac involvement includes pericarditis, endocarditis and left ventricular failure. Renal failure is common due to vasculitis, amyloidosis and drug toxicity. Chronic anaemia results from anaemia of chronic disease, upper GI bleeding from NSAIDs, bone marrow suppression from gold and penicillamine and haemolytic anaemia.

## Mucopolysaccharidoses (Hurler's, Hunter's syndromes)

A group of inherited connective tissue disorders. Enzyme defects result in the accumulation of intermediate products of degradation of mucopolysaccharides. Characterized by dwarfism, cardiac failure, abnormal airway anatomy, respiratory failure, hepatosplenomegaly and skeletal abnormalities. Associated with prolonged recovery from anaesthesia, with breath holding, bronchospasm and respiratory failure.

## Glycogen storage diseases (von Gierke's, Pompe's, McArdle's, Thompson's diseases)

A group of genetic diseases with defects in enzymes controlling glycogen metabolism, causing muscle and liver disease. Cramps, stiffness, muscle weakness and muscle pains. Hypertrophic cardiomyopathy (Pompe's) and hypoglycaemia (von Gierke's). Avoid shivering, tourniquets and suxamethonium, all of which cause muscle damage. Avoid hypoglycaemia. Risk of postoperative respiratory failure.

## Von Recklinghausen's neurofibromatosis

Autosomal dominant condition characterized by multiple neurofibromata and pigmented skin patches (café-au-lait spots). Airway difficulties due to upper airway neurofibromas. Kyphoscoliosis, undiagnosed associated malignancies, e.g. phaeochromocytoma, fibrosing alveolitis, renal artery stenosis and hypertension. Abnormal sensitivity to muscle relaxants.

### References

Jensen N F, Fiddler D S, Striepe V 1995 Anesthetic considerations in porphyrias. Anesthesia and Analgesia 80: 591–599
Peacock J E 1994 Anaesthesia and miscellaneous diseases. In: Nimmo W S, Rowbotham D J, Smith G (eds) Anaesthesia, 2nd edn. Blackwell Scientific Publications, Oxford, p 1130–1147
Roizen M F 1997 Anesthesia and medical disease. Current Opinion in Anaesthesiology 10: (5) L
Simpson K H, Ellis F R 1994 Inherited metabolic diseases and anaesthesia. In: Nimmo W S, Rowbotham D J, Smith G (eds) Anaesthesia, 2nd edn. Blackwell Scientific Publications, Oxford, p 1113–1129
Vijay V, Cavenagh J D, Yate P 1998 The anaesthetist's role in acute sickle cell crisis. British Journal of Anaesthesia 80: 820–828
Wiklund R A, Rosenbaum S H 1997 Thyroid dysfunction in the preoperative period. Current Opinion in Anaesthesiology 10: 244–247

## MAJOR INCIDENT MANAGEMENT

### DEFINITION OF A MAJOR INCIDENT

A major incident arises when any occurrence presents a serious threat to the health of the community, disruption to the service, or causes such numbers of casualties as to require special arrangements by the health service.

### CAUSES OF DISASTERS

- *Natural*
  - storms
  - floods
  - earthquakes
- *Technological*
  - transport accident
  - industrial (toxic/radioactive)
- *Social* – epidemics
- *Environmental* – air, water and land pollution
- *Hostile acts*
  - terrorist acts
  - civil disorder.

### OBJECTIVE OF THE EMERGENCY SERVICE RESPONSE TO A MAJOR INCIDENT

- To save life
- To prevent escalation of the disaster
- To relieve suffering
- To safeguard the environment
- To facilitate criminal investigation
- To restore normality as soon as possible.

The first member of the emergency services should not become involved with rescue but should make a rapid initial assessment of the disaster and report to their services control:

- nature and location
- number of dead, injured and uninjured
- hazards; actual and potential
- access to site
- which emergency services are present or required.

### INITIAL CONTROL AND COORDINATION

The successful outcome of a major incident depends on the early

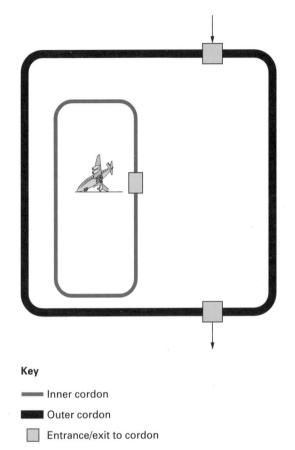

**Key**

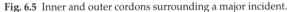 Inner cordon

▬ Outer cordon

□ Entrance/exit to cordon

**Fig. 6.5** Inner and outer cordons surrounding a major incident.

implementation of a command and control structure to manage the incident and assign control of specific duties to each emergency service.

An inner cordon is established which contains the immediate area of damage. No member of the emergency services should enter or leave the inner cordon without logging their details at a checkpoint. An outer cordon is also established which encloses the incident in its entirety. Specific entry and exit points for emergency vehicles may also be established (see Fig. 6.5).

Following establishment of the inner and outer cordons, specific areas are then designated for emergency teams. These are (Fig. 6.6):

- rendezvous point (RVP) for emergency vehicles
- joint emergency services control centre (JESCC) (fire, police and ambulance command vehicles)
- triage area

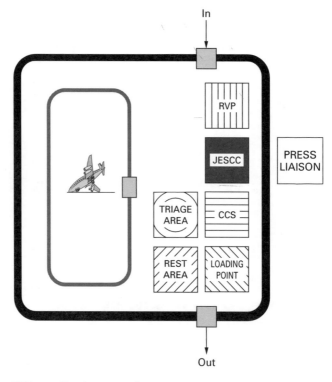

RVP     – Rendezvous point
CCS     – Casualty clearing station
JESCC – Joint emergency services control centre

**Fig. 6.6** Designated areas for emergency teams.

- casualty clearing station (CCS)
- ambulance loading point for casualties
- press liaison point.

A survivor reception centre and temporary mortuary may be established in suitable buildings nearby.

Medical teams sent from hospital to support the emergency services must always report to the ambulance control point before entering the incident. All emergency personnel must be suitably dressed in protective clothing (not white coats!), which includes the following:

- safety helmet (+/– headlamp)
- bright reflective waterproof clothing
- tabards with designation clearly displayed
- appropriate footwear.

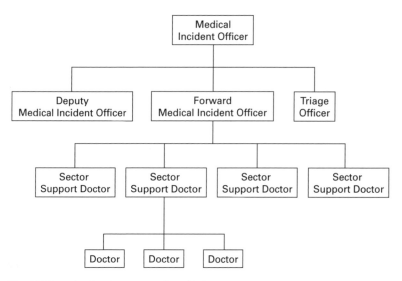

**Fig. 6.7** Organizational structure of medical support.

Medical support is organized in a similar structure to the ambulance service command structure (Fig. 6.7). A medical incident officer should be based with the ambulance incident officer in the ambulance command vehicle. A deputy medical incident officer, forward medical officer and triage officer may be appointed depending on the size and nature of the incident.

## ROLE OF THE MEDICAL INCIDENT OFFICER

### Liaison

Liaises with senior officers of all other services:

- ambulance incident officer (AIO)
- police incident officer
- fire incident officer.

Also liaises with the coordinating medical officer at receiving hospitals.

### Organization

- Appoints:
  — deputy
  — triage doctor
  — sector support doctors
- Requests mobile medical teams via AIO
- Supervises the work of all doctors on site and, in the absence of nursing incident officer, all other health care workers

- In conjunction with the AIO, establishes:
  - casualty collecting point
  - ambulance loading point
  - equipment dump
- In conjunction with the AIO, coordinates distribution of patients to appropriate hospitals.

### Communication

- Obtains regular reports from deputy, triage officer and forward medical incident officer
- Liaises continuously with the AIO
- Sends regular reports to the receiving hospitals in conjunction with the AIO
- Initially directs press inquiries to the police press officer.

## SECTOR SUPPORT DOCTOR

- Responsible to, and reports regularly to, the medical incident officer
- Liaises with ambulance crews and fire officer responsible for that sector
- Supports any doctors also committed to the rescue of casualties in that sector
- If possible, ensures that each medical team follows the patient through to the ambulance loading point and, if necessary, accompanies to hospital.

## TRIAGE

The rapid assessment of casualties to establish the severity of injuries in each patient and the priority of evacuation of the casualties – 'the most good for the most people'.

- *Immediate* – first priority, e.g. serious head injury, tension pneumothorax
- *Urgent* – second priority, e.g. fractured femur, spinal injury
- *Delayed* – third priority, e.g. superficial wounds
- *Dead.*

### Triage officer

- Responsible to and reports to medical incident officer
- Liaises with:
  - ambulance casualty clearing officer
  - ambulance loading officer
- Based at casualty collecting point and liaises with paramedics, nurses and doctors treating patients
- Allocates triage category to each patient on arrival at the casualty collecting point

- Patients should be retriaged at appropriate intervals
- Regularly updates medical incident officer of numbers in each category.

## CARE OF SURVIVORS

### Uninjured

May still be suffering from shock, anxiety and grief. May be able to provide crucial information about what happened.

*Short-term needs*
- Emotional support
- Food and drink
- First aid to treat minor injuries
- Spare clothing
- Toilet and washing facilities.

*Long-term needs*
- Help in finding temporary accommodation
- Help contacting family and friends
- Financial advice and assistance
- Social services and counselling.

### Injured

Injured survivors should be taken to the casualty clearing station for

- triage
- appropriate stabilization measures.

Casualties are then evacuated in accordance with priority.

## FATALITIES

- Dead bodies should be labelled and not moved unless it is necessary to protect them from fire or chemicals. Bear in mind the need to preserve forensic evidence.
- The authority of HM Coroner is required before those who have been pronounced dead can be removed. Arrangements are then the responsibility of the police.
- Bodies are usually taken to a temporary mortuary where autopsies can be carried out.

## POLICE CASUALTY BUREAU

- Handles enquiries from the general public about friends and relatives who may have been involved
- Collates details of survivors, their condition and whereabouts

- Gathers data to assist in identification of casualties
- Compiles a list of persons believed to have been involved but who are now missing.

**References**

Carli P, Telion C 1998 Prehospital care on scene. Current Anaesthesia and Critical Care 9: 74–77
Department of Health 1990 Emergency planning in the NHS: health services arrangements for dealing with major incidents. Health Circular (90)25
Lipp M, Paschen H, Daublander M et al 1998 Disaster management in hospitals. Current Anaesthesia and Critical Care 9: 78–85

## MECHANISMS OF ANAESTHESIA

General anaesthetic agents are not related to any specific group of compounds, but depend more upon the solubility characteristics of the molecule. Although these agents have a selective effect on CNS function, at high doses all organ systems are affected.

### MEYER–OVERTON THEORY

States that MAC × solubility = K (Fig. 6.8).

Original solvent was vegetable oil, but more accurate correlation exists using a lecithin-based oil which more closely resembles the cell membrane. Provides evidence that the site of action of the volatile agents is at a hydrophobic site, i.e. lipids within the cell membrane.

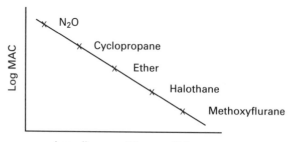

**Fig. 6.8**  Meyer–Overton theory.

**HYDRATE HYPOTHESIS** (discovered by Pauling 1961, Miller 1961)

The fact that the brain consists of 78% water led to the suggestion that

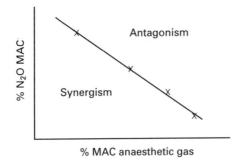

**Fig. 6.9** Hydrate hypothesis.

anaesthetics act on hydrophobic molecules. However, there is poor correlation between anaesthetic potency and water solubility. This theory also predicted that two anaesthetic agents would have a synergistic effect, but volatile agents appear only to have an additive effect (Fig. 6.9).

## CLATHRATE HYPOTHESIS

This evolved from the hydrate hypothesis to suggest that anaesthetic molecules are trapped within a sphere of water molecules. These hydrates may then act to decrease nerve conduction or stiffen lipid membranes and occlude ion channels. Little evidence now exists for any of these theories.

## CRITICAL VOLUME HYPOTHESIS (Lever 1971)

This followed on from pressure reversal studies to suggest that when cell membranes are expanded to a critical volume, cellular function is impaired. High pressures then reverse the expansion to restore normal cellular function. A 0.4% volume increase at the critical site correlates with onset of anaesthesia.

Evidence for critical volume comes from studies of pressure reversal. Light from luminous bacteria is dimmed by anaesthetic agents but returns to normal under high pressures (Johnson 1940). Tadpoles stop swimming in an anaesthetic solution, but resume swimming as the hydrostatic pressure is increased (Johnson & Flagler 1950). However, experiments to very high pressures with tadpoles show a loss of correlation of anaesthesia with pressure.

## MULTISITE EXPANSION HYPOTHESIS (Halsey 1979)

This hypothesis proposed that although anaesthetic agents expand the membrane at critical sites, the actual sites involved may vary between anaesthetic agents and have a finite size and limited capacity for the anaesthetic. Expansion at these sites may act to impair ion channel function and thus electrical activity of the cell membrane. Correctly predicts the non-additive potencies of i.v. anaesthetic agents.

## Molecular site of action

*Lipids.* Anaesthetic agents may change the fluidity of the lipid membrane, thereby altering the function of membrane proteins contained within it.

*Proteins.* Anaesthetic agents may directly block ion channels or alter the ability of protein molecules to change their shape.

## Cellular site of action

*Synapses and axons.* Local anaesthetics may act on axonal membranes to block ion channels. General anaesthetics act at synapses to reduce transmitter release and alter the interaction of the neurotransmitter with receptor. GAs may also affect presynaptic calcium channels, reducing the axonal calcium necessary for binding vesicles of neurotransmitter to the presynaptic membrane.

## Higher neuronal circuits

GA may cause loss of consciousness by blocking the reticular formation processing of sensory input to the cortex (corticothalamic-reticular loop).

## NITRIC OXIDE

Recent studies suggest that nitric oxide (NO) inhibition may be an important mechanism of action of some general anaesthetic agents. NO is involved in central nociceptive pathways and maintaining wakefulness. NO sythase inhibitors cause a dose-dependent reduction in MAC for volatile agents and impair the righting reflex in mice, suggesting that the effects involve higher integrative neuronal processes rather than analgesia alone.

### References

Bovill J G 1997 Mechanisms of actions of anaesthetic drugs. Current Opinion in Anaesthesiology 10: 261–266
Halsey M J 1994 The molecular basis of anaesthesia. In: Nimmo W S, Rowbotham D J, Smith G (eds) Anaesthesia, 2nd edn. Blackwell Scientific Publications, Oxford
Johns R A 1996 Nitric oxide, cyclic guanosine monophosphate and the anesthetic state. Anesthesiology 85: 457–459
Pocock G, Richards C D 1994 Cellular mechanisms in general anaesthesia. British Journal of Anaesthesia 66: 116–128

# ORGAN DONATION AND TRANSPLANTATION

## DIAGNOSIS OF BRAINSTEM DEATH

### A CODE OF PRACTICE FOR THE DIAGNOSIS OF BRAINSTEM DEATH Department of Health 1998

#### Definition
Irreversible loss of capacity for consciousness combined with irreversible capacity to breathe.

50% of cases are due to trauma, 30% to subarachnoid haemorrhage.

#### Brainstem testing
*Preconditions*

1. No doubt that the patient's condition is due to irremedial brain damage of known aetiology.

2. The patient is deeply unconscious, but not due to depressant drugs, hypothermia or reversible circulatory, metabolic or endocrine disturbances.

3. The patient is being maintained on a ventilator because spontaneous respiration is inadequate or has ceased.

#### Diagnosis of brainstem death
All brainstem reflexes must be absent, i.e.:

- Pupils fixed, dilated and unresponsive
- No corneal reflex
- No vestibulo-ocular reflexes to > 50 ml iced water (must view eardrums first)
- No cranial motor response to pain. No limb response to supraorbital pressure
- No gag or cough reflex
- No spontaneous ventilation on disconnection from ventilator. Give 100% $O_2$ for 10 min then disconnect and give 6 l $O_2$/min via tracheal catheter during which time observe for respiratory effort. Allow $P_aCO_2$ to rise > 6.65 kPa before cessation of test. (Alternatively, ventilate with 100% $O_2$ for 10 min, then 5% $CO_2$ in oxygen for 5 min.)

#### Repetition of testing
Diagnosis should be made by at least two doctors (of whom at least one should be a consultant) registered for more than 5 years who are competent in this field and are not members of the transplant team.

Two sets of tests should be carried out, either separately or together. Timing between the two tests should be adequate for the reassurance of all those directly concerned. Legal time of death is time of the first set of tests.

**Management**

Relatives, partners and carers must be kept fully informed.

Maintenance of treatment to sustain normal physiological parameters is allowed after diagnosis of brainstem death in order to maintain the condition of the organs. Elective ventilation solely to preserve organ function is unlawful.

**Persistent vegetative state**

Characterized by cortical damage with an intact brainstem.

## MANAGEMENT OF PATIENTS FOR ORGAN DONATION

**GUIDELINES FOR THE MANAGEMENT OF POTENTIAL ORGAN AND TISSUE DONORS** Department of Health 1998

ITU / ward staff identify brainstem death
Relatives are fully informed of the condition and prognosis for the patient
↓
Diagnosis of brainstem death
↓
Local transplant coordinator informed
↓
Lack of objection of relatives, partners or carers confirmed
↓
Virological and bacterial testing
Tissue typing
↓
Suitability confirmed
↓
UK Transplant Support Service Authority and user transplant units informed
↓
Organ retrieval and transport
↙                                              ↘
Tissue banking                          Organ transplantation

It is important to maintain normal physiological parameters to prevent end-organ damage. As many as 20% of hearts from otherwise suitable patients are lost to donation through poor management. Cerebral trauma and subarachnoid haemorrhage are common causes of brainstem death. These conditions are associated with haemodynamic instability, hypotension, neurogenic pulmonary oedema, impaired thermoregulation, diabetes insipidus and aspiration of gastric contents.

### Preoperative

Regular physiotherapy and careful fluid balance avoid deterioration in lung function. Maintain core temperature above 35°C with warming blanket and fluid warmer. Check electrolytes, full blood count, blood gases and urine/plasma osmolality. Right subclavian artery and left brachiocephalic vein are divided early in the operation, so place a left radial arterial cannula and right central venous cannula. Fluid replacement with colloid is recommended to reduce tissue oedema caused with crystalloids.

### Operative

Record ECG, central and venous pressure and core temperature. Maintain with $O_2$:$N_2O$ mixture to provide adequate $S_aO_2$. Pancuronium prevents spinal reflexes causing muscular contraction. Severe hypertension may require treatment with isoflurane or sodium nitroprusside. Cephalosporin and methylprednisolone are generally requested by transplant team. Anticipate large volume losses.

For multiple organ donation, the thorax and abdomen are opened by a longitudinal incision from the suprasternal notch to the umbilicus. The liver and kidneys are mobilized, during which compression of the inferior vena cava may cause hypotension. The patient is then anti-coagulated with heparin (3 mg/kg) and the thorax opened. Ensure each tidal breath is adequate to inflate all lobes of the lungs if lung harvest is being performed. Thoracic organs are then removed prior to removal of abdominal organs.

## MANAGEMENT OF RECIPIENTS FOR RENAL TRANSPLANTATION

(See also 'Anaesthesia and renal failure', p. 96.)

### Preoperative

Optimize fluid balance and consider preoperative dialysis. Aim to normalize electrolytes, particularly $K^+$. Use in-line leucocyte filter if blood transfusion is required. Avoid veins on forearms.

### Anaesthesia preparation

ECG (CM5), invasive BP, pulse oximetry, CVP, urinary catheter, regular blood glucose. Avoid Hartmann's as this contains $K^+$.

## Induction

Thiopentone, etomidate, midazolam and propofol are all suitable; 5–7 $\mu$g/kg fentanyl on induction provides good perioperative analgesia and reduces the hypertension from the pressor response. Neuromuscular blockade with suxamethonium (if $K^+ < 5.0$) if rapid sequence induction is required, followed by atracurium or cis-atracurium. High-dose methylprednisolone given at induction for renal transplantation may cause circulatory collapse, arrhythmias and cardiac arrest.

## Maintenance

Patients with chronic renal failure (CRF) are acidotic so avoid spontaneous respiration. Isoflurane has least metabolism to $F^-$ and minimal nephrotoxicity. $N_2O$ is safe. Keep warm and well hydrated, particularly when clamp is removed (CVP above normal). Replace fluid loss with salt-containing solutions. Aim for normotension.

## Other

Prior to removal of arterial clamp and reperfusion of transplant kidney, give mannitol 0.5 g/kg, frusemide 250 mg (omit if live, related donor) and dopamine 3 $\mu$g/kg per min.

## Postoperative

Usually extubated immediately postoperatively. Monitor CVP and renal function. Consider early postoperative dialysis if there is poor graft function. Fentanyl PCA provides good postoperative analgesia. Immunosuppression for transplantation is associated with increased infection risk. Currently 5-year organ survival is 60%.

## MANAGEMENT OF RECIPIENTS FOR CARDIAC/LUNG TRANSPLANTATION

Survival rates are improving as follows:

- heart      – 75–80% at 5 years
- lung       – 65% at 1 year
- heart–lung – 55–60% at 1 year.

Similar anaesthetic technique to that for cardiac surgery.
   Specific problems with management include:

- no SNS-mediated tachycardia, making atropine ineffective; use isoprenaline
- no ANS response to hypovolaemia, with exaggerated responses to both hypovolaemia and decreased SVR

- delayed response to circulating catecholamines (5–6 min)
- arrhythmias (mostly ventricular) common for 6 months post-transplant
- no cough reflex following stimulation distal to bronchial anastomosis and no lung lymphatic drainage.

### Anaesthesia for non-cardiac surgery after heart/lung transplant

General anaesthesia with i.v. induction, opioid, neuromuscular blocker and volatile agent with intubation and ventilation has proved suitable for most patients. Spinal and epidural techniques may cause exaggerated hypotensive responses. All cannulae should be placed using an aseptic technique and bacterial filters used on all intravenous lines. Avoid excessive airway pressures stretching suture lines in patients following lung transplant. Also avoid fluid overload in these patients because of impaired pulmonary lymphatic drainage. Use appropriate prophylactic antibiotics. Regular physiotherapy and postural drainage postoperatively.

#### References

Briegel J, Groh J, Haller M 1998 Perioperative management of patients undergoing lung transplantation. Current Opinion in Anaesthesiology 11: 51–59

Colson P 1998 Renal disease and transplantation. Current Opinion in Anaesthesiology 11: 345–348

Department of Health 1998 A code of practice for the diagnosis of brain stem death including guidelines for the identification and management of potential organ and tissue donors. Department of Health, London

Ghosh S, Bethune D W, Hardy I et al 1990 Management of donors for heart and heart-lung transplantation. Anaesthesia 45: 672–675

Jennett B 1999 Brain stem death defines death in law. British Medical Journal 318: 1755

Pallis C, Harley D H 1996 ABC of brainstem death. BMJ Publishing Group, London

Presler J, Csete M 1996 Anesthesia for liver transplantation. Current Opinion in Anaesthesiology 9: 263–266

Robertson K M, Cook D R 1990 Perioperative management of the multiorgan donor. Anaesthesia and Analgesia 70: 546–556

Shaw I H, Kirk A J B, Conacher I D 1991 Anaesthesia for patients with transplanted hearts and lungs undergoing non-cardiac surgery. British Journal of Anaesthesia 67: 772–778

## POSTOPERATIVE NAUSEA AND VOMITING (PONV)

### PHYSIOLOGY

The vomiting centre is situated in the reticular formation of the medulla within the blood–brain barrier. The chemoreceptor trigger zone is situated

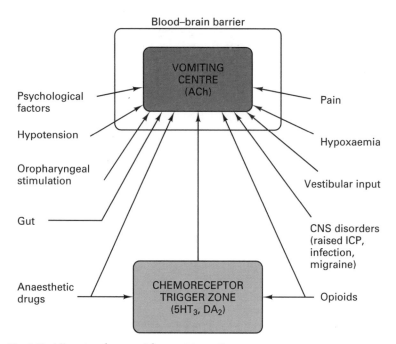

**Fig. 6.10** Afferent pathways of the vomiting reflex.

in the area postrema on the floor of the IV ventricle and receives input from many afferents (Fig. 6.10).

### Vomiting reflex

Activated by vomiting centre via glossopharyngeal, hypoglossal, trigeminal, accessory and spinal nerves. Abdominal muscles contract against a closed glottis to raise intra-abdominal pressure. The lower oesophageal sphincter then relaxes and the pyloric sphincter contracts to expel the gastric contents.

One-third of all surgical patients experience nausea and vomiting which may last for up to 24 h postoperatively. Until recently, it has been an under-estimated problem which is becoming more relevant with the rapid growth of day-case surgery.

## EFFECTS OF PONV

- Wound pain
- Distress and exhaustion
- Commonest cause of patient dissatisfaction with surgery
- Dehydration and electrolyte imbalance
- Breakdown of surgical wound

- Prevents administration of oral medication and nutrition
- Risk of aspiration if impaired upper airway reflexes
- Delays mobilization and prolongs stay in hospital
- Increases need for extra nursing
- Admission of day-case patient.

## RISK FACTORS FOR PONV

- Female
- Obese
- Young age
- Past history of PONV
- History of motion sickness or migraine
- Prolonged starvation or recent oral intake.

## SURGERY ASSOCIATED WITH PONV

- GI surgery due to bowel manipulation
- ENT surgery with pharyngeal or middle ear stimulation
- Eye surgery involving extraocular muscles
- Gynaecological surgery
- Orthopaedic surgery
- Emergency surgery.

## PERIOPERATIVE DRUGS CAUSING PONV

- Volatile agents: enflurane and halothane > isoflurane
- $N_2O$ distends bowel
- Thiopentone, etomidate and methohexitone (propofol may have intrinsic antiemetic properties due to $5HT_3$ antagonism)
- Hypotension from regional techniques (duration > degree of hypotension)
- All opioids
- Anticholinergics.

## PREVENTION

- Adequate but not prolonged fasting
- Avoid postoperative movement, e.g. bumpy trolleys
- Avoid excessive pharyngeal stimulation, e.g. suctioning
- Avoid gastric inflation
- Gentle handling of bowel because 5HT stored in enterochromaffin cells of the GI tract is released in response to surgical manipulation
- Ensure adequate oxygenation, analgesia, hydration and blood pressure.

## TREATMENT

Use antiemetic prophylaxis in high-risk patients. (Low-dose droperidol 0.005 mg/kg may be more effective than high dose.)

Use drug appropriate to neurotransmitter: anticholinergic for vagally mediated vomiting, e.g. hyoscine; antidopaminergic for opioid-mediated vomiting, e.g. phenothiazines, butyrophenones. Ondansetron ($5HT_3$ antagonist) may be useful in chemotherapy-induced vomiting and vomiting resistant to conventional drugs where it is more effective than metoclopramide or droperidol.

### References

Kenny G N C 1994 Risk factors for postoperative nausea and vomiting. Anaesthesia 49(suppl): 6–10
Naylor R J, Inall F C 1994 The physiology and pharmacology of postoperative nausea and vomiting. Anaesthesia 49(suppl): 2–5
Watcha M F 1996 Nausea and vomiting: choice of drugs and treatment. Current Opinion in Anaesthesiology 9: 300–305

## RESUSCITATION

## ADULT ADVANCED CARDIAC LIFE SUPPORT GUIDELINES

### Precordial thump

A precordial thump is now recommended for a witnessed arrest, with both VF and asystole. Mechanical energy from the blow is converted to a short-duration electrical current. The energy required for successful cardioversion rapidly rises with time and soon exceeds that delivered by a precordial blow. Conversion rates of 11–40% for VT and 2% for VF have been reported.

### Defibrillation

The chances of successful defibrillation and the long-term outcome decline rapidly after 90 seconds due to depletion of high-energy phosphate stores. Therefore, the current guidelines place emphasis upon rapid defibrillation, with three initial shocks to be given within 30 seconds without the sequence being interrupted by basic life support. One paddle should be placed below the right clavicle in the midclavicular line and the other over the lower left ribs in the mid/anterior axillary line (just outside the position of the normal cardiac apex).

The most commonly used transthoracic defibrillation waveform has a damped sinusoidal pattern. Biphasic waveforms are now being evaluated

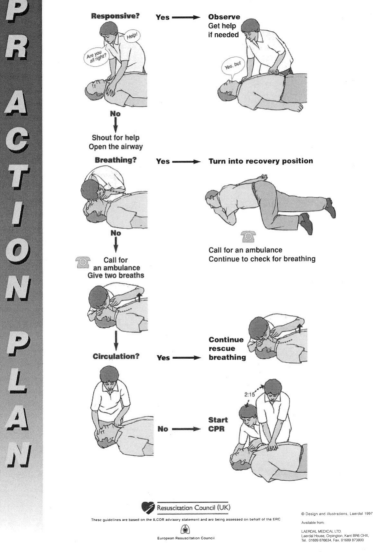

**Fig. 6.11a** Adult basic life support guidelines. European Resuscitation Council 1997 (updated 1998) Cardiopulmonary resuscitation guidelines for use in the UK. © Laerdal Medical Ltd, 1997.

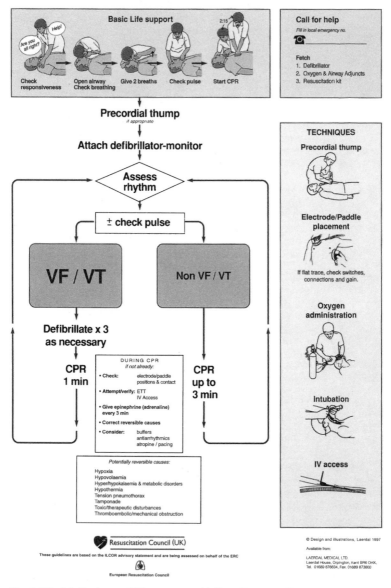

**Fig. 6.11b** Adult advanced life support guidelines. European Resuscitation Council 1997 (updated 1998) Adult advanced life support guidelines for use in the UK. © Laerdal Medical Ltd, 1997.

which have the following advantages compared with sinusoidal waveforms:

- lower energy benefits – same first shock efficacy at lower energy levels
- improved performance with anti-arrhythmic drugs – little or no increase in defibrillation threshold
- less post-shock dysfunction – 90% less post-shock ST segment changes and fewer post-shock arrhythmias.

### Cardiac massage

Closed chest compression should be performed at a rate of 100/min. Trials of active compression–decompression have not shown any improvement in long-term outcome.

### Adrenaline (epinephrine)

Adrenaline improves myocardial and cerebral blood flow. Animal studies suggest current doses in humans (1 mg or 0.015 mg/kg) may be suboptimal for maintaining a minimum cerebral and myocardial blood flow. High-dose adrenaline during cardiac arrest in humans has shown improved short-term survival but not survival to discharge from hospital. Therefore, 1 mg adrenaline remains the standard dose, but a higher dose (5 mg) may be indicated although its effect is not proven.

Experimentally, vasopressin has shown promising results with greater myocardial blood flow and return of spontaneous circulation.

### Atropine

3 mg of atropine is now thought to be necessary to completely block the massive vagal discharge associated with cardiac arrest.

### Lignocaine

Lignocaine increases the electrical threshold for defibrillation and its use in refractory VF is now not recommended until three loops have been completed. Other anti-arrhythmic drugs to be considered for refractory VF include amiodarone (300 mg loading dose) or bretylium (400 mg), but if the latter drug is given, cardiopulmonary resuscitation must be continued for at least a further 20 minutes before it has any effect.

### Bicarbonate

Although acidosis is known to depress myocardial contractility (pH < 7.2), reduce tissue oxygen delivery and increase susceptibility to VF, there is no good evidence that correction of pH improves outcome of CPR.

Side effects of bicarbonate include:

- increased osmolality through large sodium load
- increased $P_a\text{co}_2$ causing respiratory acidosis
- metabolic alkalosis
- paradoxical intracellular acidosis (limited evidence)
- decreased ionized $Ca^{2+}$
- impaired arterial oxygenation and reduced myocardial oxygen consumption
- decreased cerebral blood flow
- increased risk of neonatal intraventricular haemorrhage.

More judicious use of bicarbonate is now recommended. At venous pH < 7.1 and base excess > −10, correct with 1 mmol/kg. If arterial blood gas measurements are not possible, bicarbonate should only be administered after resuscitation has been attempted for 10–20 minutes.

### Routes of delivery

If drugs are given by the endobronchial route (lignocaine, adrenaline and atropine only), give two to three times the i.v. dose, in a volume of at least 10 ml. Following administration, give five ventilations to increase dispersion to the distal bronchial tree. However, this is still a poor route for drug delivery and causes well-documented decreases in $P_a\text{O}_2$ with little or no change in BP. Drugs administered via peripheral veins should be flushed with 20 ml of 0.9% saline.

## RESUSCITATION DURING PREGNANCY

- < 25 weeks – as above
- 25–32 weeks – use wedge to relieve aortocaval compression
- > 32 weeks – degree of aortocaval compression precludes effective CPR; therefore, perform immediate caesarean section whilst CPR is continued.

## GUIDELINES FOR PAEDIATRIC ADVANCED LIFE SUPPORT
(Fig. 6.12)

Causes of paediatric arrest are significantly different from those in adults. Cardiac arrest at birth is usually due to asphyxia; in infancy to respiratory illness or sepsis; and in later childhood to trauma (Zideman et al 1994).

Humidified oxygen with as high a $F_i\text{O}_2$ as possible should be used. Face masks should be made of soft clear plastic and have a minimum dead space. Oral endotracheal intubation with an uncuffed tube is the optimum method of securing the airway. During attempts at intubation, basic life support must not be interrupted for more than 30 seconds, after which the child must be reoxygenated before further attempts at intubation are made (Zideman et al 1994). Use 15–30 breaths/min with 100–120 compressions/

# Paediatric Advanced Life Support

1997 guidelines for use in the UK

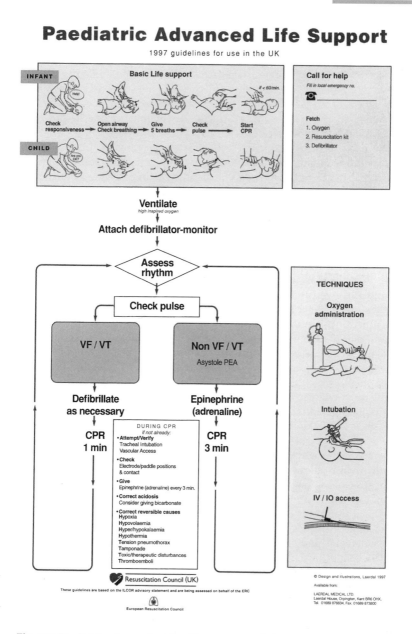

**Fig. 6.12** Paediatric advanced cardiac life support guidelines. European Resuscitation Council 1997 (updated 1998) Paediatric advanced life support guidelines for use in the UK. © Laerdal Medical Ltd, 1997.

min at a ratio of 3 compressions:1 ventilation. Massage at the junction of middle/lower third sternum and depress to one-third of the resting chest diameter. Tracheal suctioning may cause vagally mediated bradycardia.

Asystole is the commonest paediatric arrest arrhythmia and is usually preceded by an agonal bradycardia. VF occurs in only 6–9% of arrests, when two shocks at 2 J/kg should be given with subsequent shocks at 4 J/kg. Look for specific causes of VF, including hypothermia, tricyclic anti-depressants and hyperkalaemia.

The initial dose of adrenaline is 10 $\mu$g/kg, increased to 100 $\mu$g/kg for further doses. High-dose adrenaline may improve neurological outcome in asystolic arrest but animal models have shown an increased risk of neonatal intracranial haemorrhage. Bradycardia is usually due to hypoxaemia and atropine is rarely indicated. Guidelines recommend 20 $\mu$g/kg atropine with a maximum dose of 1 mg in children and 2 mg in teenagers.

Hypernatraemia secondary to sodium bicarbonate administration greatly increases the risk of intracranial haemorrhage in neonates. Current recommendations are that bicarbonate is not administered until the first dose of adrenaline has been shown to be ineffective. The initial dose is 1 mmol/kg given as a slow bolus before the second dose of adrenaline. Give further doses of bicarbonate according to arterial or mixed venous pH. Calcium chloride is more efficacious than the gluconate and should be given in a dose of 10–30 mg/kg. Lignocaine should be given as 1 mg/kg.

Hypoglycaemia is common in sick infants. Check glucose during resuscitation and treat hypoglycaemia with glucose 0.5 g/kg as a 10 or 25% solution.

The commonest causes of electromechanical dissociation are hypovolaemia, cardiac tamponade and tension pneumothorax. Correct hypovolaemia with boluses of 20 ml/kg crystalloid or colloid.

If venous access cannot be gained within 90 seconds, use an intraosseous needle which is suitable for all resuscitation drugs, colloid, crystalloid and blood. It also allows samples of marrow aspirate to be withdrawn for estimation of haemoglobin, venous pH and electrolytes. Endotracheal drugs should be administered down a fine-bore cannula inserted deep into the bronchial tree but is a poor route. The recommended dose of endotracheal adrenaline is 10 times the standard dose. Hypoxaemia, acidosis, hypercapnia, hypovolaemia and hypothermia cause reversion to a fetal circulation, which results in a right-to-left shunt and reduced absorption of drugs administered through the endotracheal tube.

## PAEDIATRIC RESUSCITATION DRUG DOSES

- Adrenaline 0.01 mg/kg. Subsequent doses 0.1 mg/kg
- Atropine 0.02 mg/kg
- Give initial dose of 1 mmol/kg bicarbonate (diluted in equal volume 5–10% dextrose). Further doses titrated against blood gases

- Calcium chloride 10–30 mg/kg
- Lignocaine 1.0 mg/kg
- Glucose 0.5 g/kg
- Frusemide 1 mg/kg
- Crystalloid 20 ml/kg if hypovolaemic. Repeat three times and then give 10 ml/kg blood if shock persists

### Apgar score

Table 6.5 Apgar score

|                    | 0           | 1                           | 2               |
|--------------------|-------------|-----------------------------|-----------------|
| Colour             | Blue, pale  | Body pink, extremities blue | All pink        |
| Pulse              | Absent      | < 100/min                   | > 100/min       |
| Reflex irritability| No response | Some motion                 | Cry             |
| Muscle tone        | Limp        | Some flexion of extremities | Well flexed     |
| Respiratory effort | Absent      | Slow, irregular             | Good strong cry |

## GUIDELINES FOR THE MANAGEMENT OF PERI-ARREST ARRHYTHMIAS (Fig. 6.13)

European Resuscitation Council guidelines cover the management of brady-arrhythmias, broad complex tachycardias and narrow complex tachycardias (supraventricular tachycardias, SVTs), including atrial fibrillation.

### Bradyarrhythmias

The definition of a bradycardia is based more upon the haemodynamic response to the rhythm rather than any specific rate. The recommended treatment of bradycardias depends upon the perceived risk of the progression of the arrhythmia to asystole. When asystole is likely and atropine (500 $\mu$g i.v. to maximum 3 mg) is not efficacious, treatment options include a transvenous ventricular pacing wire, external pacing or an isoprenaline infusion commencing at 1 $\mu$g/min.

### Broad complex tachycardia

The differential diagnosis of broad complex tachycardias lies between SVT with aberrant conduction and a ventricular tachyarrhythmia. In the context of resuscitation, it is recommended that broad complex tachycardia is assumed to be ventricular in origin until proven otherwise, because treatment of SVT as a ventricular arrhythmia is unlikely to be harmful whereas the opposite error may be fatal. Pulseless tachyarrhythmias should be treated by the same algorithm as for ventricular fibrillation. If a pulse is present,

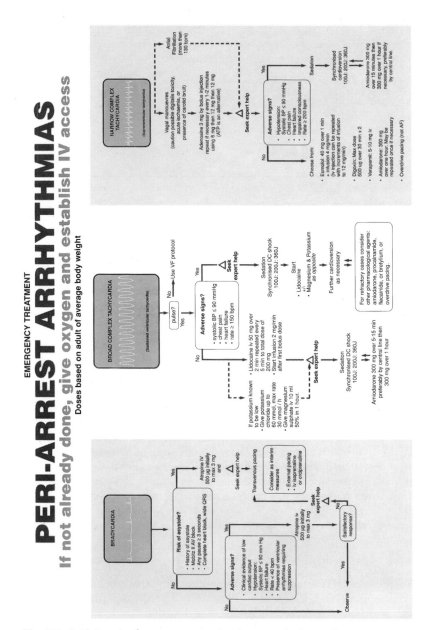

**Fig. 6.13** Guidelines for the management of peri-arrest arrhythmias. European Resuscitation Council 1997 (updated 1998). © Laerdal Medical Ltd, 1997.

with a rate of 150/min, a systolic BP of 90 mmHg or heart failure, administer synchronized DC shocks (100 J; 200 J; 360 J) followed by lignocaine and magnesium infusions if the potassium is known to be less than 3.6 mmol/l. Other drugs recommended for the treatment of refractory cases include amiodarone, flecainide, bretylium and procainamide. In the absence of adverse signs, use lignocaine (50 mg to a total of 200 mg) followed by synchronized DC shocks and amiodarone (300 mg over 15 min) as necessary.

### Narrow complex tachycardia

Narrow complex tachycardias are usually supraventricular in origin but may progress to VF. Carotid sinus massage may be effective but risks severe bradycardia triggering VF or atherosclerotic plaque rupture causing a stroke. Cardiovascular collapse requires DC cardioversion. Pharmacological treatment of choice is adenosine (3 mg increasing to 12 mg i.v.). If adenosine is unsuccessful, consider amiodarone, digoxin, esmolol or verapamil. Never use verapamil for the treatment of Wolff–Parkinson–White syndrome, ventricular tachycardias or in the presence of β-blockers.

## ADVANCES IN DEFIBRILLATION TECHNOLOGY

### Impedance-determined shocks

Delivery of a fixed energy level results in a widely variable transmyocardial current because of variations in thoracic size. New defibrillators first measure transthoracic impedance and adjust the energy delivered accordingly.

### Biphasic defibrillation waveforms

Most defibrillators use a truncated sine wave to deliver energy (Fig. 6.14). New defibrillators are being developed that deliver energy using a biphasic waveform (Fig. 6.15). This waveform has a number of advantages:

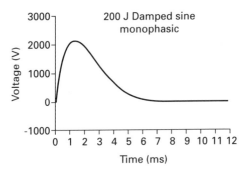

**Fig. 6.14** Truncated sine wave delivered by most defibrillators.

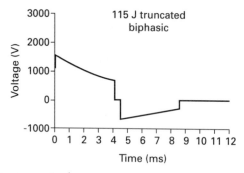

**Fig. 6.15** Biphasic waveform.

*Lower energy benefits*
- lower energy biphasic waveforms are associated with greater first shock efficacy
- 171 J biphasic shows a 21% improvement for VF compared with 215 J monophasic.

*Improved performance in VF*
- At 5 min, VF requires four times more energy using monophasic waveforms compared with biphasic
- Biphasic automatic implantable cardiac defibrillators give shorter cardiac arrest times than monophasic equivalents.

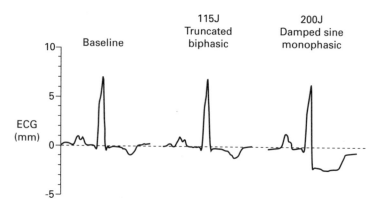

**Fig. 6.16** Post-shock ST depression comparing sine wave with biphasic waveform.

*Improved results with anti-arrhythmics*

*Lignocaine.* Monophasic requirements increase by 92%; decrease 6% with biphasic.

*Amiodarone.* Monophasic requirements increase by 22%; decrease 22% with biphasic.

### Less post-shock dysfunction

- Biphasic defibrillation produces less post-shock conduction block and fewer post-shock arrhythmias (9 vs 24%)
- Reduced post-shock ST depression – 130 J biphasic causes 12.5 times less depression than equivalent 360 J monophasic (Fig. 6.16).

## PHYSIOLOGY OF CIRCULATION DURING CLOSED CHEST MASSAGE

There are two theories of blood flow:

- *Cardiac pump theory.* Blood is ejected from the heart as it is squeezed between the sternum and spine. The AV valve prevents retrograde flow.
- *Thoracic pump theory.* Cardiac massage raises intrathoracic pressure and forces blood out of the thorax. Venous valves and venous compression prevent retrograde flow.

Both mechanisms are probably involved. Adrenaline constricts vascular beds to direct most flow to the brain and heart, so although total cardiac output is 10–30%, brain and heart flows approach 50% of normal. All flows decrease rapidly with time.

### Other techniques of cardiac massage

- *Active compression–decompression* – uses a toilet plunger-like device to actively re-expand the thoracic cavity during relaxation phase of compression; results in:
  — increased intrathoracic blood volume
  — increased LV filling during decompression
  — coronary blood flow during compression as well as relaxation
  — increased myocardial perfusion pressure
  — increased cerebral perfusion pressures
  Shown to improve short-term survival but evidence lacking for improved long-term outcome.
- *Pneumatic vest.*
- *Interposed abdominal compression.*
- *Simultaneous compression/ventilation* – increases cardiac output by increasing peak intrathoracic pressure, but intracranial pressure increases more than aortic pressure and actually decreases cerebral flow.
- *High-impulse CPR* – causes excessive thoracic trauma.

## USE OF END-TIDAL $CO_2$ MONITORING

$CO_2$ excretion during CPR is dependent upon cardiac output and not ventilation. A high correlation exists between $P_{ET}CO_2$ and cardiac output, coronary perfusion pressure and survival from cardiac arrest. $P_{ET}CO_2$ < 10 mmHg during resuscitation is associated with an unsuccessful outcome. Monitoring $P_{ET}CO_2$ during cardiac massage therefore provides feedback to optimize chest compression and may also give an early indication of operator fatigue.

### References

European Resuscitation Council 1998a Guidelines for adult advanced life support. Resuscitation 37: 81–90

European Resuscitation Council 1998b Paediatric basic life support. Resuscitation 37: 97–100

European Resuscitation Council 1998c Paediatric advanced life support. Resuscitation 37: 101–102

European Resuscitation Council Advanced Cardiac Life Support Committee 1994 Management of peri-arrest arrhythmias. Resuscitation 28: 151–159

Kattwinkel J, Niermeyer S, Nadkarni V et al 1999 Resuscitation of the newly born infant: an advisory statement from the Paediatric Working Group of the International Liaison Committee on Resuscitation. Circulation 99: 1927–1938

Rubertsson S 1999 Cardiopulmonary cerebral resuscitation – present and future perspectives. Acta Anaesthesiologica Scandinavica 43: 526–535

Zideman D, Bingham R, Beattie T et al 1994 Guidelines for paediatric life support. A statement by the Paediatric Life Support Working Party of the European Resuscitation Council. Resuscitation 27: 91–105

## STATISTICS

- Incidence = rate of occurrence of new cases
- Prevalence = total number of cases:
  — point prevalence – at a given moment in time
  — period prevalence – over a given period of time.

## NORMAL (GAUSSIAN) DISTRIBUTION

A sample of data may form a normal distribution curve which is bell-shaped and symmetrical about the mean value, e.g. height, weight, heart rate (Fig. 6.17). **Mean, median and mode**
- Mean = average of all values
- Median = the value above and below which half the observations lie
- Mode = most frequently occurring value.

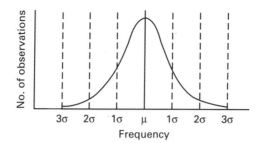

1σ either side of the mean covers 68% of the sample
2σ either side of the mean covers 95% of the sample
3σ either side of the mean covers 99% of the sample

**Fig. 6.17** Normal (Gaussian) distribution curve. $\mu$ = mean; $\sigma$ = standard deviation.

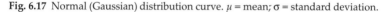

The mean, median and mode have identical values within normally distributed data (Fig. 6.18a).

Curves of normal distribution have symmetry about the mean. A curve that is not symmetrical is referred to as skewed. A curve is positively skewed if most data lie below the mean, and negatively skewed if most data lie above the mean. In a skewed distribution, mean, median and mode are not equal (Figs 6.18b and c). The amount of skewness is given by the following equation:

$$\text{Skewness} = \frac{\Sigma\,(x - \bar{x})^3}{N(SD^3)}$$

where:
x = observed mean
x̄ = expected mean
n = number of observations
n – 1 = degrees of freedom (N).

A result of zero indicates a completely symmetrical distribution; positive values indicate positively skewed distribution and vice versa. Strongly skewed data must be examined using non-parametric tests.

**Variance, standard deviation and standard error**

The variance of a sample is a measure of the scatter about the sample mean:

$$\text{Variance} = \frac{\Sigma\,(x - \bar{x})^2}{n - 1}$$

Variance is derived from a 'squared' equation, so to return to a measure of scatter about the mean that fits with original data, the square root of the variance is used. This is the standard deviation (SD):

$$SD(\sigma) = \sqrt{\text{variance}}$$

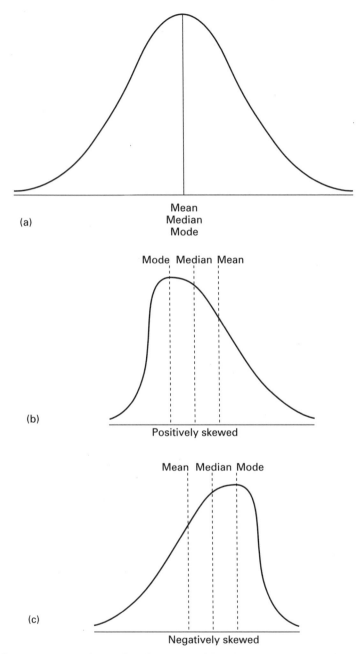

**Fig. 6.18** Mean, median and mode: (a) normal distribution; (b) positively skewed distribution; (c) negatively skewed distribution.

Therefore:

$$SD = \sqrt{\frac{\sum (x - \bar{x})^2}{n-1}}$$

Standard error (SE) is the standard deviation of the population mean:

$$SE = \sqrt{\frac{variance}{n}} \text{ or } \frac{SD}{\sqrt{n}}$$

## Standard error of the mean ($SE_m$)

Describes the deviation of the sample mean from the estimated population mean:

$$SE_m = \sqrt{\frac{variance_m}{n}} \text{ or } \frac{SD_m}{\sqrt{n}}$$

## Confidence intervals

Confidence limits express a range of values within which the true mean is likely to lie. The 95% confidence limits are given as the mean value ± 1.96 times the standard error, i.e. there is a 95% chance that the true population mean will lie within the calculated range. The limits either side of the mean are the 'confidence limits' and the interval between them is the 'confidence interval'.

For example, if the 95% confidence interval for percentage improvement between two groups following a given treatment is 15–35%, there is a 95% chance that the true difference lies between these two values.

## STATISTICAL TESTS (Tables 6.6 and 6.7)

Table 6.6 Statistical tests for comparing two or more groups

| Data type | Statistical test | | | | |
|---|---|---|---|---|---|
| | $t$-test | Mann–Whitney | Analysis of variance | Kruskal–Wallis | $x^2$ test |
| Normal distribution | | × | | × | × |
| Non-parametric distribution | × | | × | | × |
| Binary | × | × | × | × | |

**Table 6.7** Statistical tests for one or paired samples

| | Statistical test | | |
| --- | --- | --- | --- |
| Data type | t-test | Wilcoxon | McNemar |
| Normal distribution | | × | × |
| Non-parametric distribution | × | | × |
| Binary | × | × | |

## Parametric tests

Used for data fitting a normal distribution curve and for comparison of the sample mean with the population mean:

- **t-test** – Used to compare data from different groups (Student's t-test) or paired samples (paired t-test)
- **analysis of variance** (ANOVA) – similar to t-test but for three or more sample groups. Assesses whether the variability in group means is greater than that expected by chance.

## Non-parametric tests

Used for data not fitting, or assumed not to fit, a normal distribution, e.g. number of times patient pregnant, number of visits to GP/year, binomial data (true/false, heads/tails etc.).

### Chi-squared test

$$\chi^2 = \Sigma \frac{(O - E)^2}{E}$$

where:
O = observed frequencies
E = expected frequencies.

(O – E) is squared because some of the values will be negative. This value is then divided by the expected number (E) and the sum of these values is calculated to give $\chi^2$. The probability of the observed difference occurring by chance is then calculated from $\chi^2$ tables.

### Ranking tests
- Fisher's exact test
- Wilcoxon's signed rank test.

Ranking tests involve placing the data from both groups in an ascending/descending order. Numerical values are then assigned to each of the numbers of data and the sum of these numerical values calculated for each group. Probabilities are then calculated from tables.

## Significance values

Expressed as $P$-values, e.g. $P = 0.01$ means 1 chance in 100 that the results occurred by chance:

- $P > 0.05$ is taken as non-significant
- $P < 0.05$ and $> 0.01$ are significant
- $P < 0.01$ is highly significant.

## Linear correlation and linear regression

Observation of a scattergram may suggest some form of correlation between two variables (Fig. 6.19).

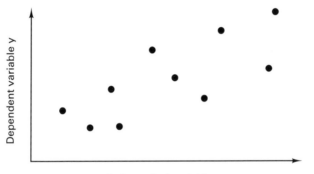

**Fig. 6.19** Scattergram of x against y.

The best-fit straight line is calculated for the data (Fig. 6.20). The position of the best-fit straight line is adjusted to minimize the sum of the distances d1–d4 so that $\Sigma d$ is a minimum.

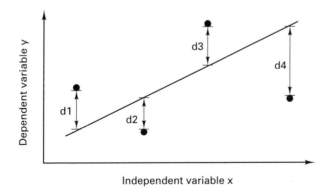

**Fig. 6.20** Linear regression for scattergram data.

The best-fit line is given by the equation:

$$y = m\,x + C$$

where:
x = independent variable
y = dependent variable
m = slope of the straight line
C = a constant.

*Multiple linear regression* is designed to establish any relationships when several variables are present within the same set of data.

## Correlation coefficient

The correlation coefficient, r, is an indication of how close the points lie to the best-fit line. As the data lie closer to the best-fit line, r tends towards 1.0 (Fig. 6.21).

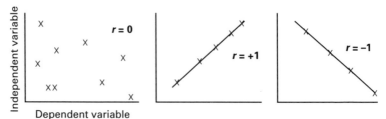

**Fig. 6.21** Correlation coefficients.

## Sensitivity and specificity

*Sensitivity* is a measure of the ability of a test to correctly select patients with a condition from an affected population, i.e. true positives:

$$\text{Sensitivity} = \frac{\text{number tested as positive}}{\text{total with condition}}$$

*Specificity* is a measure of the ability of a test to correctly select patients without the condition from an unaffected population, i.e. true negatives:

$$\text{Specificity} = \frac{\text{number tested as negative}}{\text{total without condition}}$$

## Sample size

Studies must be of sufficient size to be able to detect a difference between the study populations. Failure to show a difference between groups is only of significance if the sample size was adequate. Sample size can be calculated by equations but nomograms are easier for most studies. The power of a study is the chance of showing a difference between study populations if one exists, e.g. a study with a power of 0.80 has an 80% chance of detecting a difference if one exists.

### References

Gardner M J, Altman D G 1989 Statistics with confidence. British Medical Association, London
Swinscow T D V 1983 Statistics at square one, 8th edn. British Medical Association, London
Yentis S M 1996 The struggle for power in anaesthetic studies. Anaesthesia 51: 413–414

## TRAUMA MANAGEMENT

A Royal College of Surgeons Working Party (RCS 1988) highlighted serious deficiencies in trauma patient management.

A Major Trauma Outcome Study (MTOS) was published in 1992 with similar conclusions:

- worse outcome when comparing 6111 UK patients with USA data
- 21% patients with major trauma took > 1 h to reach hospital
- SHO in charge of resuscitation for 57% patients with major trauma.

Trunkey has described a trimodal pattern of death seen after major trauma (Fig. 6.22). The first peak comprises patients with serious, generally non-survivable injuries. The second peak comprises patients with life-threatening injuries in whom prompt, appropriate treatment may be life-saving. It is these patients to which the Advanced Trauma Life Support (ATLS) protocol is directed. The third peak comprises patients who die several days/weeks later from sepsis or multiple organ failure.

### Advanced Trauma Life Support

- Introduced from USA in 1988
- Some controversial aspects, e.g. no anaesthetic input to first edition, nasal vs. oral intubation, colloids vs. crystalloids
- Introduced concept of trauma team
- Limited data to suggest any improvement in outcome following its introduction
- Focuses on 'golden hour'.

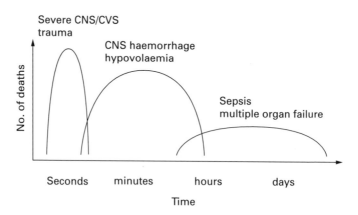

**Fig. 6.22** Trimodal distribution of death.

## PRIMARY SURVEY

**1. Airway** with cervical spine control

- Assess the airway for patency. Avoid neck extension / flexion if there is a risk of cervical spine injury.
- Assume cervical spine injury in multisystem trauma and, in particular, in patients with impaired consciousness or blunt injury above the clavicle.
- Stabilize the cervical spine with manual in-line stabilization or hard collar + head blocks.

**2. Breathing** with ventilatory support

- Look, listen and feel
- Tension pneumothorax, haemothorax or flail chest may require immediate treatment.

**3. Circulation** and haemorrhage control

*Pulses*
- Radial – present if systolic BP > 80 mmHg
- Femoral – present if systolic BP > 70 mmHg
- Carotid – present if systolic BP > 60 mmHg.

*Classification of hypovolaemic shock* (Table 6.8)

**Table 6.8** Classification of hypovolaemic shock

|  | Class I | Class II | Class III | Class IV |
|---|---|---|---|---|
| % blood loss | < 15 | 15–30 | 30–40 | > 40 |
| Volume | < 750 | 800–1500 | 1500–2000 | > 2000 |
| Systolic | Normal | Normal | Reduced | Very low |
| Diastolic | Normal | Raised | Reduced | Very low |
| Pulse | Normal | > 100/min | > 120/min | > 120/min |
| Capillary refill | Normal | > 2 s | > 2 s | Absent |
| Respiratory rate | Normal | Normal | > 20/min | > 20/min |
| Urine (mL/h) | > 30 | 20–30 | 10–20 | 0–10 |
| Mental state | Alert | Anxious | Drowsy | Confused |

*Intravenous access*
- ATLS recommends insertion of two 14 G cannulae.
- Remember flow $\propto r^4/l$, so a small increase in cannula radius (r) results in large increase in flow. Doubling the length (l) of an infusion set halves the flow.
- There is now increasing evidence that attempting to establish normovolaemia *before* surgical haemostasis dislodges any blood clots and accelerates the rate of bleeding. Intravenous fluids at this stage also cause dilution of clotting factors and hypothermia, increasing overall morbidity and mortality.

Until haemostasis is secured, aim for systolic of 80 mmHg, which is thought to be adequate to perfuse vital organs.

**4. Disability** – a rapid assessment of neurological function

- Assess GCS and pupils.
- Check cord function by observing arms and legs for spontaneous movement.
- A GCS < 8 is associated with impaired gas exchange. Therefore consider intubating head-injured patients to reduce 2° injury.

**5. Exposure** – completely undress the patient, but prevent hypothermia

- Hypothermia correlates with mortality.

## SECONDARY SURVEY

Involves a systematic head-to-toe survey:

- Head
- Maxillofacial

- Cervical spine and neck
- Chest
- Abdomen
- Perineum / rectum / vagina
- Musculoskeletal
- Neurological
- Don't forget to examine the back (log roll).

### References

Brussel T 1998 Anaesthetic considerations for acute spinal cord injury. Current Opinion in Anaesthesiology 11: 467–472

Meyer P-G 1998 Paediatric trauma and resuscitation. Current Opinion in Anaesthesiology 11: 285–288

Nolan J P, Parr M J A 1997 Aspects of resuscitation in trauma. British Journal of Anaesthesia 79: 226–240

Royal College of Surgeons of England 1988 Report of the Working Party on the Management of Patients with Major Injuries. RCS, London

# 7. Intensive care

## ACUTE RESPIRATORY DISTRESS SYNDROME (ARDS)

First described in Denver, Colorado, in 1967 by Ashbaugh. North American–European consensus group has changed the definition to '*acute*' (as opposed to 'adult') respiratory distress syndrome, since the syndrome can occur in children. It is often the pulmonary component of the systemic inflammatory response syndrome (SIRS) and is characterized by severe hypoxia refractory to oxygen, low compliance, high airway pressure, bilateral diffuse alveolar infiltrates and microscopic atelectasis. It has an annual incidence of about 3.5:100 000.

### CAUSES

**Table 7.1** Causes of ARDS

| Direct injury | Indirect injury |
| --- | --- |
| Pulmonary contusion | Septicaemia |
| Gastric aspiration | Major trauma |
| Fat and amniotic fluid embolus | Cardiopulmonary bypass |
| Infection | Massive blood transfusion |
| Cytotoxic drugs | Prolonged hypotension |
| Smoke inhalation | Hepatic and renal failure |
| Oxygen toxicity | Disseminated intravascular coagulation |

### PATHOPHYSIOLOGY

Activated neutrophils adhere to endothelial cells and release inflammatory mediators, including oxygen-free radicals and proteases, to cause lung damage. Direct lung damage or endotoxins alone are sufficient to damage endothelial cells with cytokine release and an inflammatory cascade (Fig. 7.1).

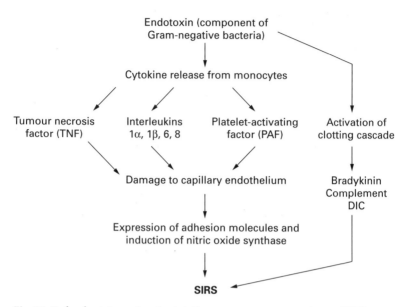

**Fig. 7.1** Pathophysiology of systemic inflammatory response syndrome (SIRS).

Endothelial damage results in increased capillary permeability and formation of protein-rich alveolar exudate rich in neutrophils. Type I alveolar cells are damaged and type II cells proliferate. As the disease progresses, fibroblast infiltration and collagen proliferation cause microvascular obliteration and widespread fibrosis. Areas of lung involvement are not fixed but shift to dependent areas. Within areas of reduced lung volume, some alveoli remain open and capable of gas exchange whereas others are filled with alveolar exudate.

IPPV may cause damage more through excess volume ('volutrauma') than through pressure itself. The significance of oxygen toxicity is controversial.

## TREATMENT

*Treat underlying cause.*

*Ensure adequate resuscitation.* Guided by invasive pulmonary artery pressure monitoring to prevent multiple organ failure. Aim for the lowest PCWP producing an adequate cardiac output to prevent high levels of lung water which are associated with a poor outcome.

*Ventilatory support.* Maintain peak airway pressures $< 40$ cmH$_2$O, mean airway pressures $< 30$ cmH$_2$O and limit PEEP $< 15$ cmH$_2$O to avoid barotrauma. Achieved by:

- inverse ratio ventilation (risks autoPEEP)
- pressure-controlled ventilation (better distribution of gas)

- permissive hypercapnia and hypoxaemia
- HFJV
- ventilation in the prone position.

However, there is no evidence that any of these techniques improve outcome.

Supranormalization of oxygen delivery does not improve survival as it does in high-risk surgical patients.

Increased PEEP is controversial. May avoid cyclic closure/reopening of atelectatic alveolar units, but it has been suggested that PEEP only fails to recruit units filled with alveolar exudate and overdistends open alveoli causing further damage.

Standard tidal volumes of 10–12 ml/kg are inappropriate in the presence of reduced functional lung volume and cause a significant increase in airway pressure. $F_iO_2 > 0.6$ may cause oxygen toxicity and does little to improve oxygenation in the presence of large shunts.

*Other methods of improving oxygenation:*
- Patients with ARDS have profound pulmonary vasoconstriction and ↑ PAP due to loss of endothelium-derived relaxing factor (EDRF). Nitric oxide (NO) can selectively vasodilate the pulmonary vascular bed at < 40 ppm, improving $V/\dot{Q}$ and arterial oxygenation. Long-term benefits have not been proven.
- Artificial surfactant is of benefit in neonates with idiopathic respiratory distress syndrome but results in adults with ARDS are disappointing.
- Extracorporeal membrane oxygenation (ECMO) and intravascular oxygenation (IVOX) have produced poor results.

*Reduce oedema formation.* Decreasing hydrostatic pressure, increasing colloid osmotic pressure and reducing capillary leak with NSAIDs all show disappointing results.

*Cardiovascular support.* Naturally occurring nitric oxide causes systemic vasodilatation seen with SIRS. Preliminary studies show vasodilatation may be reduced by inhibitors of nitric oxide synthetase.

*Gut-derived endotoxin.* May initiate and maintain SIRS. Gut failure may be reduced by early parenteral feeding with glutamine-rich substrates. Selective decontamination of the gut may reduce the incidence of nosocomial pneumonia.

*Anti-inflammatory mediators.* Platelet-activating factor (PAF) antagonists, IL-1 and IL-6 antagonists and tumour necrosis factor antagonists are experimental but may have a role to play in terminating the inflammatory cascade.

Corticosteroids may reduce production of inflammatory mediators but increase risk of infection. May benefit some patients in the fibroproliferative stage of the disease with no associated infection. Overall benefit is unclear.

*Secondary infection.* High risk of secondary infection reduced with prophylactic antibiotics.

*Outcome.* In early reports, ARDS was associated with a 60% mortality, but recent studies have documented mortality rates of 34–36%. In survivors, pulmonary dysfunction is rare, consisting principally of mild lung restriction, but progressive pulmonary fibrosis has been reported.

### References

Bigatello L M, Zapol W M 1996 New approaches to acute lung injury. British Journal of Anaesthesia 77: 99–109

Froese A B 1997 High-frequency oscillatory ventilation for adult respiratory distress syndrome. Critical Care Medicine 25: 906–908

Hall R I, Smith M S, Rocker G 1997 The systemic inflammatory response to cardiopulmonary bypass: pathophysiological, therapeutic and pharmacological considerations. Anesthesia and Analgesia 85: 766–782

Matthay M A, Pittett J F 1998 Just say NO to inhaled nitric oxide for the acute respiratory distress syndrome. Critical Care Medicine 26: 1–2

Sair M, Evans T W 1998 ARDS: are we winning at last? Anaesthesia 53: 831–832

## CARDIOVASCULAR SYSTEM

### INOTROPES

If shock persists despite adequate volume replacement and vital organ perfusion is jeopardized, inotropic drugs may be required to improve blood pressure and cardiac output (Table 7.2).

**Table 7.2** Receptor actions of inotropes

|  | $\alpha_1$ | $\alpha_2$ | $\beta_1$ | $\beta_2$ | $DA_1$ | $DA_2$ |
|---|---|---|---|---|---|---|
| Adrenaline |  |  |  |  |  |  |
|   Low dose | + | ± | + | + | 0 | 0 |
|   Moderate dose | ++ | + | ++ | + | 0 | 0 |
|   High dose | ++++ | +++ | +++ | +++ | 0 | 0 |
| Noradrenaline | +++ | +++ | ++ | 0 | 0 | 0 |
| Isoprenaline | 0 | 0 | +++ | +++ | 0 | 0 |
| Dopamine |  |  |  |  |  |  |
|   Low dose | ± | + | ± | 0 | ++ | + |
|   Moderate dose | ++ | + | ++ | + | ++ | + |
|   High dose | +++ | + | +++ | ++ | +++ | + |
| Dopexamine | 0 | 0 | + | +++ | ++ | + |
| Dobutamine | ± | 0 | ++ | + | 0 | 0 |

*Cardiogenic shock.* Characterized by low cardiac output, high filling pressures and increased systemic vascular resistance (SVR). Inodilators (dobutamine, enoximone, milrinone, dopexamine) improve cardiac contractility and decrease SVR. Specific vasodilators (nitroprusside, GTN) may reduce afterload further, increasing stroke volume and decreasing cardiac work by decreasing systolic wall tension.

*Septic shock.* Characterized by high cardiac output (if hypovolaemia corrected) and decreased SVR. Vasoconstrictors (noradrenaline) reduce SVR. Dobutamine or adrenaline may be required to improve myocardial contractility.

## PULMONARY ARTERY CATHETERS

It has recently been suggested that pulmonary artery catheter (PAC) use increases mortality. Although there is limited evidence to show improved outcome with PAC use, the general consensus is that their use in appropriate patients by clinicians skilled in their insertion and data interpretation is of benefit.

A recent USA pulmonary artery consensus conference (1997) (broadly in line with UK views) concluded:

- There is no basis for a moratorium of PAC use at this time.
- Clinicians should carefully weigh the risks and benefits of the PAC and patients should be fully informed before use.
- Criteria for appropriate use in specific situations should be developed.
- Clinicians' knowledge about PAC use and complications should be improved.

### Indications

- Haemodynamic instability with unknown diagnosis
- Major trauma – as a guide to volume replacement and haemodynamic support
- Myocardial infarction – to differentiate hypovolaemia from cardiogenic shock
- Pulmonary oedema – to differentiate cardiogenic from non-cardiogenic causes
- Hypotension when right atrial pressure may not equal that of the left atrium, e.g. right heart failure, chronic obstructive airway disease, pulmonary hypertension
- Pre-eclampsia with hypertension, oliguria and pulmonary oedema
- High-risk surgical patients
- Pulmonary embolism to assist in diagnosis and guide haemodynamic support.

### Pressure changes during PAC insertion (Fig. 7.2)

Place catheter so that it does not wedge until at least 1.2 ml air is in the

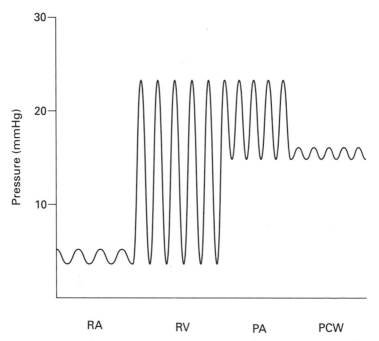

**Fig. 7.2** Pressure changes during pulmonary artery catheter insertion. RA, right atrium; RV, right ventricle; PA, pulmonary artery; PCW, pulmonary capillary wedge.

balloon (1.5 ml max.). Greatest degree of accuracy if tip of catheter is placed in West's zone III. Zone I tends to measure airway pressure, particularly with hypovolaemia. Measure wedge from 'a' wave at end of expiration.

### Complications

**Table 7.3** Complications of pulmonary artery catheter insertion

| Associated with insertion | Associated with catheter presence |
| --- | --- |
| Pneumothorax/haemothorax | Infection of catheter or site |
| Haematoma | Pulmonary thrombosis/infarct |
| Cardiac arrhythmias | Cardiac arrhythmias |
| Arterial puncture | Valve damage/endocarditis |
| Pulmonary artery perforation | Pulmonary artery erosion |
| Catheter knotting | Thrombocytopenia |
| Cardiac valve damage | |

# CARDIAC OUTPUT MONITORING

## Invasive techniques

- *Intermittent thermodilution.* Calculated from the Stuart–Hamilton equation:

$$CO = \frac{VI(BT - IT)}{(BT_0 - BT)}$$

where:
CO = cardiac output,
VI = volume of injectate,
BT = blood temperature after injection,
$BT_0$ = blood (pulmonary artery) temperature before injection
IT = injectate temperature.

- *Continuous thermodilution.* Calculated from a modified Stuart–Hamilton equation.
- *Indocyanine green dilution*

$$CO = \frac{\text{milligrams of dye injected} \times 60}{\begin{array}{l}\text{Average concentration of dye in}\\ \text{blood for the duration of the curve}\end{array} \times \text{duration of the curve}}$$

- *Fick calculated cardiac output*

$$CO = \frac{O_2 \text{ consumption}}{\text{arteriovenous } O_2 \text{ content difference}}$$

## Non-invasive techniques

- *Transthoracic/oesophageal Doppler ultrasonography.* Measurement of aortic cross-sectional area and blood flow velocity allows calculation of cardiac output. Acceleration and peak velocity indicate myocardial performance, while flow time is related to circulating volume and peripheral resistance.
- *Transthoracic impedance.* Can be measured across externally applied electrodes. Small changes in impedance ($< 1\ \Omega$) occur with the cardiac cycle as the blood volume in the heart increases during diastole and decreases during systole. Rate of change of impedance can be used to estimate cardiac output.

# TRANSOESOPHAGEAL ECHOCARDIOGRAPHY (TOE)

Increasing use in critical care. Uses the physical principle that sound is reflected from tissue interfaces. Piezoelectric crystals transmit and receive acoustic signals to build a two-dimensional image. TOE provides better cardiac views than transthoracic echocardiography, particularly of valves, contractility and filling status.

TOE is of particular use for assessment of:

- left ventricular systolic function
- left ventricular filling
- wall motion abnormalities
- cardiac tamponade
- valve function
- chest trauma (limited views of ascending aorta).

TOE has shown a poor relationship between PCWP and left ventricular end-diastolic volume, particularly in septic patients and those on high doses of inotropes. In these patients, mean pulmonary capillary pressure may be a more accurate measure.

### References

Cholley B P 1998 Benefits, risks and alternatives of pulmonary artery catheterization. Current Opinion in Anaesthesiology 11: 645–650

Dalen J E, Bone R C 1996 Is it time to pull the pulmonary catheter? Journal of the American Medical Association 276: 916–918

Edwards J D 1997 Continuous thermodilution cardiac output: a significant step forward in hemodynamic monitoring. Critical Care Medicine 25: 381–382

Hinds C J, Watson D 1999 ABC of intensive care. Circulatory support. British Medical Journal 318: 1749–1752

Koobi T 1999 Non-invasive cardiac output determination: State of the art. Current Opinion in Anaesthesiology 12: 9–13

Poelaert J, Schmidt C, Colardyn F 1999 Transoesophageal echocardiography in the critically ill. Anaesthesia 54: 55–68

Porembka D T 1997 Transesophageal echocardiography in the trauma patient. Current Opinion in Anaesthesiology 10: 130–144

Pulmonary artery catheter consensus conference 1997 Consensus statement. Critical Care Medicine 25: 910–925

Sandham J D, Hull R D, Brant R F 1998 The pulmonary artery catheter takes a great fall. Critical Care Medicine 26: 1288–1289

Townend J N, Hutton P 1996 Transoesophageal echocardiography in anaesthesia and intensive care. British Journal of Anaesthesia 77: 137–139

Vincent J-L, Dhainaut J-F, Perret C 1998 Is the pulmonary artery catheter misused? Critical Care Medicine 26: 1283–1287

## FLUID AND ELECTROLYTE BALANCE

The neonate has a greater proportion of body water and in a different distribution than the adult (Fig. 7.3). More fluid is distributed within the extracellular compartment (interstitial and plasma volume) compared with the adult, resulting in a larger volume of distribution for water-soluble

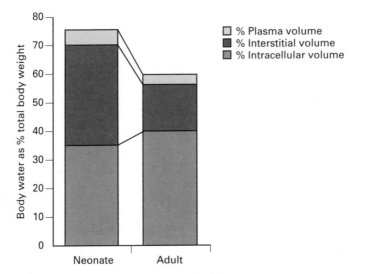

**Fig. 7.3** Body water distribution in neonate and adult.

drugs. A large proportion of interstitial fluid is excreted within the first few weeks after birth and adult levels are attained by adolescence.

A 70 kg male has about 42 kg of water distributed through three body compartments.

- extracellular fluid – 20% (plasma volume 4%, interstitial fluid 16%)
- intracellular fluid – 40%

$$= 60\% = 42\,l$$

Plasma volume expansion is least effective with fluids that are distributed throughout all body compartments and most effective with those that remain within the intravascular compartment. Therefore:

- 1000 ml 5% dextrose expands plasma by $1000 \times 4/60 = 67$ ml
- 1000 ml normal saline expands plasma by $1000 \times 4/20 = 200$ ml
- 1000 ml colloid expands plasma by $1000 \times 4/4 = 1000$ ml.

## STARLING EQUATION

$$Q = K\,[(P_c - P_i) - \sigma(\pi_c - \pi_i)]$$

where:
Q = fluid flux out of capillary bed
K = capillary filtration coefficient (permeability of membrane to water)
$P_c$ = capillary hydrostatic pressure
$P_i$ = interstitial hydrostatic pressure
σ = reflection coefficient of albumin (permeability of membrane to protein)

$\pi_c$ = capillary colloid osmotic pressure
$\pi_i$ = interstitial colloid osmotic pressure.

*Osmolality* is the number of osmotically active particles per kg of solvent:

$$= 2\,Na^+ + glucose/18 + urea/2.8$$

## HOMEOSTATIC CONTROL

A rise in serum osmolality stimulates osmoreceptors in the anterior hypothalamus to release ADH from the supraoptic nuclei. ADH release is also stimulated by volume receptors in the left atrium and carotid sinus baroreceptors in response to hypovolaemia.

ADH increases permeability of the distal collecting ducts, resulting in more fluid reabsorbtion and a reduction in the osmolality of body fluids.

Aldosterone is produced by the adrenal cortex in response to ACTH, renin, hyponatraemia or hyperkalaemia. It acts on the distal tubules and collecting ducts to increase $Na^+$ resorption and $K^+$ excretion.

Renin is secreted by the juxtaglomerular apparatus in response to a fall in extracellular volume or BP and acts on angiotensinogen to form angiotensin I which is converted to angiotensin II by passage through the lungs. Vasoconstriction produced by angiotensin II produces a marked rise in both systolic and diastolic blood pressures.

## NORMAL FLUID REQUIREMENTS

### Loss

- Insensible loss (skin and lungs) – 1000 ml/24 h
- Urine (minimum)                – 300 ml/24 h
- Faeces                         – 500 ml/24 h.

### Electrolyte requirements per 24 hours

- $Na^+$: 0.7–1.4 mmol/kg
- $K^+$: 0.8–1.4 mmol/kg.

### Postoperative fluid requirements

Intravenous fluids administered perioperatively during minor gynaecological surgery reduce morbidity, particularly nausea and dizziness. However, blood coagulation appears to be accelerated by haemodilution with saline, and in patients undergoing elective abdominal surgery, the incidence of DVT was four times greater than in the fluid-restricted group (Janvrin et al 1980).

Despite this latter study, it is generally agreed that the advantages of perioperative fluids outweigh any disadvantages. Campbell et al (1990) suggest Hartmann's 15 ml/kg per h for major surgery. This rate has been shown to improve postoperative renal function. Septic patients or those with lung trauma have raised extravascular lung water, and lesser rates may be necessary to avoid pulmonary oedema. In addition, give blood to maintain Hb > 10 g/dl.

Surgical stress causes release of ADH, renin and aldosterone, resulting in sodium and water retention, potassium excretion and an inability to excrete a hypotonic urine. Postoperative catabolism increases the minimum metabolic demand for water from 20 to 30 ml/kg per day, i.e. 2000 ml/day. The addition of 100 g/day of glucose reduces nitrogen loss by up to 60%. Therefore, give maintenance fluids of 2000 ml 5% dextrose/24 h postoperatively with 30 mmol KCl added to each 1 l bag to provide daily $K^+$ requirements. Hidden losses are difficult to judge so titrate fluids according to urine output (> 0.5 ml/kg per h).

Sodium retention is greatly reduced by 48 h so then add $Na^+$ to maintenance fluids and reduce KCl supplements.

## COLLOID VERSUS CRYSTALLOID CONTROVERSY (Table 7.4)

There is some evidence to suggest that crystalloid resuscitation is associated with a lower mortality in trauma patients.

**Table 7.4** Comparison of crystalloids and colloids

|  | Advantages | Disadvantages |
| --- | --- | --- |
| Crystalloid | Cheap | Larger volumes needed |
|  | Replaces extravascular loss | Small ↑ in plasma volume |
|  | Increased GFR | Peripheral and pulmonary oedema |
|  | Minimal effect on clot quality |  |
| Colloid | Smaller volumes needed | Risk of anaphylaxis |
|  | Prolonged ↑ in plasma volume | Relatively expensive |
|  | Reduced peripheral oedema | Coagulopathy |
|  |  | Poor clot quality |

## ALBUMIN

Single polypeptide of 585 amino acids. Synthesized in the endoplasmic reticulum of hepatocytes at 9–12 g/day but can increase 2–3 times in states of maximum synthesis. Stimulus to production is colloid osmotic pressure, osmolality of the extravascular liver space, insulin, thyroxine and cortisol. Catabolized by vascular endothelium. 5% of albumin is removed from the intravascular space per hour. Clinical properties of albumin include:

- *binding and transport* – strong negative charge binds $Ca^{2+}$ (40%), $Cu^{2+}$,

thyroxine, bilirubin and amino acids; also binds warfarin, phenytoin, NSAIDs and digoxin
- *maintenance of colloid osmotic pressure* (COP) – contributes to 80% of COP
- *free radical scavenging* – thiol groups scavenge reactive oxygen and nitrogen species
- *platelet inhibition and antithrombotic effects*
- *effects on vascular permeability* – may bind within the subendothelium to alter capillary membrane permeability.

Serum albumin decreases due to dilutional effects with crystalloid/colloid solutions, redistribution due to altered capillary permeability (fivefold increase during sepsis), decreased synthesis in septic patients, and increased loss from kidney or gut.

Correlation between COP and serum albumin is poor. Therefore, oedema associated with hypoalbuminaemia is not necessarily related and may be related more to lymphatic dysfunction. The acute-phase response is initially associated with a decrease in albumin synthesis, possibly due to IL-6-mediated inhibition of synthesis. A later hypermetabolic phase results in increased albumin synthesis.

Benefits of correcting hypoalbuminaemia are unclear. A prospective randomized study of 475 ICU patients comparing albumin and gelatin solutions failed to show any benefit (Stockwell et al 1992). In 70 children with burns, albumin supplementation failed to improve morbidity or mortality (Greenhalgh et al 1995). In septic patients, albumin infusions will only increase COP for a relatively short period. Increased capillary permeability results in > 60% of albumin leaving the intravascular compartment within 4 h, potentially worsening oedema.

A controversial systematic review by the Cochrane Group of 23 randomized controlled trials found that the risk of death was 6% greater in the group treated with albumin compared with those receiving crystalloids or no treatment (Cochrane Injuries Group 1998). The Committee on Safety of Medicines now advises doctors to restrict the use of, and take special care when using, human albumin, but states that there is 'insufficient evidence of harm to warrant withdrawal of albumin'. Hypoalbuminaemia in itself is not an appropriate indication. Risks of hypervolaemia and cardiovascular overload warrant monitoring in patients receiving albumin.

## INTRAVENOUS FLUIDS

### 0.9% normal saline (per 1000 ml)

- Sodium          150 mmol
- Chloride        150 mmol
- Osmolality      308

## Hartmann's (per 1000 ml)

- Sodium          131 mmol
- Chloride        111 mmol
- Lactate         29 mmol
- Potassium       5 mmol
- Calcium         2 mmol
- Osmolality      280

## Dextrose saline (per 1000 ml) (4% dextrose, 0.18% saline)

- Sodium          30 mmol
- Chloride        30 mmol
- Osmolality      300
- Calories        160 (40 g CHO)

## 5% Dextrose (per 1000 ml)

- Osmolality      278
- Calories        200 (50 g CHO)

## Gelofusine (per 1000 ml)

- Sodium          154 mmol
- Chloride        125 mmol
- Calcium         0.4 mmol
- Magnesium       0.4 mmol
- Gelatin         40 g with MW 30 000

## Haemaccel (per 1000 ml)

- Sodium          145 mmol
- Chloride        145 mmol
- Potassium       5 mmol
- Calcium         6.25 mmol

### References

Campbell I T, Baxter J N, Tweedie I E, Taylor G T, Keens S J 1990 IV fluids during surgery. British Journal of Anaesthesia 65: 726–729

Choi P T L, Yip G, Quinonez L G, Cook D J 1999 Crystalloids vs colloids in fluid resuscitation: a systematic review. Critical Care Medicine 27: 200–210

Cochrane Injuries Group 1998 Human albumin administration in critically injured patients: systematic review of randomised controlled trials. British Medical Journal 317: 235–240

Greenhalgh D G, Housinger T A, Kagan R J, Rieman M, James L, Novak S, Farmer L, Warden G D, Ferrara J J, Petersen S R, Hartford C E, Hauser C, Farrell K J, Dries D J

1995 Maintenance of serum albumin levels in pediatric burn patients: A prospective, randomized trial. Journal of Trauma 39: 67–74

Janvrin S B, Davies G, Greenhalgh R M 1980 Postoperative deep vein thrombosis caused by intravenous fluids during surgery. British Journal of Surgery 67: 690–693

Margarson M P, Soni N 1998 Serum albumin: touchstone or totem? Anaesthesia 53: 789–803

Shearer E S, Hunter J M 1992 Perioperative fluid and electrolyte balance. Current Anaesthesia and Critical Care 3: 71–76

Steward D J 1994 Fluid management for the paediatric patient. Canadian Journal of Anaesthesia 41: R87–90

Stockwell M A, Soni N, Riley B 1992 Colloid solutions in the critically ill. A randomised comparison of albumin and polygeline. 1. Outcome and duration of stay in the intensive care unit. Anaesthesia 47: 3–6

# NITRIC OXIDE

In 1987, nitric oxide (NO) was identified as an endothelium-derived relaxing factor. It is a free radical acting as a local transcellular messenger through binding to transition metals within enzymes such as guanylate cyclase. It is involved in:

- regulation of smooth muscle tone
- antimicrobial defence by its free radical action
- platelet and neutrophil adherence and aggregation
- peripheral and central neurotransmission
- regulation of smooth muscle proliferation.

The synthesis and action of NO are shown in Figure 7.4.

## CARDIOVASCULAR EFFECTS

Intracellular calcium is thought to play an important role in activating nitric oxide synthase. Increasing shear stress increases endothelial cell calcium with a resulting reduction in vascular tone. NO synthesis is also increased by acetylcholine, bradykinin, hypoxia and α-adrenergic stimulation, although the degree of vasodilation induced by these factors is uncertain. Excess NO produced in the presence of ischaemia may contribute to ischaemic damage through its free radical damage to myocardium. Inhibitors of NO synthesis may protect against myocardial reperfusion injury. Inadequate NO production increases platelet aggregation and adhesion.

### Hypertension

Basal production of NO continuously vasodilates the peripheral circulation.

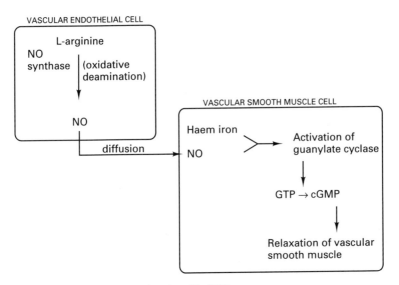

**Fig. 7.4** Synthesis and action of nitric oxide (NO).

Basal NO release is greater in arteries than in veins. Untreated hypertension in humans is associated with reduced NO synthesis. L-arginine supplementation alone does not restore NO levels to normal, suggesting that other mechanisms in addition to substrate depletion are involved. Excess end-products of glycosylation and oxidized lipoproteins in atherosclerosis have been proposed to inactivate nitric oxide synthetase.

### Synthetic vasodilators

Organic nitrates such as GTN and nitroprusside undergo enzymatic reduction, releasing NO within vascular smooth muscles. Small vessels, e.g. coronary arteries, lack the capacity for this metabolism and only large capacitance vessels and coronary vessels > 100 $\mu$m dilate in response to clinical doses of nitroglycerine. This selective vasodilation is less likely to cause coronary steal and contributes to the anti-anginal effects of nitrates. Tolerance to organic nitrates occurs due to a reduction in the biotransformation of the drug.

## RESPIRATORY EFFECTS

Normal pulmonary vascular tone is very low and exogenous NO has little effect on pulmonary vascular resistance. However, in disease states where pulmonary vascular tone is increased (pulmonary hypertension, ARDS, chronic respiratory failure), NO selectively vasodilates pulmonary vasculature around functioning alveolar units. This local vasodilation diverts blood towards functioning alveoli, reduces intrapulmonary shunting and may improve oxygenation. Significant systemic vasodilation does not occur because NO is rapidly inactivated by binding to haemoglobin.

Although NO improves arterial oxygen tension, no studies yet show improvement in mortality in adults with ARDS. Treatment of persistent pulmonary hypertension of the newborn appears promising and may avoid the need to use extracorporeal membrane oxygenation. In infants with hypoxic respiratory failure, NO appears as effective as ECMO in reducing mortality but is cheaper and simpler to use.

## NEURONAL NO

NO acts as a neurotransmitter in both the central and peripheral nervous systems, where its release is stimulated by excitatory amino acids. Neural functions of NO include peripheral non-adrenergic non-cholinergic transmission, neurotransmission in contractile and secretory tissue, synaptic plasticity, learning and memory.

## TOXICITY OF NO

NO forms several toxic products, including nitrogen dioxide and nitric and nitrous acids. NO also reacts with free radicals to form peroxynitrite ($ONOO^{2-}$), which is highly cytotoxic. The clinical significance of these effects is uncertain. In the circulation, NO combines with iron to form methaemoglobin, which may be a problem with high levels of inhaled NO.

## NO AND SEPSIS

Inflammatory mediators such as TNF, cytokines and interferon induce nitric oxide synthase in endothelial cells, parenchymal cells and macrophages, increasing NO production. This may be the mechanism by which sepsis results in vasodilation. Some studies have shown that inhibition of NO synthesis with L-NMMA prevents these haemodynamic changes. Nitric oxide sythase inhibition may be a potential route for the treatment of sepsis.

### References

Galley H F, Webster N R 1998 Nitric oxide in a nutshell: genetics, physiology and pathology. Current Anaesthesia and Critical Care 9: 209–213

Hurford W E, Zapol W M 1994 Nitric oxide inhalation in the intensive care unit. Current Opinion in Anaesthesiology 7: 153–160

Kirkebøen K A, Strand Ø A 1999 The role of nitric oxide in sepsis – an overview. Acta Anaesthesiologica Scandinavica 43: 275–288

Quinn A C, Petros A, Vallance P 1995 Nitric oxide: an endogenous gas. British Journal of Anaesthesia 74: 443–451

Young J D 1997 Inhaled nitric oxide in acute respiratory failure. British Journal of Anaesthesia 79: 695–696

## NUTRITION

### MALNUTRITION

Malnutrition is common in hospital patients. In a recent study of 500 acute hospital admissions, 20% were malnourished and, of these, 5.4% had lost further weight during their stay in hospital (McWhirter & Pennington 1994).

Preoperative nutritional support can improve nutritional status but may only improve morbidity and mortality in severely malnourished patients. This support must be maintained for at least 7 days preoperatively to show any benefit. Prospective studies have demonstrated a benefit for postoperative nutritional support.

### Assessment of malnutrition

- Weight loss > 10%
- Skinfold thickness (lags behind nutritional status by 3–4 weeks)
  — arm muscle circumference decreased 20%
  — triceps skin fold thickness decreased 50%
- Hand grip tests – specific and reproducible measure
- Serum albumin < 35 g/l, transferrin, total iron-binding capacity (TIBC), thyroxine-binding prealbumin
- Lymphocyte count < 3.5
- Negative reaction to five skin antigens.

### Effects of malnutrition

*CVS.* Decreased HR, CO and CVP.

*Respiratory.* Decreased inspiratory force and FVC; weaning more difficult.

*GI.* Decreased gut motility, gut atrophy and increased gut permeability to intestinal bacteria.

*Other.* Decreased metabolic rate. Increased susceptibility to infection, poor wound healing, muscle weakness, oedema and impaired organ function. Increased morbidity and mortality.

Starvation and stress result in different rates of malnutrition and changes in catabolic pathways (Table 7.5).

**Table 7.5** Effect of starvation and stress on energy expenditure and malnutrition

|                      | Starvation | Stress    |
|----------------------|------------|-----------|
| Energy expenditure   | +          | +++       |
| R:Q                  | 0.7        | 0.8–0.85  |
| Malnutrition         | +          | +++       |
| Rate of malnutrition | +          | +++       |

## R:Q

R:Q = $CO_2$ output/$O_2$ consumption

- CHO = 1.0
- Protein = 0.83
- Fat = 0.71.

## NUTRITIONAL SUPPORT

### Indications for nutritional support

- Albumin < 30 g/l
- Marked weight loss, muscle wasting and oedema
- Dietary history showing decreased intake for > 1 week
- Medical and surgical disorders likely to result in malnutrition
- Postoperative starvation for > 10 days.

### Composition

Optimal combination of water, carbohydrate, protein, fat, vitamins and trace elements. Calories as glucose or fat; protein as amino acids.

Calorie:nitrogen ratio of 200 calories:1 g $N_2$, decreasing to 100 calories:1 g $N_2$ in catabolic and septic patients.

Monitor electrolytes daily, monitor blood sugar every 48 h, monitor liver function tests weekly.

### Caloric content

- CHO – 4 kcal/g
- Protein – 4 kcal/g
- Fat – 9 kcal/g.

### Daily requirements (per 24 h)

- Calories – 30 kcal/kg
- Protein – 0.3 g $N_2$/kg (for burns = 0.5 g $N_2$/kg)
- Glucose – 2 g/kg
- Fat – 2 g/kg
- Water – 30 ml/kg
- Sodium – 1.2 mmol/kg
- Potassium – 0.8 mmol/kg.

The following are also required:

- *Glutamine.* Involved in repairing injured gut mucosa, generates substrate for renal ammonia production and supports lymphocyte proliferation. Supplementation decreases bacterial translocation, restores secretory IgA and improves $N_2$ balance.

- *Arginine*. Precursor for nitric oxide synthesis. Enhances wound healing and survival in animal models of sepsis.
- *Insulin*. Improves protein sparing and nitrogen balance.
- *Folic acid*.
- *Branch chain amino acids*. Encourage amino acid utilization and reduce oxidation.

### Enteral feeding

Requires at least 25 cm ileum.

Paralytic ileus only affects the stomach and colon. Small bowel motility and absorption often remain normal and therefore bowel sounds and flatus are not required to start enteral feeding. Early enteral feeding through a nasojejunal tube or feeding jejunostomy may prevent paralytic ileus.

#### Advantages of enteral over parenteral feeding
- Cheaper
- More efficient utilization of nutrients
- Stimulates intestinal blood flow
- Enteral feeding maintains GI mucosal barrier, preventing bacterial translocation and portal endotoxaemia. Bacterial translocation implicated in MODS
- Disuse atrophy of GI tract occurs rapidly without enteral feeding
- Postoperative enteral feeding reduces septic complications more than parenteral route
- Avoids complications of central venous cannula insertion
- Avoids TPN-induced immunosuppression
- Shorter hospital stay and greater survival compared with TPN.

#### Complications
- Infection – infusion phlebitis, mediastinitis
- Hyperglycaemia – requiring insulin
- Mineral deficiencies – especially zinc (poor wound healing), phosphate (muscle weakness)
- Thrombosis and embolism – reduced antithrombin III levels necessitate heparin
- Metabolic bone disease – osteomalacia, hypercalciuria
- Acid–base imbalance
- Hepatic dysfunction
- Fat overload.

### References

Bistrian B R, Babineau T 1998 Optimal protein intake in critical illness? Critical Care Medicine 26: 1476–1477

Kearney P A, Annis K 1994 Perioperative nutrition support in critical illness. Current Opinion in Anaesthesiology 7: 305–309

Marshall W J 1994 Perioperative nutritional support. Review. Care of the Critically Ill 10: 163–167
Nelson L D 1998 Death knell for parenteral nutrition? Critical Care Medicine 26: 4
O'Leary M J, Coakley J H 1996 Nutrition and immunonutrition. British Journal of Anaesthesia 77: 118–127

## OXYGEN TRANSPORT

## PHYSIOLOGY

**Oxygen cascade** ($P_{O_2}$) (kPa)

- Dry atmospheric gas    21.1
- Inspired tracheal gas    19.8
- Alveolar gas    14.7
- Arterial blood    13.3
- Mixed venous blood    5.3

**Table 7.6** Oxygen content of arterial and mixed venous blood

|  | Oxygen content (ml/dl) | |
|---|---|---|
|  | **Arterial** | **Mixed venous** |
| Total | 20.0 | 15.0 |
| Attached to Hb | 19.7 | 14.9 |
| Dissolved | 0.3 | 0.1 |
|  | 2.0 (100% $O_2$) |  |
| Saturation | 97% | 73% |

## HAEMOGLOBIN

- Complex compound of MW 64 500
- $O_2$-carrying capacity (Hufner's constant) = 1.39 ml/g
- Because of impurities (e.g. methaemoglobin) = 1.34–1.36 ml/g
- $P_{50}$ (50% saturation)
  — adults: 3.5–3.9 kPa
  — fetus: 2.6 kPa

### Haemoglobin dissociation curve

*Bohr effect.*  Increase $H^+$ shifts dissociation curve to right.

**2,3-DPG.** Produced by glycolysis. Reduces $O_2$ affinity.
*Temperature.* Pyrexia shifts dissociation curve to right.

## OXYGEN CONTENT

$$C_aO_2 = (1.3 \times Hb \times S_aO_2) + (0.003 \times P_aO_2)$$

where:
$C_aO_2$ = arterial oxygen content
$(1.3 \times Hb \times S_aO_2)$ – i.e. 1 g Hb, when completely saturated, binds 1.3 ml $O_2$
$(0.003 \times P_aO_2)$ = amount of $O_2$ dissolved in plasma = 0.003 ml/mmHg.

## OXYGEN DELIVERY

$$DO_2 = \dot{Q} \times C_aO_2$$

where:
$DO_2$ = oxygen delivery
$\dot{Q}$ = cardiac output.

$$DO_2 = 3 \times (1.3 \times 14 \times 0.98) \times 10$$
$$(\times 10 \text{ converts volumes \% to ml/s})$$
$$= 540 \text{ ml/min per m}^2$$

## OXYGEN UPTAKE

$$VO_2 = \dot{Q} \times (C_aO_2 - C_vO_2) \quad \text{(Fick equation)}$$

where:
$VO_2$ = oxygen uptake
$C_vO_2$ = venous oxygen content.

$$VO_2 = \dot{Q} \times (13 \times Hb) \times (S_aO_2 - S_vO_2)$$
$$= \dot{Q} \times (13 \times Hb) \times (0.97 - 0.73)$$
$$= 130 \text{ ml/min per m}^2$$

## OXYGEN EXTRACTION RATIO

The oxygen extraction ratio ($O_2ER$) is the fractional uptake of oxygen from the capillary bed.

$$O_2ER = VO_2/DO_2 \times 100$$
$$= 130/540 \times 100$$
$$= 24\%$$

### Normal response

Decreased blood flow results in increased $O_2$ extraction, i.e. drop in cardiac index is balanced by increased $(S_aO_2 - S_vO_2)$. Thus $VO_2$ remains unchanged.

All vascular beds can increase $O_2$ extraction if flow drops, *except* coronary circulation and diaphragm. Therefore it is necessary to maintain cardiac output in patients with coronary artery disease because $Do_2$ is flow dependent.

### Response in critically ill patients

Oxygen extraction from capillary beds may not increase where necessary and oxygen uptake ($Vo_2$) becomes flow-dependent (Fig. 7.5). Therefore it is imperative to maintain cardiac output to maintain oxygen supply to the tissues.

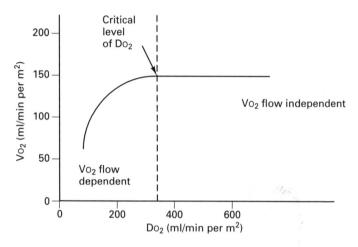

**Fig. 7.5** Oxygen delivery ($Do_2$) versus uptake ($Vo_2$) in critically ill patients.

## MIXED VENOUS OXYGEN

Under normal conditions, venous oxygen levels will vary directly with changes in cardiac output. This is the rationale for using mixed venous (pulmonary artery) oxygen saturation to monitor changes in cardiac output:

$$S_vO_2 = S_aO_2 - (Vo_2/\dot{Q} \times Hb \times 13)$$

### Causes of low mixed venous oxygen

- Hypoxaemia
- Increased metabolic rate
- Low cardiac output
- Anaemia.

### Causes of high mixed venous oxygen

- Decreased $O_2$ uptake, e.g. hypothermia, cell poisoning

- Left-to-right shunt
- Inappropriately high cardiac output, e.g. excessive use of inotropes/vasodilators.

$S_vO_2$ usually reflects cardiac output, but in seriously ill patients unable to mount a compensatory response to low blood flow, $S_vO_2$ will change little in response to changes in cardiac output. Thus, these patients show little correlation between venous oxygen and cardiac index.

## LACTIC ACID

When the metabolic rate exceeds the rate of oxygen supply, tissues will switch to anaerobic metabolism and produce lactic acid. Therefore, the serum lactate concentration reflects the balance between $VO_2$ and the metabolic demand for oxygen.

Lactate is the end-product of anaerobic glycolysis, but it is also produced under normal aerobic conditions. The lactate anion is cleared by the liver and used for gluconeogenesis. Renal clearance becomes significant once levels reach 6–7 mEq/l. Hepatic failure probably contributes little to raised lactate levels in critically ill patients. A normal serum lactate does not exclude tissue ischaemia.

Raised lactate levels not associated with organ ischaemia are found with bacterial pneumonia, thiamine deficiency, generalized seizures, respiratory alkalosis and generalized trauma.

### References

Shoemaker W C 1994 Monitoring and therapy for young trauma patients. Critical Care Medicine 22: 548–549

Soni N, Fawcett W J, Halliday F C 1993 Beyond the lung: oxygen delivery and tissue oxygenation. Anaesthesia 48: 704–711

Yu M, Burchell S, Hasaniya N W et al 1998 Relationship of mortality to increasing oxygen delivery in patients > or = 50 years of age: a prospective, randomized trial. Critical Care Medicine 26: 1011–1019

## RENAL REPLACEMENT THERAPY

In patients with severe acute renal failure, renal excretory function is lost. Resolution may take several weeks during which catabolism is marked, producing increased amounts of waste products. Requirements for intravascular space arise from intravenous drugs, fluids and feeding.

Renal replacement therapy therefore aims to remove excess water and remove unwanted solutes.

**Normal kidney**

- filters 180 l/day
- filters solutes weighing < 60 000 Da
- reabsorbs 99% filtrate.

Urea is the waste product of protein metabolism (60 Da). Creatinine is the waste product of muscle metabolism (113 Da).

## IMMEDIATE MANAGEMENT OF OLIGURIA/ACUTE RENAL FAILURE

- Assess and treat any circulatory impairment
- Assess and treat any respiratory impairment
- Treat any acute manifestations if acute renal failure (salt and water retention, hypertension, hyperkalaemia, acidosis)
- Exclude urinary tract obstruction or infection
- Establish underlying cause and begin treatment as soon as possible
- Ensure patient is not taking nephrotoxic drugs.

## INDICATIONS FOR DIALYSIS

### Absolute

- $K^+ > 6.5$ mmol/l
- Pulmonary oedema unresponsive to diuretics
- Uraemic encephalopathy / pericarditis / neuropathy.

### Relative

- Urea > 35 mmol/l
- Creatinine > 600 mmol/l
- Oliguria (< 5 ml/kg per day)
- Metabolic acidosis (pH < 7.2)
- To create intravascular volume for feeding, drugs etc.
- Hyperpyrexia.

## HISTORY

Intermittent haemofiltration was introduced in the 1950s and remained the only form of renal replacement therapy until the introduction of intermittent haemodialysis in 1967. Technical problems delayed the introduction of continuous techniques until the 1980s with continuous arteriovenous haemofiltration (CAVH) followed by continuous arteriovenous haemo-diafiltration (CAVHD).

### Filters

- Clear molecules < 60 000 Da

- Filter surface area approx 70 m$^2$
- Low resistance to enable high flow.

## PRINCIPLES

### Water removal

Water is removed by a process called ultrafiltration. This process is similar to that performed by the glomerulus in the kidney. It requires a hydrostatic driving force to overcome oncotic pressure and move water across a semi-permeable membrane.

In the artificial kidney, this can be achieved by:

- applying a positive pressure (patient's blood pressure/pump pressure) across a semi-permeable membrane
- using a hyperosmolar solution (e.g. peritoneal dialysis)
- applying a negative pressure to the dialysate side of the membrane (e.g. haemodialysis).

### Solute removal

This can be achieved by either diffusion or ultrafiltration.

*Diffusion across a semi-permeable membrane.* This is movement of solutes across a semi-permeable membrane from an area of high concentration to one of low concentration. A concentration gradient is therefore always necessary for diffusion to occur. Molecules of a smaller MW will move across the membrane more readily than those with a larger MW (Fig. 7.6). A semi-permeable membrane has a defined pore size; any molecule exceeding this will not be able to pass through.

This is the principle utilized for dialysis.

*Ultrafiltration* (convective transport) is the bulk movement of water molecules containing permeable solutes through a semi-permeable membrane (Fig. 7.7). Water molecules are small and can pass through all semi-permeable membranes. The driving force for ultrafiltration can be either an osmotic gradient or hydrostatic pressure. Haemofiltration is based on the principle of ultrafiltration.

The volume of filtrate removed can be in excess of 2 l/h, and to maintain CVS stability, fluid must be replaced concurrently. The fluid used as replacement should be isotonic and should aim to replace the solutes lost as filtrate that would otherwise be selectively reabsorbed by the 'normal' kidney

## TYPES OF FILTRATION CIRCUIT

### Continuous arteriovenous haemofiltration (CAVH) (Fig. 7.8a)

Blood flows from an artery (A) into the filter to produce an ultrafiltrate

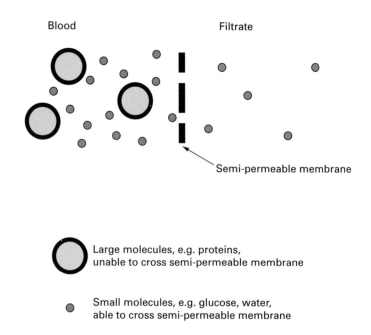

Fig. 7.6 Diffusion across a semi-permeable membrane.

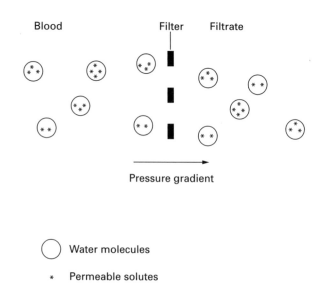

Fig. 7.7 Ultrafiltration through a semi-permeable membrane.

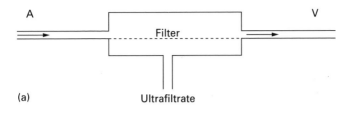

(a)

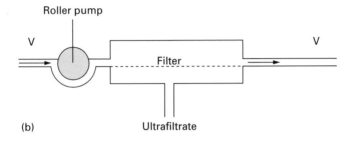

(b)

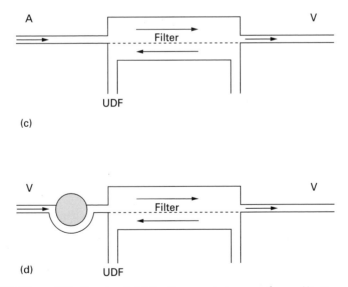

(c)

(d)

**Fig. 7.8** Types of filtration circuit. (a) Continuous arteriovenous haemofiltration (CAVH). (b) Continuous venovenous haemofiltration (CVVH). (c) Continuous arteriovenous haemodiafiltration (CAVHD). (d) Continuous venovenous haemodiafiltration (CVVHD).

before return to the body via a vein (V). Used as an intermittent technique, this was the earliest method of renal replacement therapy. A systolic BP > 90 mmHg is adequate for a driving pressure.

### Continuous venovenous haemofiltration (CVVH) (Fig. 7.8b)

A similar technique to CAVH, except that because venous pressure is inadequate to overcome resistance of a filter and circuit tubing, a roller pump is used to generate a perfusing pressure. This is a commonly used technique in ITU patients.

### Continuous arteriovenous haemodiafiltration (CAVHD) (Fig. 7.8c)

The circuit is the same as that for CAVH, but ultrafiltrate is added as a countercurrent across the membrane to generate diffusive and convective clearance. This produces an ultradiafiltrate (UDF).

### Continuous venovenous haemodiafiltration (CVVHD) (Fig. 7.8d)

This is the same circuit as for CVVH but with the addition of dialysate to increase clearance of waste products.

## FACTORS AFFECTING THE EFFICACY OF HAEMOFILTRATION

- Driving pressure
- Blood flow rate
- Haematocrit
- Oncotic pressure (glucose, protein)
- Arterial/venous access/flow
- Height of filter in relation to:
  — heart (CAVH)
  — filtrate collection bag
- Countercurrent dialysis
- Filter surface area.

  Filtration may be increased by:

- improving arterial flow from access site
- CVVH – increasing pump speed (normal range 150–250 ml/min)
- CAVH – increasing cardiac output
- adding suction to filter
- increasing anticoagulation
- changing filter if volumes are poor.

## INTERMITTENT VERSUS CONTINUOUS FILTRATION

Fluid removal in intermittent dialysis has to occur over a short period of time, but if it is too rapid or too large a volume, hypotension will result. A longer duration of dialysis at a lesser ultrafiltration rate is more appropriate for ITU patients, who are often haemodynamically unstable.

Intermittent dialysis is less effective than continuous dialysis because waste products and water in the interstitial compartment do not have time to equilibrate with blood. Following a short period of dialysis, urea and creatinine levels are initially low, but will rise relatively quickly as these waste products equilibrate with the lower levels in the blood.

Intermittent, large-volume dialysis also risks a disequilibrium syndrome in which a relatively high intracellular concentration of urea and creatinine following dialysis causes an osmotic effect, drawing water into cells.

Techniques using dialysate fluid reduce the chance of electrolyte imbalance as serum electrolyte levels equilibrate with the dialysate fluid; for example, if the dialysate fluid's $K^+$ is 4.6 mmol/L and the serum $K^+$ falls below that level, $K^+$ will diffuse across the membrane until the level reaches 4.6 mmol/L. Equally, the reverse would happen if the patient's level was greater than that of the dialysate.

## VASCULAR ACCESS

- *Arterial*
  - — large-bore single-lumen catheter
  - — cutdown and direct arterial cannulation
  - — exiting AV shunt (Cimino) fistula
- *Venous*
  - — double-lumen catheter
  - — large-bore single-lumen catheter.

## ANTICOAGULATION

Contact of blood with plastic surfaces and filter activates clotting cascade. Anticoagulation is therefore required to prevent thrombus deposition in the circuit. Usually with heparin (5–10 u/kg per h), aiming to keep APTR 2.0–2.5. Prostacyclin (2.5–10 ng/kg per min) may be used as an alternative to prevent heparin-induced thrombocytopenia, but it can cause hypotension.

Many ITU patients have coagulopathies and do not require further anti-coagulation.

## POTENTIAL PROBLEMS

- Arterial/venous access
- Infection
- Bleeding
- Heat loss
- Emboli – air/thrombus

- Disconnection
- Intravascular fluid depletion
- Drug/colloid clearance.

## DRUG CLEARANCE

The effect of renal failure and renal replacement therapy on drug levels is variable and difficult to predict. Many factors affect drug levels in these patients, such as whether the drug is normally eliminated entirely or partly by renal excretion and the effect of plasma protein levels (often low) on drug binding. For many drugs with minor or no side-effects, no modification to dose is required. For more toxic drugs with a low therapeutic index, monitoring of drug levels is required. The loading dose should be the same as that used in a patient with normal renal function, but subsequent doses should be given according to drug levels. It is important to try to avoid nephrotoxic drugs in patients with renal failure, or if they are used, care should be taken to prevent doses reaching nephrotoxic levels.

Elimination of aminoglycosides, vancomycin, aminophylline and digoxin is greatly reduced in patients with renal failure; they require dosing based on drug levels to prevent toxicity.

### References

Mallick N P, Gokal R 1999 Haemodialysis. Lancet 353: 737–742
Short A, Cumming A 1999 ABC of intensive care. Renal support. British Medical Journal 319: 41–44

# SCORING SYSTEMS

## PROBLEMS OF PREDICTIVE SCORING SYSTEMS

*Physiological reserve.*  Prior health is an important predictor of outcome in acute illness. Best correlation with age.

*Selection bias.*  Errors in predictive power if patients used to create the database are different to those being evaluated.

*Lead-time bias.*  Patients delayed in their arrival to ITU may fare worse than those admitted earlier, despite having the same disease.

## APACHE (ACUTE PHYSIOLOGY AND CHRONIC HEALTH EVALUATION)

Designed to predict outcome in groups of ITU patients, such as risk of death, ICU length of stay, type and amount of therapy, and nursing intensity. Standardized mortality rate (actual vs. predicted mortality rate) can also be used to assess unit performance. Daily APACHE risk predictions are a precise measure of the patient's condition and may aid in patient treatment decisions. An increasing score is associated with increasing risk of death.

APACHE I was developed in 1981 based on 34 variables, age and previous health. Criticisms that it considered unmeasured variables as normal and that it involved too many variables led to the development of APACHE II in 1985.

APACHE II was simplified to 12 physiological variables, age and chronic health evaluation and one of 34 admission diagnoses. Its main criticisms are failure to compensate for lead-time bias and the ability to select only one diagnostic criterion. This led to poor performance when applied to trauma victims, patients receiving TPN, severely ill postoperative patients, patients with myocardial infarction and those with congestive cardiac failure.

APACHE III was developed in 1991 and is now based on multiple regression values from a database of approximately 300 000 patients.

The APACHE III system consists of three scores:

- age – maximum score 24 points
- chronic health evaluation – maximum score 23 points
- acute physiology score – 17 variables using the worst value in 24 h, giving a maximum score of 252 points. The variables are:

| | | |
|---|---|---|
| Mean blood pressure | Respiratory rate | Temperature |
| Pulse | Glasgow Coma Scale | Urine output |
| Haematocrit | White cell count | Blood pH |
| $P_aO_2$ | $P_aCO_2$ | Serum sodium |
| Serum albumin | Serum bilirubin | Serum glucose |
| Serum creatinine | Blood urea nitrogen | |

The total APACHE score is then determined by the total of the above three categories multiplied by a specific weight for one of 78 diagnostic categories. APACHE III also allows estimation of length of ICU stay, amount and type of therapy required and the intensity of nursing care. In a sample of 37 668 ICU admissions, it has been shown to predict hospital mortality accurately.

## TISS (THERAPEUTIC INTERVENTION SCORING SYSTEM)

Scores the severity of illness by analysing degree of nursing care required in a 24-h period. Each therapeutic intervention is scored from 1 to 4, e.g. PA catheter monitoring, transfusion of blood products, inotropic support etc. Total score is used to calculate severity of illness, required staff:patient ratio and costs of patient care.

## MORTALITY PROBABILITY MODEL (MPM)

Predicts probability of hospital mortality on admission to ITU before treatment is commenced ($MPM_0$) and after 24 h of treatment ($MPM_{24}$).

$MPM_0$ is based on 13 variables, with $MPM_{24}$ based on seven of these variables plus another eight to allow assessment of the effects of ICU treatment. It does not require a diagnosis. Now revised to the MPM II model following analysis of 12 610 patients treated in 139 ICUs in 12 countries. MPM II coefficients have been developed for patients at 48 and 72 h. These have shown that if a patient's physiological condition is remaining static, the patient is actually deteriorating with a decreasing chance of survival.

## SIMPLIFIED ACUTE PHYSIOLOGY SCORE (SAPS)

SAPS II is based on 12 997 patients from 137 European centres. It uses 12 physiological variables, age, type of admission and three underlying disease variables. The risk of death is estimated without having to specify an underlying diagnosis. It appears to be one of the most accurate systems for estimating the risk of mortality.

### References

Beck D H, Taylor B L, Millar B, Smith G B 1997 Prediction of outcome from intensive care: a prospective cohort study comparing Acute Physiology and Chronic Health Evaluation II and III prognostic systems in a United Kingdom intensive care unit. Critical Care Medicine 25: 9–15

Le Gall J R, Lemeshow S, Saulnier F 1993 A new Simplified Acute Physiology Score (SAPS II) based on a European/North American multicenter study. Journal of the American Medical Association 270: 2957–2963

Le Gall J R 1994 Scoring systems and prognostic indexes. Current Opinion in Anaesthesiology 7: 166–168

Lemeshow S, Teres D, Klar J, Avrunin J S, Gehlbach S H, Rapoport J 1993 Mortality Probability Models (MPM II) based on an international cohort of intensive care patients. Journal of the American Medical Association 270: 2478–2486

Ridley S 1998 Severity of illness scoring systems and performance appraisal. Anaesthesia 53: 1185–1194

Steele A, Bocconi G A, Oggioni R, Tulli G 1998 Scoring systems in intensive care. Current Anaesthesia and Critical Care 9: 8–15

Tunnell R D, Millar B W, Smith G B 1998 The effect of lead time bias on severity of illness scoring, mortality prediction and standardised mortality ratio in intensive care – a pilot study. Anaesthesia 53: 1045–1053

Zimmerman J E, Wagner D P, Draper E A, Wright L et al 1998 Evaluation of Acute Physiology and Chronic Health Evaluation III predictions of hospital mortality in an independent database. Critical Care Medicine 26: 1317–1326

## SEDATION

## AIMS

- To reduce awareness and stress of the patient in intensive care
- To facilitate treatment, e.g. ventilation and weaning, physiotherapy

- To reduce awareness during invasive or painful procedures
- To aid management of acute confusional and withdrawal states.

Consider whether better analgesia would reduce sedation requirements, the effects of disease pathology on pharmacokinetics and unwanted side-effects of the sedative drugs. Sedative drugs must have a short half-life, enabling rapid reversal to assess the patient.

### Side-effects of sedation

- Impaired respiratory effort, if excessive
- Accumulation of active metabolites in hepatic / renal failure
- Altered sleep patterns may paradoxically produce sleep deprivation
- Paralytic ileus
- Withdrawal symptoms when the drug is stopped.

## SEDATIVE DRUGS

*Opioids.* Dependence does not occur when used for short-term pain relief. Morphine and pethidine result in accumulation of metabolites (morphine 6-glucuronide and norpethidine, respectively). Alfentanyl has the shortest half-life of all opioids. Beware of side-effects, particularly respiratory depression, decreased cough reflex, gastric stasis and hypotension.

*Benzodiazepines.* Cause anxiolysis, sleep, amnesia and muscle relaxation. Diazepam is unsuitable because of accumulation of long-acting metabolites (desmethyldiazepam). Midazolam has a shorter duration of action and is metabolized to inactive metabolites. Accumulation of midazolam and opioids may result in prolonged sedation on cessation of the infusion.

*Propofol.* Approved for sedation of ITU patients. Propofol allows regular waking of the patient to assess neurological status. If the patient is well filled and the infusion rate titrated carefully, hypotension is not usually a problem. Propofol has also been shown to decrease $O_2$ requirements and decrease requirements for vasodilators in hypertensive patients. Also used on ITU for patient-controlled sedation. Propofol infusion for sedation at 25–75 $\mu g$ / kg per min.

*Ketamine.* May be useful for bronchodilator properties in sedation of asthmatics and analgesic properties for sedation of burns patients. Fewer hallucinations if combined with benzodiazepine infusion.

*Volatile agents.* Isoflurane has been studied as a sedative agent but it is expensive, requires low flow circle systems and scavenging.

## ASSESSING SEDATION

*Scoring systems, e.g. Ramsay sedation score*
1 – patient anxious, restless or agitated
2 – patient cooperative, orientated and calm

3 – patient responds to commands only
4 – brisk response
5 – sluggish response
6 – no response.

*Plasma drug concentrations.* But interpatient variation in pharmacodynamics and it does not take into account levels of active metabolites.

*EEG.* Difficult to interpret and correlates poorly with depth of sedation. Different drugs alter the EEG in different ways.

*Lower oesophageal contractility.* Wide variation between patients and between drugs.

*Evoked responses.* Lack of agent specificity.

*Sinus arrhythmia.* Reflects autonomic activity. Being investigated as a monitor of depth of sedation.

### References

Peruzzi W T 1997 Sedation of the critically ill: goals, plans and cost effectiveness. Critical Care Medicine 25: 1942

Shelly M P 1994 Assessing sedation. Care of the Critically Ill 10: 118–121

Szalados J E, Boysen P G 1998 Sedation in the critically ill patient. Current Opinion in Anaesthesiology 11: 147–155

Willatts S M, Spencer E M 1994 Sedation for ventilation in the critically ill. Anaesthesia 49: 422–428

## SYSTEMIC INFLAMMATORY RESPONSE SYNDROME

The systemic inflammatory response syndrome (SIRS) and multiple organ dysfunction syndrome (MODS) are two recently introduced terms aimed at facilitating standardization of terminology for research into critically ill patients. The systemic inflammatory response is triggered by sepsis, burns, trauma or hypovolaemia, and may be driven by bacterial and endotoxin translocation across an ischaemic, damaged gut (Fig. 7.9).

SIRS is defined as the presence of two or more of the following:

- temperature > 38°C or < 36°C.
- heart rate > 90/min.
- tachypnoea > 20/min.
- leucocytosis < $4 \times 10^9/l$ or > $12 \times 10^9/l$.

Inflammatory mediators include:

- stress hormones – steroids, catecholamines, insulin, glucagon, growth hormone

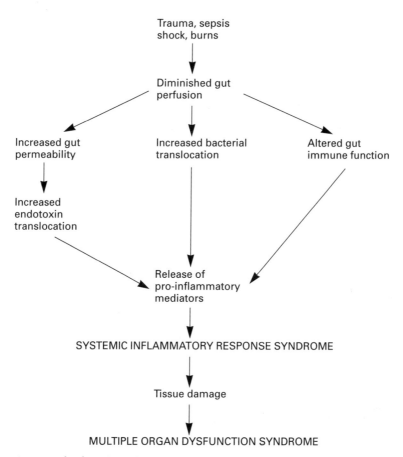

**Fig. 7.9** Pathophysiology of systemic inflammatory response syndrome (SIRS) and multiple organ dysfunction syndrome (MODS).

- archidonic acid derivatives – interleukins, prostaglandins, thromboxanes, leucotrienes
- histamine, serotonin, neuropeptides, myocardial depressant factor
- macrophage-derived growth factor, platelet-activating factor.

Multiple organ dysfunction syndrome (MODS) frequently develops in previously healthy patients following resuscitation from the initial insult. It is commonly associated with sepsis, trauma, ARDS and acute renal failure. Pathophysiology involves tissue hypoperfusion with a failure of $O_2$ supply, intense inflammatory mediator activity, tissue catabolism, activation of leucocytes, macrophages and platelets and ischaemia-reperfusion injury. If the resulting cellular dysfunction is of sufficient magnitude, cell death occurs.

MODS develops as a progressive deterioration of two or more organ systems, usually cardiovascular, respiratory, renal, hepatic, gastrointestinal or haematological, to a state in which the organ cannot maintain homeostasis without intervention. Risk factors for the development of MODS include the severity of pathology at the time of ITU admission, presence of sepsis at the time of ITU admission and age.

### References

Blackwell T S 1996 Sepsis and cytokines: current status. British Journal of Anaesthesia 77: 110–117

Galley H F, Webster N R 1996 The immuno-inflammatory cascade. British Journal of Anaesthesia 77: 11–16

Marik P E 1998 Total splanchnic resuscitation, SIRS, and MODS. Critical Care Medicine 27: 257

Muckart D J, Bhagwanjee S 1997 American College of Chest Physicians/Society of Critical Care Medicine Consensus Conference definitions of the systemic inflammatory response syndrome and allied disorders in relation to critically injured patients. Critical Care Medicine 25: 1789–1795

Sheeran P, Hall G M 1997 Cytokines in anaesthesia. British Medical Journal 78: 201–219

# 8. Obstetrics

## REGIONAL ANAESTHESIA FOR OBSTETRICS

Epidurals give excellent/satisfactory analgesia in 91% of mothers. Increased use of regional techniques probably accounts for the continuing reduction in maternal mortality by avoiding risks of failed intubation and aspiration.

Table 8.1 Advantages and disadvantages of epidural anaesthesia

| Advantages | Disadvantages |
| --- | --- |
| Maternal participation at delivery | May take too long to perform if there is fetal distress |
| Avoids risk of failed intubation | Hypotension |
| Reduced risk of aspiration | Risk of patchy, incomplete block |
| Avoids morbidity from GA drugs | Backache |
| Avoids risk of awareness | Urinary retention |
| Earlier breast feeding | |
| Good postoperative analgesia | |
| Less postnatal depression | |

### INDICATIONS FOR EPIDURAL

- Slow or painful labour
- Pregnancy-induced hypertension
- Cardiac or respiratory disease
- Premature or high risk fetus
- Multiple pregnancy
- Breech delivery
- Trial of labour.

### PAIN PATHWAYS (Fig. 8.1)

- *First stage*
  - — pain due to cervical dilatation and uterine contractions
  - — pain transmitted via uterine sympathetic nerves to $T_{10}$–$T_{12}$
  - — some transmission via tubo-ovarian vessels

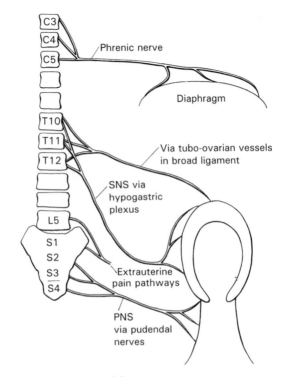

**Fig. 8.1** Pain pathways during labour.

- *Second stage*
  — pain due to vaginal and perineal stretching and tearing
  — pain transmitted via pudendal nerves to $S_2$–$S_4$.

Extrauterine pelvic structures supplied by $L_5$/$S_1$. Particularly stimulated by the fetal head in the occipitoposterior position to cause backache.

LSCS stimulates sensory nerves to $T_{10}$ in addition to phrenic. Aim to block from $T_8$ to $S_5$.

Aortocaval compression may occur from 20 weeks onwards. In the presence of acute blood loss, cardiovascular compensation may be seriously impaired if the block is extensive. Delivery of the baby relieves the compression.

## EPIDURAL TEST DOSE

Recommended to avoid complications of inadvertent intravenous injection of bupivacaine. Usually use a dose insufficient to cause total spinal anaesthesia if injected into the intrathecal space.

### Catecholamines

Addition of adrenaline (> 15 $\mu$g) or isoprenaline to the test dose may cause tachycardia within 1 min following intravenous injection. However, this sign may be unreliable because pregnancy may alter physiological changes to catecholamines and the pain of contraction may also cause sudden tachycardia. Catecholamines have also been shown to reduce placental blood flow in animal studies. Therefore, their use is controversial. If used, give between contractions and avoid in hypertensive or pre-eclamptic patients.

### Opioids

The addition of 100 $\mu$g fentanyl to a test dose has been reported as a reliable indicator of intravascular injection by causing sedation and altered perception.

### Air

Air (1 ml) injected intravenously and detected by parasternal Doppler has been proposed as an effective marker of inadvertent intravenous injection. There appear to be no adverse maternal or fetal effects from this small dose of air.

## FETAL AND MATERNAL EFFECTS OF EPIDURALS

- Improve coordination of uterine contraction by reducing noradrenaline levels
- Relief of pain reduces maternal hyperventilation
- Improve placental blood flow in pre-eclampsia and reduce fetal acidosis in the second stage of labour
- Fetal acidosis accelerates transfer of LA across placenta
- General anaesthesia is associated with lower Apgar scores at 1 min compared with regional techniques, but both techniques have similar scores by 5 minutes. Therefore, use a regional technique if possible when delivering a baby with fetal distress, but remember further fetal deterioration may occur whilst epidural is inserted.

See 'Epidural and spinal anaesthesia' for further details (p. 292).

### References

Birnbach D J, Chestnut D H 1999 The epidural test dose in obstetric patients: has it outlived its usefulness? Anesthesia and Analgesia 88: 971–972

Capogna G, Celleno D 1998 Regional blocks for cesarean section. Current Opinion in Anaesthesiology 11: 507–509

Crowhurst J A 1994 Analgesia for labour. Current Opinion in Anaesthesiology 7: 224–230

Santos A, Pedersen H 1994 Current controversies in obstetric anesthesia. Anesthesia and Analgesia 78: 753–760

# OBSTETRICS

## ANAESTHESIA FOR NON-OBSTETRIC SURGERY DURING PREGNANCY

1% of patients require GA during pregnancy. In the first trimester, there is a risk of organogenesis; in the third trimester there is a risk of premature labour. Therefore, the second trimester is the safest.

In descending order of preference:

- spinal – method of choice
- epidural – higher doses of LA required and block less effective
- other regional blocks
- combined epidural and GA – lower doses of inhalational agents and narcotics, good postoperative analgesia and can avoid $N_2O$
- GA (NB – delayed gastric emptying present from first trimester onwards).

*Known teratogenic drugs in humans include:*

- tetracycline – bone defects, dental enamel staining
- warfarin – bone malformations
- alcohol – craniofacial abnormalities
- thalidomide – limb abnormalities
- synthetic progestagens – masculinization of female genitalia
- cocaine
- ACE inhibitors
- possibly diazepam.

## EFFECT OF ANAESTHESIA AND SURGERY ON THE FETUS DURING LSCS

- Maternal catecholamine levels are lower with epidural/spinal than with GA.
- IPPV lowers cardiac output and reduces placental flow, especially with hypovolaemia. Minimize effects by reducing mean intrathoracic pressure.
- Hyperventilation shifts maternal $O_2$ dissociation curve to the left, reducing placental $O_2$ transfer and umbilical blood flow, and causes fetal

acidosis. Slight maternal hypercapnia may benefit the fetus by improving oxygen delivery.

• Maternal $P_aO_2 < 13$ kPa reduces fetal oxygenation and delays onset of spontaneous ventilation in the newborn. A maternal $F_iO_2 > 0.65$ was shown to improve Apgar scores and reduce fetal acidosis at delivery, but the study did not control for aortocaval compression or $F_iN_2O$.

• Aortocaval compression occurs in 15% of women at term. When lying supine, the pregnant uterus at term almost completely obstructs the inferior vena cava. Reduced with lateral tilt, more effective to the left.

• Degree of fetal acidosis on delivery is related to the time from uterine incision to delivery. Induction–delivery time has little effect on acidosis if using left lateral tilt.

## EFFECT OF ANAESTHETIC DRUGS ON THE FETUS DURING LSCS

• Placental transfer of drugs is influenced by protein binding, high lipid solubility, low ionization and kPa.

• Fetus is not anaesthetized by i.v. induction agents because hepatic extraction and dilution of drugs with blood from the lower limbs and upper body reduce the concentration of drug delivered to the fetal CNS.

• Injection of induction agent at the onset of a contraction reduces the dose delivered to the fetus. Fetal plasma levels of induction agents follow the same pattern as in adults by 2–3 min.

• Thiopentone reduces placental blood flow and may reduce fetal $O_2$ delivery. Ketamine increases placental flow, but increased force of uterine contraction may worsen cord prolapse or abruptio placentae.

• $N_2O$ may reach equilibrium in the fetus with a possible risk of diffusion hypoxia in the fetus upon delivery which should therefore have $O_2$. There is no evidence of methionine synthetase depression when $N_2O$ is used for LSCS. Less than 1.0 MAC halothane, enflurane or isoflurane does not increase perioperative blood loss and is not detrimental to the fetus. Minimal fetal fluoride levels with enflurane.

• Neuromuscular blocking drugs are large highly ionized molecules with minimal placental transfer. However, fetal paralysis has been reported following extremely high doses of non-depolarizing drugs, e.g. when given in error. Suxamethonium administration to patients with homozygous plasma cholinesterase deficiency may result in fetal paralysis.

• Opioids rapidly cross the placenta to achieve fetal levels equal to those of the mother. Fentanyl 1 $\mu$g/kg at induction does not affect fetal Apgar score, neurobehavioural scores or acid–base status. Opioids may reduce the maternal stress response and lessen catecholamine-induced placental vasoconstriction.

## CARDIOTOCOGRAPH

• Type I decelerations (early) – head compression causing vagal reflex

- Type II decelerations (late) – uteroplacental insufficiency
- Type III decelerations (variable) – umbilical cord compression.

## FAILED INTUBATION

Difficult intubation occurs in 1:300 (1:2000 in normal population). More common in Africans and Afro-Caribbeans.

It is the commonest cause of anaesthetic-related maternal deaths (it is not failure of intubation but subsequent failure of oxygenation that kills). Difficult intubation is due to left lateral tilt, increased weight, increased breast size, full dentition, laryngeal oedema, incorrect application of cricoid pressure, minimum dose of induction agent and attempted intubation before onset of neuromuscular blockade.

Perform no more than three attempts at intubation. Know the failed intubation drill which is being modified in many hospitals to use the laryngeal mask (but maintain cricoid pressure, which reduces aspiration risk and stops gastric distension if the patient is being bagged).

## ASPIRATION

### Incidence

In 1946 Mendelson described an asthma-like syndrome in 0.15% of deliveries using GA by mask due to aspiration of gastric contents. In more recent studies, the incidence of pulmonary aspiration syndrome is reported as 0.01%. More common with coughing during direct laryngoscopy and emergency surgery, even with cricoid pressure.

### Symptoms

63% of patients who aspirate are asymptomatic. Commonest symptoms are cough, bronchospasm, hypoxaemia and X-ray changes.

### Gastric volumes

It is traditionally taught that > 0.4 ml/kg aspirate of pH < 2.5 is needed to cause symptoms, but these figures were based on a study from a single Rhesus monkey. Now thought to be a larger volume of at least 0.8 ml/kg.

### Prophylaxis

30 ml 0.3 M sodium citrate has replaced magnesium-based antacids, which did not mix with gastric contents and caused pneumonitis themselves if aspirated. Also give $H_2$ antagonist (not cimetidine, which increases blood levels of bupivacaine) and gastric prokinetic, e.g. metoclopramide. Avoid prolonged fasting which is associated with increasing gastric volume and

decreased pH. Anticholinergics only inhibit vagal stimulation and have little effect on gastric pH.

### Anaesthetic manoeuvres reducing risk

Pre-oxygenation, rapid sequence induction with cricoid pressure (44 N), avoid bagging following suxamethonium, avoid attempts at intubation before patient is fully paralysed and extubate awake.

### Postpartum

Assuming no opioids are present, rate of emptying, gastric pH and volume of stomach contents rapidly return to normal values within about 6–8 hours. However, reflux (80% of women at term) may persist for up to 48 hours. Therefore, anti-aspiration measures necessary for 48 hours postpartum.

## PREGNANCY-INDUCED HYPERTENSION

### Incidence

- Pre-eclampsia – 5% all pregnancies
- Eclampsia – 0.05% all pregnancies.

### Associations

Associated with positive family history, young primiparous, elderly, multiparous, diabetes, pre-existing hypertension, renal disease and collagen vascular disease. There is some evidence to suggest that there is an autosomal recessive predisposition to an immune response within the placenta.

Characterized by a *triad* of:

- *hypertension* – ↑ BP > 30/15mmHg; ↑ systolic above 160 mmHg,
  ↑ diastolic > 15 mmHg
- *oedema*
- *proteinuria* – > 0.3 mg/kg; severe > 5 g/day.

### Pathophysiology

Thought to be triggered by an autoimmune reaction against the placenta (Fig. 8.2).

*Airway.* Facial and laryngeal oedema may make intubation difficult. Consider awake fibreoptic intubation in elective patients undergoing GA.

*Cardiovascular.*  In untreated patients, cardiac index (CI) is low/normal, SVR is normal/high and PCWP is low/normal due to contraction of intravascular volume by as much as 30–40% in severe cases. Fluid challenge may improve cardiovascular stability, increase CI and reduce SVR to more normal levels. PCWP becomes normal/high, but CVP correlates poorly.

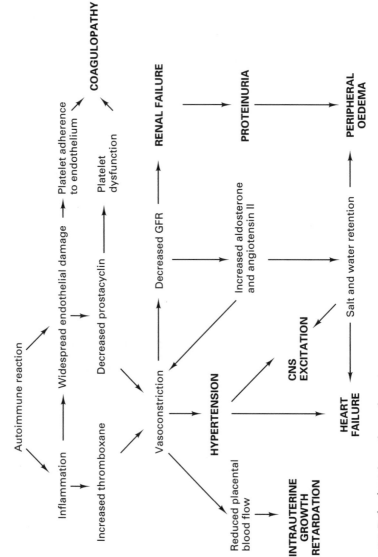

**Fig. 8.2** Pathophysiology of pre-eclampsia.

Consider invasive monitoring if oliguria persists following 500 ml fluid challenge.

Treat hypertension with hydralazine 5–10 mg i.v. boluses or 5–40 mg/h infusion. Causes headache, tremor and vomiting, mimicking symptoms of eclampsia. Also consider labetolol up to 1 mg/kg (reports of fetal bradycardia if used in the presence of fetal distress) or sodium nitroprusside 0.3–8 μg/kg/min. Nifedipine may cause severe hypotension if used with magnesium.

*Central nervous system.* Cerebral vasospasm, microinfarcts, petechial haemorrhage and oedema cause CNS irritability, visual disturbance and headache. May be worsened by hypertension following pressor response to intubation. Fits are more common in teenage mothers and multiple pregnancies. CNS haemorrhage is a major cause of maternal deaths.

Treat CNS irritability with magnesium sulphate 4 g loading dose then 1–3 g/h which suppresses EEG excitatory activity, aiming for therapeutic blood level of 2–4 mmol/l. Titrate against deep tendon reflexes. Also vasodilates uterine vessels and attenuates uterine vascular response to catecholamines. May accumulate in renal failure. Excess (> 4mmol/l) causes respiratory paralysis, heart block and fetal weakness. Treat with calcium gluconate 1 g i.v.

*Coagulation.* Thrombocytopenia < 100 000 is common. Normal platelet counts are associated with prolonged bleeding times in 10–25% of pre-eclamptics; 34% of patients with severe eclampsia have prolonged bleeding times. Low-grade DIC is common.

Recent Collaborative Low Dose Aspirin Study (CLASP) cast doubt on the efficacy of aspirin in reducing the incidence of pre-eclampsia.

*Hepatic.* Abnormal LFTs due to oedema and hepatic congestion. Associated with HELLP syndrome (Haemolysis, Elevated Liver enzymes, Low Platelets).

*Renal.* Decreased glomerular filtration, acute tubular necrosis and increased permeability to proteins causing proteinuria.

### Anaesthetic management

*Epidurals.* Are best established early and are the technique of choice for labour or LSCS in pre-eclamptic toxaemia (PET). Advantages are better control of blood pressure and improved uteroplacental flow, with avoidance of intubation risks from laryngeal oedema. Epidurals do not alter cardiac output as long as hydration is maintained. Antihypertensive drugs may be augmented by the epidural but the use of ephedrine may result in rebound hypertension.

Spinals are best avoided because of risks of sudden refractory hypotension and unpredictable spread.

Platelet count < 100 000, abnormal clotting or prolonged bleeding time is a relative contraindication to regional anaesthesia.

*General anaesthesia.* Probably safer than an epidural if there is severe hypertension, uncorrected hypovolaemia, fetal distress, coagulopathy or risk of convulsions. Short-acting antihypertensive drugs may be necessary to prevent intubation-induced hypertension, which causes CVA, pulmonary oedema and reduced placental blood flow. Beware of laryngeal oedema. Magnesium increases sensitivity to non-depolarizing neuromuscular blockers by inhibiting presynaptic calcium-facilitated neurotransmitter release.

*Postoperative.* Pre-eclampsia may not begin to resolve until 3–4 days post-delivery. Therefore monitor BP and urine output carefully; 60% of patients who develop pulmonary oedema do so > 48 h after delivery.

---

### GUIDELINES FOR OBSTETRIC ANAESTHESIA SERVICES
Association of Anaesthetists of Great Britain and Ireland and the Obstetric Anaesthetists Association 1998

Anaesthetists are involved in as many as 60% of labours in some units, demonstrating the importance of anaesthetists in maternity care.

1. **Staffing of units.** Each obstetric unit should have a nominated consultant in charge of obstetric anaesthesia. A consultant anaesthetist should be on call and responsible for the unit at all times. A duty anaesthetist and resuscitation team shold be availble at all times.
2. **Regional anaesthesia service.** Ideally, units should be able to provide a regional anaesthesia service on request at all times. The duty anaesthetist is responsible for the regional block; the midwife is responsible for providing care and monitoring of the mother for the duration of the epidural.
3. **Acceptable anaesthesia response times.** If it is essential for the anaesthetist to leave the patient to deal with a life-threatening emergency nearby, he/she should instruct another person to observe the patient's vital signs and should delegate overall responsibility to another registered medical practitioner. Anaesthetic response to fetal distress should be less than 30 minutes and may need to be much less. Anaesthetic response to a request for an epidural should ideally not exceed 30 minutes.
4. **Monitoring of the mother and fetus with regional anaesthesia.** BP and pulse should be recorded every 5 minutes for the first 20 minutes and at least every 30 minutes throughout labour. The midwife may be asked by the anaesthetist to perform hourly assessments of motor and sensory levels. The anaesthetist should assess the woman at regular intervals throughout the duration of regional anaesthesia. Attending the woman only when called by the midwife is not sufficient.
5. **Anaesthesia for caesarian delivery.** The patient should be visited by the anaesthetist preoperatively if possible. When elective cases

are postponed for more than 4 hours, the mother should be given the option of an intravenous infusion. Monitoring for operative delivery under regional block should include pulse oximetry, non-invasive BP, ECG and fetal heart rate. Monitoring for general anaesthesia should be in accordance with the recommendations of the AAGBI (see p. 349).

6. **Obstetric theatre, recovery, HDU and ICU facilities.** Every unit should have at least one dedicated emergency theatre and fully equipped recovery area. Midwifery staff caring for postoperative patients should be trained in monitoring, care of the airway and resuscitation and be supervised by an anaesthetist at all times.

7. **Requirements for blood availabity.** All units should have at least 2 units of uncross-matched 'O' negative blood available within 5 minutes. Cross-matched blood should be available within 30 minutes.

8. **Consent for obstetric anaesthesia services.** Consent must be obtained from all patients. Efforts must be made to improve the quality of information provided. All explanations should be documented and witnessed.

9. **Assessment of the sick obstetric patient.** Anaesthetists should liaise with midwives, obstetricians and physicians to agree management for successful delivery. The anaesthetist must become involved in the management of the 'at risk' patient at an early stage and can provide the liaison with high dependency/ICU on behalf of the management team.

10. **Assistance for the anaesthetist in obstetric anaesthesia.** This should be provided by an ODP or anaesthesia nurse trained to appropriate national standards.

11. **Departmental guidelines.** These should be drawn up for the management of major haemorrhage, pre-eclamptic toxaemia, failed intubation drill and management of regional anaesthesia.

## AMNIOTIC FLUID EMBOLUS

Amniotic fluid may cause amniotic fluid embolus characterized by sudden cardiorespiratory collapse and coagulatory abnormalities. It is thought that the amniotic fluid itself is relatively non-toxic, even in volumes as large as 500 ml. Toxicity appears to be determined by the meconium content. In a pig model, 10 ml/kg of meconium-free amniotic fluid caused few problems, whereas just 3 ml/kg of meconium-contaminated amniotic fluid caused severe cardiorespiratory and coagulatory abnormalities.

**References**

American Society of Anesthesiologists 1999 Practice guidelines for obstetrical anesthesia. A report by the American Society of Anesthesiologists' Task Force on Obstetrical Anesthesia. Anesthesiology 90: 600–611

Association of Anaesthetists of Great Britain and Ireland and the Obstetric Anaesthetists Association 1998 Guidelines for obstetric anaesthesia services. AAGBI and OAA, London

Benhamou D 1995 Complications of obstetric anaesthesia. Current Opinion in Anaesthesiology 8: 216–219

Bogod D G 1994 The postpartum stomach – when is it safe? Editorial. Anaesthesia 49: 1–2

Duley L, Neilson J P 1999 Magnesium sulphate and pre-eclampsia. British Medical Journal 319: 3–4

Malek W H, Petroianu G A 1999 Autologous blood transfusion and amniotic fluid embolism. British Journal of Anaesthesia 82: 154

Morgan B M 1994 Pregnancy, hypertension and pre-eclampsia. Current Opinion in Anaesthesiology 7: 221–223

Morgan M 1994 Obstetric anaesthesia and analgesia. In: Nimmo W S, Rowbotham D J, Smith G (eds) Anaesthesia, 2nd edn. Blackwell Scientific Publications, Oxford, p 1000–1028

Mushambi M C, Halligan A W, Williamson K 1996 Recent developments in the pathophysiology and management of pre-eclampsia. British Journal of Anaesthesia 76: 133–148

Nimmo W S, Rowbotham D J, Smith G 1994 Anaesthesia, 2nd edn. Blackwell Scientific Publications, Oxford

Stackhouse R A, Hughes S C 1994 Caesarian section. Current Opinion in Anaesthesiology 7: 231–239

Stuart J C, Kan A F, Rowbottom S J, Yau G, Gin T 1996 Acid aspiration prophylaxis for emergency Caesarian section. Anaesthesia 51: 415–421

## MATERNAL AND FETAL PHYSIOLOGY

## MATERNAL PHYSIOLOGY

### Cardiovascular

- Cardiac output 30–40% above normal by 32 weeks. Aortocaval compression is sufficient to reduce cardiac output from 20 weeks
- ↑ heart rate of 15%, ↑ stroke volume of 30%. Fall in SVR results in unchanged BP
- Cardiac hypertrophy and dilation cause ECG changes of left axis deviation, ST depression and flattening/inversion of T wave in III
- Albumin is diluted, reducing plasma oncotic pressure and predisposing to pulmonary oedema at lower pressures
- ↑ progesterone due to pregnancy and reduced protein binding increases myocardial sensitivity to bupivacaine
- Aortocaval compression significant from mid-pregnancy.

## Respiratory

- Reduction in lung volume by a 4 cm elevation of diaphragm compensated for by increased transverse and AP diameter of the chest due to hormonal effects that loosen ligaments
- Increased minute volume by 40%, ↑ tidal volume and 15% ↑ respiratory rate. Causes respiratory alkalosis and shifts $O_2$ dissociation curve to the left. Increase in $P_{50}$ from 3.5 to 4.0 facilitates oxygen unloading across the placenta
- ↑ tidal volume with ↓ FRC results in faster pre-oxygenation in 2 min of tidal breathing (more effective than four vital capacity breaths) and quick gas induction, accelerated by reduced MAC
- Increased CC which may exceed FRC
- Increased $O_2$ consumption.

## Gastrointestinal

- Uterine pressure increases intragastric pressure and distorts lower oesophageal sphincter, causing incompetence
- Delayed gastric emptying and increased acid production.

## Blood

- Increased red cell mass by 20–30% and increased plasma volume by 40–50% at term, causing dilutional anaemia
- Hypercoagulable state with increased fibrinogen and factors VII, VIII, X, and XIII. Platelet, clotting and fibrinolytic systems all activated.

## Renal

Increase in GFR of 60% reduces plasma urea and creatinine by 40%.

## Epidural

Volume of epidural space is decreased due to distended venous plexus, reducing the volume of LA needed for epidurals by 30% and increasing the risk of epidural vein catheterization.

## Metabolism

- Increased volume of distribution of intravenous agents prolongs their elimination half-lives. Elimination $t_{1/2}$ for thiopentone is doubled at term
- Serum cholinesterase levels fall by 25% during the first trimester and fall further by 33% during the first 7 postpartum days. The decreased levels of enzymes are adequate for normal hydrolysis of suxamethonium

during gestation, but may prolong duration of action in 10% of patients in the postpartum period.

## FETAL PHYSIOLOGY

• Fetus exists in a hypoxic environment. Oxygenation enhanced by left shift of $O_2$ dissociation curve with fetal $P_{50} = 2.6$ compared with maternal value of 4.0.

• Uterine vascular bed is maximally dilated at term but remains responsive to the effects of catecholamines. Ephedrine acts on $\beta > \alpha$ receptors and has less effect on placental flow than other vasopressors which act by $\alpha$ stimulation, e.g. methoxamine.

• Fetal acidosis results in more local anaesthetic taken up by the fetus with increased risk of toxicity.

### References

Gaiser R R 1998 Old concepts applied to new problems: the fetus as a patient.
   Current Opinion in Anaesthesiology 11: 251–253
Morgan M 1994 Obstetric anaesthesia and analgesia. In: Nimmo W S, Rowbotham D J,
   Smith G (eds) Anaesthesia, 2nd edn. Blackwell Scientific Publications, Oxford
Telfeyan C, Santos A C 1995 Pharmacology of local anaesthetics during pregnancy.
   Current Opinion in Anaesthesiology 8: 196–199

# 9. Paediatrics

## DEFINITIONS

- *Neonate* – first 28 days of life or < 44 weeks post-conception
- *Infant* – 1 month to 1 year
- *Child* – > 1 year to adolescence
- *Low birth weight* – 2500 g at birth
- *Premature* – less than 37 weeks.

## PHYSIOLOGICAL CHANGES AT BIRTH

- Tactile stimulus triggers respiratory centre. Inflation of lungs reduces pulmonary vascular resistance.
- Increased flow to lungs increases left atrial pressure, closing the foramen ovale.
- Cessation of placental flow increases SVR. Combined with decreased PVR, flow through ductus arteriosus reverses. High $P_aO_2$ causes ductal smooth muscle to constrict, and closure occurs (reversible for several days).

Fetal circulation is shown in Figure 9.1.

## NEONATAL PHYSIOLOGY

### CVS

- Tendency to revert to fetal circulation for 2 weeks is triggered by acidosis and $\uparrow P_aCO_2$.
- Relatively little contractile tissue in heart (30%), so increased cardiac output achieved by increased heart rate rather than stroke volume. Ventricular thickness equal by 6 months.
- Cardiac index is 2–3 times that of an adult.
- Heart rate at term is 120/min. Rises to 160/min by 1 month and decreases to adult rates by 15 years.

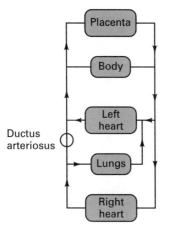

**Fig. 9.1** Fetal circulation.

- PNS more developed than SNS. Therefore there is a tendency to bradycardia. Response to adrenergic drugs is diminished.
- Ductus arteriosus reopens following fluid overload.

**Respiratory**

- Obligatory nasal breathing until 5 months. Nasal passages account for 30–50% of airway resistance. May be unable to convert to mouth breathing if there is nasal obstruction.
- Large tongue obstructs the airway and makes laryngoscopy difficult. Epiglottis is longer, narrower and angled away from the axis of the trachea.
- Larynx is higher ($C_3$–$C_4$) and more anterior than in adults ($C_4$–$C_5$).
- Narrowest part of upper airway is cricoid cartilage. Even minimal oedema causes a large increase in airway resistance (Hagen–Poiseuille law).
- Short trachea at term: ≈ 4 cm.
- Tendency to apnoea if < 50 weeks post-conceptual age, due to immature respiratory centre.
- Negative pressure of 40–80 $cmH_2O$ is required for initial lung expansion.
- Surfactant produced from 32 weeks by type II alveolar pneumocytes.
- No bucket handle rib movement, therefore increased minute volume is achieved by increasing respiratory rate.
- Diaphragmatic > intercostal respiration. Fewer type I muscle fibres used in prolonged work so earlier diaphragm fatigue.
- Rapid respiratory rate of 32 breaths/min.
- FRC < CC due to decreased outward recoil of chest wall.
- Small FRC, high $O_2$ consumption; therefore rapid desaturation.

- Increased laryngeal irritability with susceptibility to laryngospasm.
- Increased susceptibility to respiratory infection.

## GI

- Acute gastric dilatation is common, so consider a NG tube.
- Lower oesophageal sphincter incompetence predisposes to aspiration pneumonia.
- Immature hepatic function and reduced blood flow, increasing half-life of drugs excreted by hepatic metabolism. Phase I reactions attain adult levels within 1 week; phase II reactions within 3–4 months.

### Renal

- Immature renal function with reduced GFR; therefore reduced ability to excrete drugs, dependent upon renal clearance.
- Reduced concentrating ability.
- 50% $N_2$ forms new tissue; therefore less renal $N_2$ load.

## CNS

- Immature blood–brain barrier with increased permeability to lipid-soluble drugs.
- Motor nerve endings differentiate to form end plates at 26–28 weeks, but process still incomplete at term.
- Increased proportion of low-affinity $\mu_2$ opiate receptors (mediate respiratory depression).
- Increased sensitivity to volatiles due to increased progesterone, increased β-endorphins, immature blood–brain barrier and decreased protein binding.

### Blood

- 70% HbF at term; $P_{50}$ = 2.7 kPa (3.5–4.0 kPa in adult) with leftward shift of $O_2$ dissociation curve.
- Blood volume 80 ml/kg at term.
- Physiological anaemia is greatest at 3–4 months, with Hb = 10 gm/dl.

  Change of haematocrit with age is shown in Figure 9.2.

### Temperature

- Increased surface area:body weight ratio. Therefore increased heat loss.
- Thermoneutral temperature at term = 33°C.
- Noradrenaline > adrenaline released with stress to trigger non-shivering thermogenesis in brown fat. Brown fat stores are limited. Shivering does not occur before 3 months.

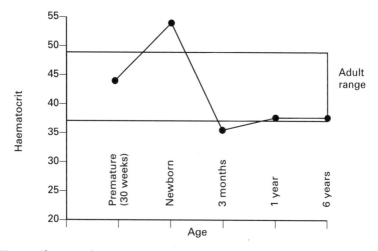

**Fig. 9.2** Changes in haematocrit with age.

- Immature thermoregulatory mechanisms, further inhibited by GA.
- Hypothermia causes acidosis, persistent fetal circulation, hypoxia, diaphragm fatigue, intraventricular haemorrhage and coagulopathy.

### Glucose

- Minimal glycogen reserves for gluconeogenesis.
- Poorly developed glucose homeostasis.
- High glucose requirements at term. Tendency to hypoglycaemia in small-for-dates babies, infants of diabetic mothers and sick neonates.

### Pharmacokinetic and pharmacodynamic differences

- Decreased lean body mass.
- Increased total body water (increased central volume by 50%).
- Decreased total body fat. Therefore, increased $V_D$ of water-soluble drugs, decreased $V_D$ of fat-soluble drugs.
- Decreased protein binding.

## GENERAL ANAESTHESIA

### NCEPOD RECOMMENDATIONS FOR PAEDIATRIC ANAESTHESIA

- Anaesthetist must have sufficient paediatric experience
- One anaesthetist in each hospital must be responsible for paediatric anaesthesia
- Most problems occur in children < 3 years
- Neonates (< 28 days) must be anaesthetized in specialist units

## Weight (kg)

- 1–8 years = (age + 4) × 2
- > 9 years = age × 3

## Preoperative fasting

Half-life of gastric fluid (saline) is 11 min, prolonged by fat and glucose. Recent studies show that prolonged fasting may actually decrease gastric pH and increase volume. Clear fluids administered 2–3 h preoperatively do not alter gastric residual volume and cause less distress. A recent study suggests that breast milk can be given safely up to 3 h preoperatively (Seth et al 1999).

Fasting recommendations to reduce the risk of pulmonary aspiration are given in Table 9.1.

**Table 9.1** Summary of fasting recommendations to reduce the risk of pulmonary aspiration (American Society of Anesthesiologists 1999)

| Ingested material | Minimum fasting period (h) |
| --- | --- |
| Clear liquids | 2 |
| Breast milk | 4 |
| Infant formula | 6 |
| Non-human milk | 6 |
| Light meal | 6 |

## Preoperative assessment

Examine for congenital defects, cardiorespiratory pathology due to prematurity, hypoglycaemia and hypocalcaemia.

## Premedication

Bradycardia secondary to cholinergic effects of drugs (halothane, suxamethonium) and upper airway stimulation is reduced with anticholinergic premedication.

## Intubation

- Tracheal tube size (> 1 year) = age/4 + 4 mm
- Tracheal tube length = age/2 + 12 cm.

## Volatiles

MAC is lower in the neonate. Gas induction is fast because alveolar ventilation is large compared with FRC, high cardiac output and lower blood:gas solubility of volatiles in neonates. Single breath gas induction has been described using 5% halothane in 70% nitrous oxide with oxygen.

Volatiles depress respiration, depress intercostal muscles and ventilation becomes diaphragmatic. Therefore intubate if < 5 kg or < 44 weeks post-conceptual age. Volatiles reduce SVR, worsening a right-to-left shunt if persistent fetal circulation is present.

Age-related change in MAC of sevoflurane is less pronounced. Sevoflurane produces less laryngeal irritation than desflurane and is more suitable for gas induction. Baroreflex response is maintained with isoflurane and sevoflurane but not with halothane or desflurane.

MAC of nitrous oxide is not related to age. $N_2O$ may cause marked cardiovascular depression in neonates and diffusion into bowel may impair ventilation.

Variation in MAC of isoflurane with age is given in Figure 9.3.

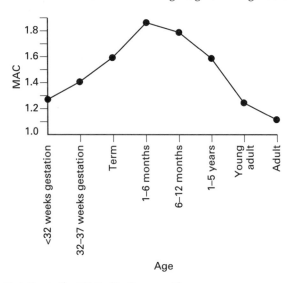

**Fig. 9.3**  Variation in the MAC of isoflurane with age.

## Barbiturates

Reduced $V_D$ of lipid-soluble drugs reduces redistribution of thiopentone, thus prolonging recovery. Induction doses: 2–4 mg/kg in neonates; 7–8 mg/kg in infants; 5–6 mg/kg in older children.

## Propofol

Pain on induction, more excitatory phenomenon and less postoperative nausea and vomiting than with thiopentone. Greater depression of laryngopharnygeal reflexes than with thiopentone so more suitable for use with laryngeal mask. Larger $V_D$, faster metabolism and clearance. Therefore, a larger induction dose of 2.5–3.5 mg/kg is required.

Only licensed as an induction agent in children > 3 years because of case reports of a syndrome of lactic acidaemia, bradyarrhythmias, hypotension, lipaemia and oliguria.

### Benzodiazepines

Diazepam has similar $V_D$ to adult values but greatly prolonged $t_{1/2}$ (20–50 h in neonates; 8–14 h in children). Midazolam is more suitable in children, with a $t_{1/2}$ of 1.5 h.

### Opioids

Increased sensitivity due to immature blood–brain barrier, reduced protein binding and decreased glucuronidation. Reduced clearance of all opioids. High doses reduce stress response and prevent pulmonary hypertension associated with airway instrumentation.

### Muscle relaxants

*Depolarizing.* Decreased plasma cholinesterase but minimal effect on hydrolysis. Decreased sensitivity to suxamethonium due to increased $V_D$ and immature neuromuscular junction. Therefore use a higher dose of 2 mg/kg.

*Non-depolarizing.* Atracurium has an increased $V_D$ but increased clearance, so elimination half-life is unchanged and thus little change in overall pharmacokinetics. Sensitivity to, and action of, vecuronium is increased in children < 1 year.

Ensure complete reversal before extubation with glycopyrrolate 0.01 mg/kg.

### Local anaesthetics

Reduced protein binding and reduced metabolism increase risk of toxic side-effects.

## OXYGEN TOXICITY

Neonates < 2 kg or < 35 weeks are particularly susceptible to retinal damage by exposure to high $P_aO_2$. It is related to the level and duration of raised oxygen tension. Other risk factors are prematurity, twins, hypoxaemia, hyper/hypocarbia, sepsis and transfusion. $S_aO_2$ of 90–94% is considered optimal.

## FLUID MANAGEMENT

Insensible losses are greater due to:

- increased surface area:body ratio, increasing evaporation
- immature skin – loses more water
- increased alveolar ventilation – increases water lost via the lungs
- kidneys less able to concentrate urine.

Short operations < 1 h in healthy children do not usually require fluids if preoperative fasting was not excessive. For longer procedures, an i.v. infusion is necessary. When calculating perioperative fluid requirements, add fluid lost during preoperative fasting to the operative regime.

### Replacement therapy

- 0–10 kg  –  4 ml/kg per h +
- 11–20 kg –  2 ml/kg per h +
- > 21 kg  –  1 ml/kg per h.

Aim for a urine output of at least 1 ml/kg per h.

Maintain haematocrit in infants above 0.30 with packed red cells warmed to 37°C.

## ANALGESIA IN NEONATES

### Opioids

Traditional i.m. administration of opioids in children has generally been abandoned for less traumatic techniques. Subcutaneous administration through a cannula placed during GA avoids unpleasant repeated i.m. injections. Use of i.v. techniques is tempered by the risk of respiratory depression. Monitoring of respiratory frequency is an insensitive indicator of respiratory depression, and pulse oximetry in a high-dependency unit should be used when administering i.v. opioids. Patient-controlled analgesia has been used successfully in children as young as 5 years of age. Use of NSAIDs and regional/local blocks is becoming much more widespread.

Use morphine infusion 5–30 $\mu$g/kg/min.

### Non-steroidal anti-inflammatory drugs

These appear to provide analgesia in children as young as 3 years. Ketorolac, indomethacin, diclofenac and ibuprofen have all been shown to reduce postoperative opioid requirements. The degree of gastric irritation, renal impairment and fluid retention is not known. Immature renal and hepatic function may impair excretion.

### Regional techniques

Nerves are less myelinated, resulting in a faster onset of block and an adequate block at lower concentrations of LA. Reduced plasma protein results in higher blood levels of LA. All routes cause less hypotension than in adults because of an immature SNS and less developed capacitance vessels. Postoperative numbness over wide areas may cause confusion and restlessness (3% of patients).

Spinal cord ends at $L_3$; dura ends at $S_4$.

### Spinal

- Consider atropine premedication (20 $\mu$g/kg)
- 0.5% heavy bupivacaine at $L_{3/4}$ or $L_{4/5}$
    < 4kg: 0.13 ml/kg
    > 4kg: 0.07 ml/kg
    + 0.1 ml needle deadspace.

### Caudal

- 0.25% plain bupivacaine ± 0.05 mg/kg morphine
    — block to lumbosacral region: 0.5 ml/kg
    — block to thoracolumbar region: 1.0 ml/kg
    — block to low thoracic region: 1.25 ml/kg
- Urinary retention in up to 65% of patients and persistent motor block in up to 30%.

### Epidural

- 0.5% bupivacaine at 0.5 ml/kg ± 0.05 mg/kg morphine.

## PREMATURITY (37 WEEKS)

Associated with:

- aspiration pneumonia, respiratory distress syndrome
- apnoea
- hypoglycaemia, hypocalcaemia, hypomagnesaemia
- congenital defects.

### Ex-premature baby for surgery

Preoperative assessment should include respiratory system, venous access and frequency of any apnoeic attacks. Assess gestational and chronological age.

Pulmonary function is often abnormal, with a higher respiratory rate, lower compliance and impaired gas exchange which may persist for several years. Risk of life-threatening apnoea is present until 45 weeks post-conceptual age. Use apnoea alarm for at least 24 h postoperatively.

Risk of postoperative apnoea in 30–40% of babies due to immature respiratory control mechanisms, impaired respiratory function, airway obstruction, anaemia and the residual effects of anaesthetic gases (reduced chemoreceptor response to hypoxia, increased paradoxical chest wall movement, depressed intercostal muscle activity). Caffeine 10 mg/kg i.v. at induction may reduce the risk of apnoea. Regional anaesthesia reduces but does not remove the risk of postoperative respiratory depression and apnoea.

Infections and sudden death more common.

## TRACHEO-OESOPHAGEAL FISTULA (Fig. 9.4)

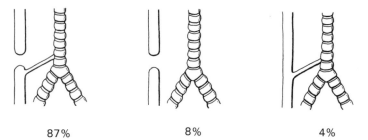

87%                              8%                              4%

**Fig. 9.4** Anatomical variants of tracheo-oesophageal fistulae.

### Presentation

Incidence of 1:3000 live births. Presents as excess oral secretions causing frothing at mouth, regurgitation of first feed and later as recurrent pneumonia. 30% are born prematurely, and 25% with major CVS abnormalities.

Associated with VATER syndrome (**V**ertebral abnormalities, **A**nal atresia, **T**racheo-oesophageal fistula, **R**adius abnormalities) and musculoskeletal and craniofacial malformation.

### Diagnosis

- Inability to pass NG tube
- Barium swallow.

### Preoperative

- Nurse head-up to reduce risk of aspiration
- Continuous suction of upper oesophageal pouch
- Physiotherapy and antibiotics if there is evidence of aspiration
- If IPPV is planned, gastrostomy under LA may be necessary preoperatively.

### General anaesthesia

Right-sided thoracotomy. Left precordial stethoscope detects ETT displacement. Awake intubation or gas induction with spontaneous respiration avoids IPPV, which causes gastric distension and respiratory impairment. IPPV may also be ineffective in patients with a gastrostomy tube as gas escapes through the tube. Intravenous induction is safe if a fistula is not present because IPPV is effective. If a fistula is present, allow the baby to breathe spontaneously until the fistula is closed.

The opening of the fistula is usually located on the posterior distal wall of the trachea. Intubate the right main bronchus and withdraw the ETT until breath sounds are heard in both lungs so that the tip of the ETT then occludes the fistula.

Aim for early extubation postoperatively to minimize suture line stress.

## CONGENITAL DIAPHRAGMATIC HERNIA

Incidence of 1:5000 live births. 50% mortality within 6 hours. Caused by early gut return or delayed diaphragm closure.

### Sites of herniation (Fig. 9.5)

- Posterolateral foramen of Bochdalek (L>>R) – 85%
- Anterior foramen of Morgagni – 10%
- Oesophageal hiatus – < 5%.

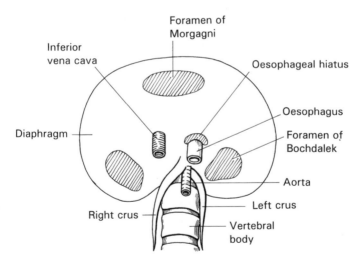

**Fig. 9.5** Sites of congenital diaphragmatic herniation.

### Embryology of diaphragm

Comprises three structures:

- septum transversum
- pleuroperitoneal membrane
- thoracic myotomes.

**Sequelae**

Ipsilateral alveolar and bronchial hypoplasia and decreased surfactant. Contralateral lung may also be affected. Usually presents as cyanosis, dyspnoea and cardiac dextroposition. Bowel sounds in thorax with reduced breath sounds.

23% are associated with cardiovascular abnormalities. Abnormalities of most other organ systems are also described; also trisomy 18 and 21.

Symptoms depend upon degree of hypoplasia:

- severe – hypoplasia incompatible with life
- moderate – respiratory distress, tachypnoea and cyanosis
- mild – less severe symptoms, not always presenting immediately.

Pulmonary hypoplasia and pulmonary artery hypertension worsen any right-to-left shunt and cause respiratory acidosis, which predisposes to persistent fetal circulation. The degree of shunting may be reduced with bicarbonate infusion:

$$NaHCO_3 \text{ (mEq) required} = \text{body weight (kg)} \times \text{base deficit} \times 0.3$$

(Dilute in equal volume of 10% glucose prior to i.v. administration.)

**General anaesthesia**

- Emergency surgery is no longer recommended as mortality is reduced by preoperative resuscitation
- Monitoring: $S_aO_2$, ECG, invasive BP (one preductal, one post-ductal to assess shunt), urinary catheter
- Good venous access above IVC which is compressed postoperatively by gut
- NG tube to decompress stomach
- Avoid IPPV which inflates the stomach and worsens respiratory distress. Therefore, awake intubation. Ventilate by hand to detect sudden changes in compliance, e.g. pneumothorax
- Avoid $N_2O$, which distends bowel. SNS stimulation worsens pulmonary vasoconstriction and is reduced by opioids, e.g. fentanyl
- Pulmonary vasodilators (tolazoline ($\alpha$-antagonist), $PGE_1$, nitroprusside, nitroglycerine) improve oxygenation and acidosis, reducing airway pressure and risk of barotrauma
- Some success with ECMO, but mortality from anticoagulation causing bleeding
- Necessity for postoperative ventilation depends upon severity of abnormalities
- Successful *in utero* surgical correction reported!

## HYPERTROPHIC PYLORIC STENOSIS

Incidence 1:5000 live births. Occurs in males > females. Due to hypertrophy of muscularis layer of pylorus. Usually presents in weeks 2–6 with non-bilious projectile vomiting. Results in:

- dehydration
- metabolic disturbance
- aspiration risk.

Characterized by hypochloraemic hypokalaemic metabolic alkalosis with acidic urine. Due to bicarbonate initially excreted with $K^+$ and $Na^+$. Once $K^+$ becomes depleted, the kidneys excrete $H^+$ in an attempt to save $Na^+$, worsening the alkalosis. Increased urinary $H^+$ acidifies the urine. Prerenal renal failure and metabolic acidosis occur in severe cases.

Resuscitate preoperatively with normal saline 0.9%:

deficit (mmol) $\times$ body wt (kg) $\times$ 0.6 = mmol $Na^+$ needed to correct deficit

Aspirate stomach with large-bore NG tube preoperatively.

Gaseous induction risks vomiting and aspiration. Therefore use awake intubation or rapid sequence induction. Balanced anaesthesia during surgery. Extubate awake.

## UPPER AIRWAY OBSTRUCTION

Resulting large negative inspiratory intrathoracic pressure may cause pulmonary oedema. If bronchoscopy is required, intubate first to establish airway then exchange ETT for a ventilating bronchoscope. If child desaturates, remove bronchoscope back into trachea and re-oxygenate.

### Epiglottitis

Usually 1–7 years. Of rapid onset and progression. Upper airway obstruction (inspiratory stridor, tachypnoea, intercostal recession) and difficulty swallowing with drooling. Systemically unwell.

Usually caused by *Haemophilus influenzae* type B. Chloramphenicol now superseded by third-generation cephalosporin, e.g. cefuroxime.

Keep the child and parents calm. No preoperative X-ray. Establish i.v. access only if the child is calm.

Perform a gas induction in the sitting position with halothane in 100% $O_2$. Then establish i.v. and give atropine 0.2 mg/kg before laryngoscopy. Use oral ETT one size smaller than usual. If unable to pass, try intubating bronchoscope or cricothyroidotomy. Change to nasal ETT if easy intubation. Steroids are controversial. Intubate for 24–48 h. Examine larynx before extubation.

### Laryngotracheobronchitis (Croup)

Occurs at 6 months–6 years. Slow onset with inspiratory stridor and intercostal recession. Mild pyrexia. Usually viral.

Treat with cool humidified air and $O_2$; nebulized adrenaline as appropriate (may initially improve, then worsen obstruction).

If there is still no improvement, it is probably due to inspissated secretions (6% of cases). If so, treat as for epiglottitis.

### Foreign body aspiration

Often a history of coughing, choking or cyanosis whilst eating. Most foreign bodies are not radiopaque. Hyperinflation and atelectasis on CXR. Specific problems are:

- potential loss of airway
- risk of full stomach
- $\dot{V}/\dot{Q}$ mismatch prolonging gas induction.

Give atropine premedication. Avoid opioids. Gaseous induction as for epiglottitis. *Gentle* bagging if necessary to avoid driving foreign body distally. Insert Storz ventilating bronchoscope once airway is secured.

Peanut oil causes intense inflammation with rapid airway obstruction if not removed early. Consider possibility of airway obstruction due to foreign body in oesophagus compressing trachea.

### References

American Society of Anesthesiologists' Task Force on Preoperative Fasting 1999 Practice guidelines for preoperative fasting and the use of pharmacologic agents to reduce the risk of pulmonary aspiration: application to healthy patients undergoing elective procedures. Anesthesiology 90: 896–905

Anon 1994 Mini-symposium: paediatric anaesthesia. Current Anaesthesia and Critical Care 5: 190–217

Anon 1995 Managing acute pain in children. Drug and Therapeutics Bulletin 33: 41–44

Finley G A 1998 Paediatric pain: a year in review. Current Opinion in Anaesthesiology 11: 295–299

Habre W 1998 Pediatric anesthesia and recent developments in asthma in children. Current Opinion in Anaesthesiology 11: 305–309

Hatch D, Fletcher M 1992 Anaesthesia and the ventilatory system in infants and young children. British Journal of Anaesthesia 68: 398–410

Marsh D F, Hatch D J, Fitzgerald M 1997 Opioid systems in the newborn. British Journal of Anaesthesia 79: 787–795

Meakin G 1994 Drugs in paediatric anaesthesia. Current Opinion in Anaesthesiology 7: 251–256

Rowney D A, Doyle E 1998 Epidural and subarachnoid block in children. Anaesthesia 53: 980–1001

Seth A K, Chatterji C, Bhargava S K, Narang P, Tyagi A 1999 Safe pre-operative fasting times after milk or clear fluid in children. Anaesthesia 54: 51–58

Steward D J 1997 Pediatric anesthesia. Current Opinion in Anaesthesiology 10: 27–29

Strunin L 1993 How long should patients fast before surgery? Time for new guidelines. British Journal of Anaesthesia 70: 1–3

Susla G M 1996 Propofol toxicity in critically ill pediatric patients: show us the proof. Critical Care Medicine 26: 1959–1960

## PAEDIATRIC CARDIOLOGY

## ANAESTHESIA FOR CONGENITAL CARDIOVASCULAR DISEASE

Approximately 8000 infants born in the UK each year have some form of congenital heart disease, of which one-third will require cardiac surgery.

- *Cyanotic lesions* – Fallot's tetralogy, transposition of great vessels, tricuspid atresia, Eisenmenger's syndrome.
- *Acyanotic lesions* – ASD, VSD, PDA, aortic coarctation.

### ASSESSMENT

*History*
- Ability to play with peers usually suggests adequate cardiac reserve
- Cyanosis, squatting, syncope, exercise/feeding intolerance, tachypnoea and failure to thrive all suggest varying degrees of cardiac failure.

*Examination*
- Previous scars
- Respiratory rate and pattern (nasal flaring, recession, grunting)
- Peripheral pulses, e.g. coarctation
- Pulse pressure, e.g. aortic regurgitation, PDA
- Enlarged liver/spleen
- Respiratory system for signs of LVF.

*Investigation*
- ECHO, cardiac catheterization
- Haematocrit is the best indicator of severity of right-to-left shunt (increased haematocrit causes renal, pulmonary and CNS thrombosis, especially with dehydration)
- Clotting – coagulopathies are common.

### GENERAL ANAESTHESIA

**General aims**

- Maintain adequate perfusion of systemic and pulmonary circulation
- If pulmonary hypertension is present, aim to reduce pulmonary artery pressures
- In the presence of an obstructive lesion, maintain filling pressures, HR and coronary perfusion pressure
- Careful purging of air bubbles from all lines to avoid systemic embolization.

## Premedication

- None for babies < 6 months or if there is minimal anxiety
- Morphine 0.1 mg/kg is well tolerated
- Glycopyrrolate as antisialogogue.

## Monitoring

- ECG, precordial/oesophageal stethoscope, NIBP, +/− arterial line, CVP, temperature, pulse oximeter, capnograph and urinary catheter
- Consider pre- and post-ductal pulse oximeters to detect degree of right-to-left shunt.

## Induction

- Intravenous is best for cardiovascular disease
- Gaseous induction risks desaturation, especially with severe disease. Slow if right-to-left shunt. If there is no venous access with severe disease, use 100% $O_2$, i.m. ketamine and i.m. suxamethonium.

## Maintenance

High-dose fentanyl, 100% $O_2$, pancuronium technique provides good cardiovascular stability and decreases the stress response. (Pancuronium offsets the vagotonic effects of fentanyl.)

Degree of shunting in PDA, ASD and VSD depends upon the pressure difference between the systemic and pulmonary circulations:

- increase PVR by decreasing $F_iO_2$, use of PEEP and high $P_aCO_2$
- decrease PVR by increasing $F_iO_2$, no PEEP, alkalosis, decreasing $P_aCO_2$ and nitric oxide
- increase SVR by vasoconstrictors and flexing hips
- decrease SVR by inhalational agents and vasodilators.

IPPV can reverse left-to-right shunt and therefore cause air bubbles to enter the arterial circulation.

## VENTRICULAR SEPTAL DEFECT (Fig. 9.6)

Commonest congenital heart lesion (2 per 1000 births); 50% close spontaneously within 1 year. Often associated with more complex lesions. Results in gradually increasing left-to-right shunt as RV pressure falls below LV pressure after birth. High pulmonary blood flow causes heart failure and pulmonary oedema. Treat with digoxin and diuretics or pulmonary artery banding to reduce pulmonary blood flow if severe.

## PATENT DUCTUS ARTERIOSUS

Similar pathophysiology to VSD. Pulmonary function is compromised

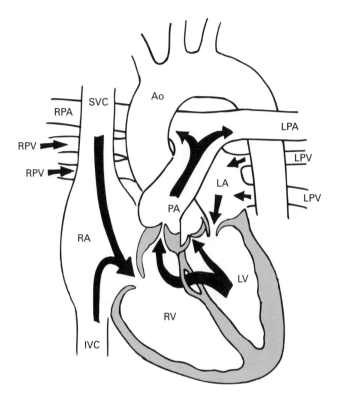

**Fig. 9.6** Ventricular septal defect – pulmonary blood flow increased by systemic vasoconstriction or pulmonary vasodilation.

because of pulmonary oedema, and reduced systemic flow may impair renal function. Give indomethacin, avoid fluid overload and consider digoxin.

## TRANSPOSITION OF THE GREAT ARTERIES (Fig. 9.7)

Aorta arises from RV and pulmonary artery arises from LV. Unless there is a shunt present (ASD, VSD, PDA), there is no communication between the two circuits and closure of the ductus arteriosus results in death. Balloon septostomy creates an atrial septal defect as a temporary measure. Definitive surgery involves switching PA and aorta or creating shunts to establish single circulation (Blalock shunt followed by Rastelli procedure).

## TETRALOGY OF FALLOT (Fig. 9.8)

- Overriding aorta

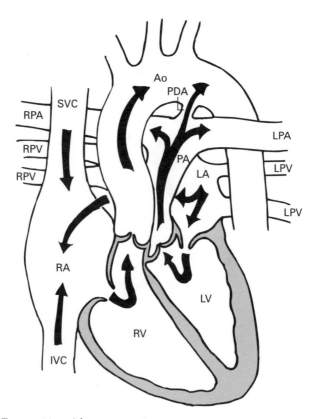

**Fig. 9.7** Transposition of the great vessels – communication between pulmonary and systemic circulations provided by the ASD and PDA.

- Right ventricular hypertrophy
- VSD with right-to-left shunt
- Pulmonary stenosis.

Both ventricles are at the same (systemic) pressure. Increasing systemic vascular resistance (SVR) reduces right-to-left shunt and increases pulmonary blood flow. Acidosis and hypoxia cause infundibular spasm and worsen shunt. Squatting increases SVR and reduces return of acidotic venous blood from the IVC. Hyperviscosity from raised haematocrit is common. Avoid dehydration, which may cause hypotension and thrombotic complications. Cyanotic spells may be reversed with propanolol 0.025–0.1 mg/kg i.v.

## PULMONARY HYPERTENSION

Common problem associated with VSD, total anomalous pulmonary

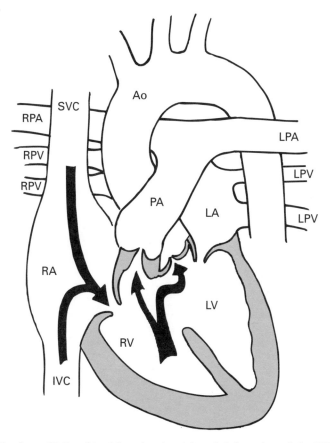

**Fig. 9.8** Tetralogy of Fallot – blood flow showing right-to-left shunt through the VSD.

venous drainage, truncus arteriosus, atrioventricular septal defect and hypolastic left heart. Defined as PAP greater than 50% of the systemic pressure. Usually associated with excess pulmonary blood flow and poor arborization of the pulmonary vasculature.

Minimize all stimuli which cause a rise in PAP, e.g. physical contact, suctioning, physiotherapy, hypoxaemia, hypercapnia and metabolic acidosis. Ensure baby is well sedated and paralyse if ventilatory pressures are high. Hyperventilate to achieve a moderate respiratory alkalosis ($P_a\mathrm{CO}_2$ = 3.5 kPa, pH 7.50) and aim for $P_a\mathrm{O}_2$ of 15–25 kPa. The only specific pulmonary vasodilator is nitric oxide (NO) at 2–10 ppm. Other vasodilators (prostacyclin, phenoxybenzamine, milrinone) all cause systemic as well as pulmonary vasodilation.

## References

Greenley W J, Kern F H 1994 Anesthesia for pediatric cardiac surgery. In: Miller R D (ed) Anesthesia. Churchill Livingstone, Edinburgh, p 1811–1850

Javorski J J, Burrows F A 1995 Pediatric cardiac anesthesia. Current Opinion in Anaesthesiology 8: 62–67

Long T J 1997 Pediatric cardiology and cardiac surgery update. Current Opinion in Anaesthesiology 10: 221–226

# 10. Pain

## OBSERVATION OF THE PATIENT

### Behavioural

- Time to sit/stand
- General activity
- Time to get in/out of bed.

### Analgesic requirements

- Time to first dose of analgesia
- Total dose of analgesia over a given period
- Number of demands from PCA pump.

## MEASUREMENT OF THE PATIENT

### Physiology

- Autonomic – BP, heart rate, respiratory rate
- Stress response – cortisol, ACTH, adrenaline
- Neuropharmacological – endorphins, skin temperature
- Neurological – nerve conduction, PET scan of CNS blood flow, skin conduction.

## MEASUREMENT BY THE PATIENT

### Self-reporting

- Verbal, numerical tests
- Visual analogue scale
- McGill Pain Questionnaire – rows of words, each with a specific score. Add up scores from each section (sensory, emotive, evaluative)
- Minnesota Pain Inventory Score (for chronic pain)
- Pain diary.

## ASSESSMENT OF CHILDREN

- Motor indicators – crying, rocking, withdrawal, kicking
- Visual analogue scale
- Objective pain score (crying, movement, agitation, posture, verbal)
- Visual scales:
  — Oucher Scale (picture scale)
  — Faces Pain Rating Scale
  — Colour matching charts
- Voice spectral analysis (research tool only).

### References

Chapman C R, Dunbar P J 1998 Measurement in pain therapy: is pain relief really the endpoint? Current Opinion in Anaesthesiology 11: 533–537

Ready L B 1994 Acute postoperative pain. In: Miller R D (ed) Anesthesia. Churchill Livingstone, Edinburgh, p 2327–2344

Wilson G A M, Doyle E 1996 Validation of three paediatric pain scores for use by parents. Anaesthesia 51: 1005–1007

## PHYSIOLOGY AND TREATMENT OF PAIN

**Definition of pain** International Association for the Study of Pain

An unpleasant sensory or emotional experience associated with actual or potential tissue damage.

## PATHOPHYSIOLOGY

Acute pain is only the initiation phase of an extensive, persistent nociceptive and behavioural cascade triggered by tissue injury. Failure to suppress acute pain may lead to amplification of tissue responses and development of chronic pain. Mechanical, thermal or chemical damage causes nociceptive neurones to increase their firing rate. Local inflammatory cascades sensitize these neurones and may recruit dormant ones. Sensitized neurones increase their basal discharge rate, have a lowered stimulus threshold and an exaggerated response to a stimulus.

- *Nociceptive pain* – activation of somatic or visceral sensory nerve fibres by noxious stimuli
- *Neuropathic pain* – due to abnormalities or damage to nerve fibres, e.g. mononeuropathies, polyneuropathies, deafferentation or reflex sympathetic dystrophy.

## PAIN PATHWAYS

C and Aδ fibres convey nociceptive information from visceral and somatic sites to the dorsal horn of the spinal cord. Ascending fibres then relay nociceptive information to thalamic, limbic and cortical structures. Descending noradrenergic pathways release noradrenaline to cause analgesia directly and to stimulate acetylcholine release to produce analgesia.

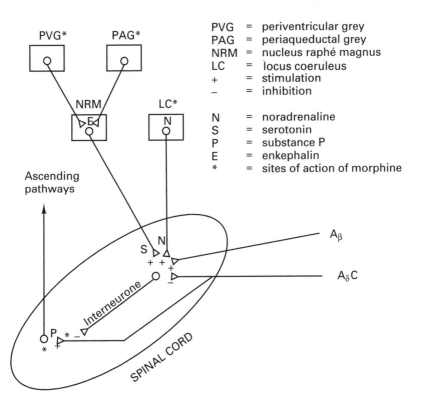

| PVG | = | periventricular grey |
| PAG | = | periaqueductal grey |
| NRM | = | nucleus raphé magnus |
| LC | = | locus coeruleus |
| + | = | stimulation |
| − | = | inhibition |
| N | = | noradrenaline |
| S | = | serotonin |
| P | = | substance P |
| E | = | enkephalin |
| * | = | sites of action of morphine |

**Fig. 10.1** Pain pathways and neurotransmitters.

**Gate control theory of pain** (Melzack & Wall)

Proposes that pain pathways (Aδ + C) are blocked by the stimulation of touch fibres (Aβ), which inhibit transmission to ascending pathways via an interneurone in the substantia gelatinosa (Fig. 10.2).

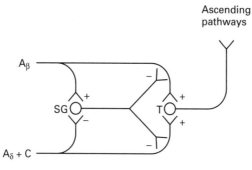

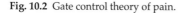

SG = substantia gelatinosa

T = intermediate transmission cell

**Fig. 10.2** Gate control theory of pain.

## EFFECTS OF PAIN

- Patient discomfort and distress
- Hyperventilation, causing respiratory alkalosis (reduces placental flow)
- Increases $O_2$ demand, causing metabolic acidosis
- Thoracic pain impairs lung expansion and reduces compliance
- Increases neuroendocrine stress response
- Reduces immunological function
- Delays postoperative mobilization
- Increases DVT risk
- Prolongs hospital stay.

## PAIN IN NEONATES

Neonates are thought to have reduced sensitivity due to incomplete myelination, high levels of endogenous endorphins and underdeveloped pain pathways. However, several studies now show that analgesia is important in neonates:

- Neonates undergoing PDA ligation anaesthetized with fentanyl in addition to $N_2O/O_2$/pancuronium show less stress response and less post-operative bradycardia, apnoea and poor perfusion.
- Neonatal heel lancing produces weeks of local sensitivity.
- Infant circumcision without analgesia is associated with altered behavioural responses to pain months later.

**ANAESTHETISTS AND NON-ACUTE PAIN MANAGEMENT**
Association of Anaesthetists 1993

Pain management is poorly taught, at both undergraduate and postgraduate levels, as a result of which it is poorly funded and not available to many patients who may benefit from its provision. Pain treatment and management should be available to all patients who require it.

## TECHNIQUES IN PAIN TREATMENT

### Pre-emptive analgesia

Concept introduced by Crile in 1913. High-intensity noxious stimuli cause altered sensory processing by mechanisms including:

- expansion of receptive fields
- decrease in thresholds of dorsal horn neurones
- enhanced release of excitatory amino acids and neuropeptides from dorsal horn neurones caused by repetitive C-fibre stimuli (wind-up)
- altered central processing.

Pre-emptive analgesia to prevent these changes may be of benefit in reducing postoperative pain but studies have produced variable results. This may be due to insufficient afferent blockade, partial pre-emptive effects in control groups (from opioids and nitrous oxide), variations in intensity of noxious stimuli and poor measurement of outcome variables.

- Preoperative intraperitoneal lignocaine is more effective than postoperative lignocaine in reducing pain from laparoscopic cholecystectomy.
- Optimal analgesia before surgery reduces the incidence of phantom limb pain following elective limb amputation.
- Pre-emptive nerve block reduced late hyperalgesia after thermal injury in human volunteers.
- Pre-emptive epidural + morphine + diclofenac + metamizole reduces postoperative morphine consumption after major abdominal surgery. Multimodal techniques, blocking pain pathways at several levels, may be a more effective method of pre-emptive analgesia.

### Combination analgesia

Combinations of opioids, NSAIDs and nerve blocks result in improved pain relief and fewer adverse side-effects.

### Interruption at specific sites

Reduced peripheral stimulus (e.g. NSAIDs), interrupted peripheral pain transmission (e.g. local anaesthetic), interrupted central pain transmission (e.g. anterolateral cordotomy), stimulation of inhibitory pathways (e.g. acupuncture, opioids), or alteration of emotional or behavioural response.

## SPECIFIC DRUGS

### NSAIDS

NSAIDs are analgesic, anti-inflammatory and antipyretic. They inhibit cyclo-oxygenase in the spinal cord and periphery to decrease prostanoid synthesis and diminish post-injury hyperalgesia at these sites. NSAIDs reversibly inhibit cyclo-oxygenase to reduce prostaglandin and thromboxane synthesis. Type 1 cyclo-oxygenase (COX-1) is present in gastric mucosa to produce protective prostaglandins and modulates renal function and platelet adhesiveness. Type 2 cyclo-oxygenase (COX-2) is responsible for inflammatory prostaglandins. Drugs which inhibit only COX-2 may therefore cause fewer gastric, renal and haemorrhagic side-effects. NSAIDs also inhibit neutrophil activation by inflammatory mediators and act centrally on the thermoregulatory centre. There is minimal protein binding with subsequent large volume of distribution.

Not generally as effective as opioids for acute pain, but reduce opioid requirements by 30–50%. May be useful in day-case surgery to avoid opioids.

### Side-effects
- GI bleeding, fluid retention, asthma
- Renal failure ($PGI_2$ enhances $Na^+$, $Cl^-$ and water excretion; $PGE_2$ vasodilates to maintain GFR)
- Inhibit platelet function
- Blood dyscrasias
- Bowel enteropathy
- Pancreatitis
- Erythema multiforme
- Reye's syndrome
- Anaphylaxis, urticaria
- Aseptic meningitis
- Delayed spontaneous labour.

There is no evidence that i.m. or rectal preparations reduce risk of side-effects. Advice from the Committee on Safety of Medicines recommends using the lowest possible doses to reduce the risk of GI complications.

### GUIDELINES FOR THE USE OF NON-STEROIDAL ANTI-INFLAMMATORY DRUGS IN THE PERIOPERATIVE PERIOD
Royal College of Anaesthetists 1998

**Usage**
NSAIDs are not sufficiently effective as the sole agent after major surgery in most patients, but are often effective after minor or moderate surgery. NSAIDs are the drug of choice after many day-case procedures.

NSAIDs often decrease opioid requirements and enhance the quality of opioid-based analgesia.

### Gastrointestinal effects
GI bleeding or ulceration should be a prominent differential diagnosis in all patients receiving NSAIDs. NSAIDs should not be given to patients with a history of GI ulceration or bleeding.

### Haematological effects
NSAIDs increase bleeding time and may increase blood loss. The clinical significance of a tendency to increased bleeding is unclear. It should not inhibit the use of NSAIDs in most cases if there are no specific contraindications. However, NSAIDs should not be given prior to surgery if there is an increased risk of intraoperative bleeding.

### Renal effects
NSAIDs are contraindicated in renally compromised patients. Renal function should be monitored regularly in all patients taking NSAIDs after major surgery. Any increase in urea, creatinine or potassium or decreased urine output is an indication for discontinuing NSAIDs.

### Other contraindications
NSAIDs are contraindicated in patients with hypovolaemia, pre-eclamptic toxaemia or uncontrolled hypertension. NSAIDs are contraindicated in aspirin-sensitive asthmatics and should be used with caution in other asthmatics. NSAIDs should be used with caution in the elderly, in patients with diabetes or vascular disease and after cardiac, hepatobiliary, renal or major vascular surgery.

### Epidural anaesthesia
It is impossible to give meaningful recommendations on the safe use of NSAIDs with epidural anaesthesia.

### Drug interactions
Patients taking NSAIDs should be monitored closely if they are also taking antihypertensive medication, cyclosporin (renal function) or lithium (lithium levels). NSAIDs used in the perioperative period have little clinical effect on warfarin, but INR should be checked after the start or withdrawal of treatment. Low-molecular-weight heparin may be affected by NSAIDs.

## Opioids

- Narcotic – from Greek *narco*, meaning deaden/numb
- Morphine – from Greek *Morpheus*, god of dreams, son of the god of sleep.

  *Pharmacology.* Protein binding is a major determinant of drug distribution. Albumin binds acidic drugs (e.g. morphine); $\alpha_1$ acid glycoprotein (AAG) binds basic drugs (e.g. fentanyl, alfentanyl, sufentanyl). Neonatal albumin and AAG levels reach adult levels by 1 year.

Opioid receptors are found in high concentrations in the limbic system and spinal cord:

- $\mu$ (mu) – analgesia ($\mu_1$), respiratory depression ($\mu_2$), constipation
- $\delta$ (delta) – analgesia, respiratory depression, euphoria
- $\kappa$ (kappa) – spinal analgesia, miosis, sedation, dysphoria, diuresis.

These opioid receptors have recently been reclassified by the International Union of Pharmacology (IUPHAR) as $OP_1$ ($\delta$), $OP_2$ ($\kappa$) and $OP_3$ ($\mu$).

*Actions*
- Cardiovascular – $\downarrow$ SNS drive, direct effect on vagal nucleus to $\downarrow$ HR, direct effect on SA node
- Respiratory – $\downarrow$ rate, dyscoordination, respiratory depression mediated by $\mu$ receptors. $CO_2$ response curve shifted to right. Depression of cough reflex
- Analgesia
- Anxiolysis (shift towards $\delta$ rhythm on EEG)
- Euphoria/dysphoria
- Histamine release via opioid receptors on mast cells. Blocked by naloxone
- GI – smooth muscle spasm, $\downarrow$ lower oesophageal sphincter tone, nausea and vomiting
- Miosis via opioid receptors on Edinger–Westphal nucleus
- Hormonal effects via $D_2$ receptors in hypothalamus – $\uparrow$ ADH, $\uparrow$ GH, $\uparrow$ prolactin; $\downarrow$ ACTH, $\downarrow$ FSH, $\downarrow$ LH
- Muscle rigidity via (?) opioid receptors in substantia nigra.

*Routes of administration.* Up to eightfold variation in minimum analgesic blood levels between patients. Therefore no one regime is suitable for all patients.

*Oral.* Delayed postoperative gastric emptying results in delayed absorption followed by large bolus absorbed when motility returns. May be of more use in the late postoperative period once bowel motility returns.

Nausea and vomiting prevent oral intake. Poor bioavailability because of first pass.

*Sublingual.* Systemic absorption avoids first pass. Dry mouth reduces absorption.

*PR.* Systemic absorption avoids first pass. Not affected by GI motility or nausea and vomiting. Slow absorption delays onset.

*Transdermal.* Rate of absorption $\propto$ lipid solubility. Reduced absorption with vasoconstriction.

*Inhalational.* Used for relieving symptoms of dyspnoea and postoperative pain. Some lost on expiration, widely variable absorption, nasal pruritis and cough limit its clinical application.

*Intra-articular.* Action via intra-articular opioid receptors.

*Intranasal.* Rapid onset of lipid-soluble drugs. Systemic absorption avoids first pass. Useful route for postoperative pain in children.

*Subcutaneous.* Useful for pain relief in children since small cannulae can be inserted with minimal distress. Use with continuous infusion or intermittent bolus.

*Intramuscular.* Pain of injection, erratic uptake if poor tissue perfusion, wide fluctuations in blood levels and thus degree of analgesia and side-effects. Often administered too infrequently if 'prn'.

*Intermittent intravenous injections.* Avoids pain of injection but has similar problems to i.m. route. Needs 1:1 nursing care to monitor respiratory depression.

*Continuous intravenous infusion.* May need initial i.v. bolus dose since steady state takes five half-lives to establish. More stable blood levels, but risk of insidious onset of respiratory depression and obstructive apnoea greater than that with PCA.

*Patient controlled analgesia* (Schzer, 1968). Route of choice. Less overall opioid requirements than other routes. Patient acts as feedback to prevent overdose. Patients do not have to wait after onset of pain to receive analgesia, and immediate administration gives patients a greater sense of control. Requires loading dose and correct settings of lockout time (5–10 min), dose per bolus (0.01–0.025 mg/kg) and maximum dose/hour. Suitable for most children over 5 years. Background dose does not affect total dose.

*Intrathecal/extradural.* Most effective when combined with local anaesthetics. Side-effects are common, especially pruritis. Respiratory depression up to 24 h.

### $\alpha_2$-Agonists (clonidine)

$\alpha_2$-adrenergic receptors are located at peripheral (primary afferent terminals), spinal (neurones in the superficial laminae of the spinal cord) and brainstem sites (brainstem nuclei) where they are involved in nociceptive modulation.

$\alpha_2$-agonists have the following characteristics:

- Haemodynamic stabilizing properties decrease arrhythmias caused by halothane and reduce labetolol requirements in hypotensive anaesthesia
- Sedative and anxiolytic (via activation of postsynaptic $\alpha_2$-adrenoceptors in the locus coeruleus of the brainstem)
- Analgesic – inhibit substance P release at dorsal root ganglia, enhance and prolong duration of epidural
- Reduced sympathetic tone (via activation of postsynaptic $\alpha_2$-adrenoceptors in the nucleus tractus solitarius and locus coeruleus of the brainstem) and reduced cortisol release
- Decreased volatile and i.v. induction agent doses, decreased intraocular pressure and attenuated rise in IOP with intubation, decreased shivering.

### NMDA receptor antagonists

NMDA receptors on the postsynaptic membrane of dorsal horn neurones are activated by glutamate to stimulate ascending pathways. Ketamine blocks the open calcium channel of the NMDA receptor. Psychotomimetic side-effects, salivation and cardiac stimulation limit its use.

## TRANSCUTANEOUS ELECTRICAL NERVE STIMULATION (TENS)

May act through the gate control theory of pain and by release of endorphins. Usually applied at 70 Hz. May take several days of use to achieve maximal effect. Most effective with neurogenic pain such as phantom limb pain, postherpetic neuralgia or nerve damage.

## CHRONIC PAIN

Defined as pain which persists past the time when healing is expected to be complete, usually more than 6 months.

---

**Definition of pain terms**

- *Allodynia* – pain due to a stimulus which does not normally cause pain
- *Dysaesthesia* – an unpleasant abnormal sensation, whether spontaneous or evoked
- *Hyperpathia* – a painful syndrome, characterized by increased reaction to a stimulus, as well as increased threshold
- *Hyperalgesia* – an increased response to a stimulus which is normally painful

---

## REFLEX SYMPATHETIC DYSTROPHY

Reflex sympathetic dystrophy (RSD) is now classified by the International Association for the Study of Pain as complex regional pain syndrome (CRPS) type I, and when associated with nerve injury (i.e. causalgia) it is known as CRPS type II.

*CRPS type I (RSD).* A syndrome that usually follows an initiating noxious event, with spontaneous pain or allodynia/hyperalgesia occurring in a regional distribution and not limited to the territory of a single peripheral nerve. Results in continuous pain in a portion of an extremity (not involving nerve damage), associated with sympathetic hyperactivity.

Characterized by:

1. *Pain.* Initial pain and burning become more diffuse and aching. Hyperalgesia and allodynia may be present.

2. *Autonomic dysfunction.* Abnormal skin blood flow causes both warm red skin and cold, cyanotic changes. Oedema occurs in 50% due to postcapillary vasoconstriction. Following nerve damage, C-polymodal nociceptors in the dorsal horn of the spinal cord develop increased sensitivity to sympathetic stimulation. Stimulation of these causes excess firing, which then causes

increased pain and discharge of sympathetic neurones to the traumatized tissue. The increased sympathetic tone sensitizes peripheral chemoreceptors to such an extent that they fire without a stimulus, causing chronic sympathetically mediated pain. (This concept of central sensitization of the CNS may also be involved with mechanisms of pre-emptive analgesia.)

3. *Trophic changes.* Muscle wasting, thin shiny skin, coarse hair and thickened nails are late manifestations.

4. *Motor impairment.* Weakness and tremor (not necessary for diagnosis). Traditionally divided into three stages, but may not progress beyond the second:

- *Acute stage* – days to months after injury. Pain and oedema. Warm, dry red skin. Treatment most effective at this stage: physiotherapy, NSAIDs, antidepressants and sympathetic nerve block.
- *Dystrophic stage* – 3–6 months after onset of symptoms. Burning pain may spread to involve whole limb. Muscle wasting, pale cyanotic skin associated with increased sympathetic activity. Decreased hair and nail growth, muscle wasting and disuse osteoporosis.
- *Atrophic stage* – 6–12 months after onset of symptoms. Pain may diminish. Cool limb, contractures and severe osteoporosis. Physiotherapy is the most effective treatment at this stage.

**CRPS type II** (*causalgia* – Greek: *kausis* = burning; *algos* = pain). Similar to RSD but associated with traumatic nerve injury. Onset may be delayed for several months. Commonest nerves are median, sciatic, tibial and ulnar.

## POSTHERPETIC NEURALGIA

Pain in the area of acute herpes zoster for at least 1 month after the initial infection. Incidence increases with age; female > male. Pain intensity during acute herpes zoster predicts severity of postherpetic neuralgia. Predilection for thoracic dermatomes and ophthalmic division of trigeminal nerve. Sharp, burning pain. Due to damage of large myelinated fibres which removes inhibition to nociceptive input. Central neurones also expand receptor fields to produce allodynia and hyperpathia.

Early aggressive treatment reduces incidence of pain. Use antidepressants, anticonvulsants, neuroleptics, TENS, sympathetic blocks and topical local anaesthetics. Capsaicin cream enhances release and prevents reaccumulation of substance P from central and peripheral nerve terminals and may be of benefit.

## TRIGEMINAL NEURALGIA

Usually a primary neuralgia, but 3% of cases are due to MS, tumours, vascular malformation or dental lesions. Paroxysmal lancing pain, triggered by tactile stimulation, lasting a few seconds. Increasing severity and frequency of attacks as disease progresses. Anticonvulsants such as carbamazepine block sodium channels to reduce neuronal firing. Phenytoin, sodium valproate and clonazepam may also be effective. Vascular decompression and radiofrequency ablation may benefit some patients.

## POSTOPERATIVE PAIN

In a recent UK study (Kuhn et al 1990), 93% of patients described their post-operative pain as moderate (53%) or very painful (40%). Attempts have therefore been made to improve pain services.

---

**PAIN AFTER SURGERY** Royal College of Surgeons of England and College of Anaesthetists 1990

**Recommendations**
- Extension of acute pain services needed
- Improve education of doctors, nurses and patients
- Designate a person in charge of acute pain services and set up pain team
- Monitor pain, including pain charts
- Encourage use of PCA
- Further research needed into pain management

---

**ANAESTHESIA UNDER EXAMINATION – THE EFFICIENCY AND EFFECTIVENESS OF ANAESTHESIA AND PAIN RELIEF SERVICES IN ENGLAND AND WALES** Audit Commission 1997

**Findings**
- Many patients still suffer postoperative pain and some hospitals are better at controlling it than others
- Some hospitals do not have guidelines regarding postoperative pain management and those that do often do not follow them
- The availability of PCA pumps varies between hospitals. The majority of patients are more satisfied with PCA than with conventional administration of analgesics. There are, however, significant numbers of patients using PCA experiencing poor analgesia or nausea and vomiting
- The use of epidural analgesia for major abdominal and thoracic surgery is increasing, but its use is limited by inadequate numbers of nurses trained in its management
- Patients' analgesia is often changed too quickly from strong opioids to minor analgesics, allowing breakthrough of pain

**Recommendations**
- Develop specific targets to reduce the number of patients in severe pain after an operation, e.g. the Welsh Office has aimed for this to be < 5% by 2002

- Identify one doctor with specialist knowledge of pain relief techniques to promote good practice
- Carry out regular audit of pain relief targets
- Develop evidence-based guidelines on effective analgesic therapies
- The acute pain team should provide written information and guidelines, coordinate and educate staff, and provide leadership and a focus for improved team working
- Develop a programme of continuing education in pain management for trainee doctors and nurses

### References

Association of Anaesthetists 1993 Anaesthetists and non-acute pain management. Guidelines of The Association of Anaesthetists. Association of Anaesthetists, London

Audit Commission 1997 Anaesthesia under examination. The efficiency and effectiveness of anaesthesia and pain relief services in England and Wales. Audit Commission, London

Carr D B, Goudas L C 1999 Acute pain. Lancet 353: 2051–2058

Cervero F, Laird J M A 1999 Visceral pain. Lancet 353: 2145–2148

Eisenach J C, de Kock M, Klimscha W 1996 $\alpha_2$ adrenergic agonists for regional anesthesia. Anesthesiology 85: 655–674

Emery P, Griffiths B, Langman M 1999 Choice of non-steroidal anti-inflammatory drug. Prescribers' Journal 39: 102–108

Kehlet H 1994 Post-operative pain relief – what is the issue? Editorial. British Journal of Anaesthesia 72: 375–377

Khan Z P, Ferguson C N, Jones R M 1999 Alpha-2 and imidazoline receptor agonists. Their pharmacology and therapeutic role. Anaesthesia 54: 146–165

Kissin I 1996 Pre-emptive analgesia. Why its effect is not always obvious. Anesthesiology 84: 1015–1019

Korpela R, Olkkola K T 1999 Paracetamol – misused good old drug? Acta Anaesthesiologica Scandinavica 43: 245–247

Kuhn S, Cooke S, Collins M, Jones L M, Mucklow J C 1990 Perceptions on pain relief after surgery. British Medical Journal 300: 1687–1690

Lambert D G 1998 Recent advances in opioid pharmacology. Postgraduate educational issue. British Journal of Anaesthesia 81: 1–93

Lehmann K A 1997 Update of patient-controlled analgesia. Current Opinion in Anaesthesiology 10: 374–379

McQuay H 1999 Opioids in pain management. Lancet 353: 2229–2232

Royal College of Anaesthetists 1998 Guidelines for the use of non-steroidal anti-inflammatory drugs in the perioperative period. Royal College of Anaesthetists, London

Royal College of Surgeons of England and Royal College of Anaesthetists 1990 Commission on the Provision of Surgical Services. Report of the Working Party on Pain after Surgery. HMSO, London

Symposium 1993 Modern approaches to pain management. Prescribers' Journal 33: 221–266

Walker S M, Cousins M J 1997 Complex regional pain syndromes: including 'reflex sympathetic dystrophy' and 'causalgia'. Anaesthesia and Intensive Care 25: 113–125

# EPIDURAL AND SPINAL ANAESTHESIA

## ANATOMY

Spinal dura is continuous with the meningeal layer of the dura mater of the brain. Vertebral canal periosteum is continuous with the outer layer of the cerebral dura.

Boundaries of the epidural space are:

- superior – foramen magnum
- inferior – sacrococcygeal membrane
- lateral – intervertebral foramina and pedicles
- anterior – posterior longitudinal ligament.

Epidural space contains dural sac, spinal nerve roots, spinal arteries, venous plexus, fat and lymphatics. It is widest in the mid-lumbar region (5–6 mm) and narrows cranially to 1.5–2 mm in the lower cervical spine. Veins are valveless; therefore fluid/air injected into vein passes to intracerebral vessels. Veins drain via azygous vein to IVC. Vena caval obstruction, e.g. pregnancy, distends veins. Intervertebral foramina smaller and calcified in the elderly; therefore smaller volumes of LA required.

Negative pressures in epidural space may be due to coning of the dura at the tip of the epidural needle, pressure transmitted from the thorax, drag of gut viscera on paravertebral spaces or differential growth of the subarachnoid space more than the spinal cord.

When supine, highest point on curve of spine is at $L_3$; lowest point is at $T_6$.

## INDICATIONS FOR REGIONAL ANAESTHESIA

### Patient assessment

Allows assessment of mental state during surgery, e.g. TURP, carotid endarterectomy, diabetes. Avoids risks of aspiration and management of difficult airway.

### Cardiac disease

Avoids haemodynamic response to intubation and hypotensive effects of induction and maintenance agents. Can therefore give greater haemodynamic stability than GA for patients with ischaemic heart disease or failure if managed carefully. May reduce early postoperative mortality compared

.with GA in high-risk patients. Not shown to reduce reinfarction rate compared with GA, but when used for general and vascular surgery, may reduce postoperative cardiac failure (Yeager et al 1987).

Decreased SVR increases cardiac output providing venous return is maintained. Reduced diastolic may reduce coronary artery perfusion pressure. Blockade of cardioaccelerator fibres ($T_1$–$T_4$) may cause bradycardia and impaired cardiovascular response to hypovolaemia.

Pregnant patients with severe cardiac disease, e.g. aortic stenosis, Fallot's, Eisenmenger's and pulmonary hypertension, require good analgesia during labour to prevent potentially dangerous hypertension and tachycardia. However, serious complications can occur following large decreases in systemic vascular resistance and cardiac output.

### Respiratory disease

Epidurals produce longer analgesia and better respiratory function ($FEV_1$ and PEFR) than i.v. morphine. May reduce postoperative respiratory complications by avoiding effects of systemic opioids.

### Gastrointestinal

For GI surgery, an epidural results in good operating conditions, reduces blood loss and gives good postoperative analgesia. However, any hypotension may reduce mesenteric blood flow, and sympathetic blockade may result in a relative increase in parasympathetic activity, causing anastomotic disruption.

### Obesity

Regional anaesthesia avoids managing a difficult airway with risk of aspiration. Postoperative analgesia using epidural opioids provides earlier ambulation, fewer respiratory complications and earlier discharge compared with i.m. opioids.

### Pregnancy

Avoids difficult airway, risk of aspiration and fetal depression with GA. Good postoperative analgesia avoids use of systemic opioids, which contaminate breast milk and impair maternal nursing (drowsiness, nausea and vomiting).

### Malignant hyperthermia

Local anaesthetics do not trigger malignant hyperthermia. Use of epidural avoids triggering agents used for GA.

## Muscle disease

Epidurals allow avoidance of muscle relaxants in myasthenia gravis, muscular dystrophy and myotonic dystrophy.

## Other advantages of regional anaesthesia

- Decreases neuroendocrine stress response and postoperative negative nitrogen balance with less hyperglycaemia because of reduced catecholamine release
- Decreases blood loss
- Decreases incidence of DVT and avoids morbidity of general anaesthetic
- May have a role in pre-emptive analgesia
- Reduces incidence of phantom limb pain if established > 3 days prior to limb amputation.

Yeager et al (1987) investigated 53 high-risk patients. One group had epidural with LA combined with light GA, whilst a second group had GA with high-dose fentanyl. Postoperative analgesia was given with i.m./i.v. opioids ± epidural. Those with epidural had significantly reduced postoperative complications, cardiovascular failure, infection and hospital costs.

## CONTRAINDICATIONS

### Cardiac disease

Fixed output states, e.g. aortic or mitral stenosis, are poorly tolerated if the patient is hypovolaemic or becomes hypotensive.

### Respiratory disease

Respiratory failure is worsened as more intercostal muscles are paralysed.

### Neurological

Epidural or intrathecal injections can cause transient increases in intracranial pressure. Avoid if there is any unstable neurological deficit, e.g. multiple sclerosis. Carefully document any stable deficits preoperatively. Back pain and previous back surgery are generally not contraindications.

### Gastrointestinal

Unopposed parasympathetic activity results in bowel contraction, and in the presence of a perforation, bowel contents are expelled into the peritoneal cavity.

### Septicaemia and local infection

Both contraindicate epidural and spinal anaesthesia.

## Coagulopathy

Epidural/spinal contraindicated if platelets < 100 000 or bleeding time prolonged.

## Aspirin

Low-dose aspirin (75 mg o.d.) prolongs bleeding time only slightly, so it is not necessary to perform a bleeding time. There is no evidence that aspirin at normal doses causes complications with epidurals. Normal bleeding time = 2–9 min.

## Heparin

Prophylactic doses (5000 U b.d.) should be avoided within 4 hours of insertion of a regional block or removal of an epidural catheter. There is no evidence of complications at this dose, although 10–20% of patients will have abnormal PT/PTT. In one study, 30 000 patients in whom heparin was given following epidural catheter insertion showed no adverse sequelae (Rao et al 1981). A study from India showed no complications of epidural catheter insertion in 1200 fully anticoagulated patients! Low-molecular-weight heparin does not produce any anticoagulant effects, so it may be safer.

# EFFECTS OF REGIONAL BLOCKADE

## Local sites of action

### Epidural
- Anterior and posterior spinal roots via root cuffs
- Spinal roots in paravertebral space
- Spinal cord.

### Spinal
- Lateral, anterior and posterior columns
- Dorsal roots, dorsal root ganglia.

## Regional effects

Loss of neuronal transmission occurs in the following order: B → C and Aδ → Aγ → Aβ → Aα, i.e. autonomic → temperature and pain → proprioception → touch and pressure → motor.

Aα = motor, fast sensory
Aβ = touch, vibration, pressure
Aδ = pain, temperature (laminae I and V)
Aγ = muscle spindles

B = autonomic preganglionic fibres
C = autonomic postganglionic fibres, pain (laminae II (substantia gelatinosa)).

### Systemic effects

Cardiovascular and CNS side-effects, usually following inadvertent intravenous injection.

## EPIDURAL

### Methods of detecting epidural space

- Loss of resistance to needle
- Loss of resistance to air/saline (Dogliotti 1933)
- Drip indicator (Baraka 1972) – sudden flow as epidural space entered
- Hanging drop technique (Gutierrez 1932) – withdrawal of hanging drop of fluid
- Odom's Indicator (1936) – air bubble movement in clear tube attached to needle
- Macintosh balloon (1950) – small rubber balloon attached to needle reduces in size as space entered
- Macintosh spring-loaded trocar (1953)
- Spring-loaded syringe (Iklé 1949)
- Amplification of the sound of air entering the epidural space (Sagarnaga 1971).

Midline approach results in the needle entering the epidural space where epidural veins are the least dense.

Adrenaline decreases systemic absorption and reduces the risk of toxicity. It also increases the spread, duration and intensity of the block and perhaps protects against cardiac toxicity. Adrenaline may worsen arterial hypotension through β effects on resistance vessels and increasing the intensity of the sympathetic block.

Early symptoms and signs of intravascular or intrathecal injection are missed if the patient is asleep. Therefore, insert the epidural prior to any GA.

### Factors affecting block

*Age.* Occlusion of intervertebral foraminae in patients > 60 years results in more variable, and usually smaller, doses required.

*Height.* Increased dose, but poor correlation with height.

*Weight.* Lower blocks in obese patients if performed erect, but not if performed whilst supine.

*Direction of bevel.* Spinal blocks using isobaric bupivacaine with a cranially directed bevel may result in a higher sensory block with shorter duration than when the bevel is directed caudally. Not found in all studies.

*Rate of injection.* No effect.

*Total amount (mg) of drug.* Determines level of sensory block, rate of onset and duration of block.

*Concentration of drug.* Determines level of motor block.

*Pharmacological modification.* Bicarbonate reduces the latency and increases the duration of the block by increasing extracellular pH and thus percentage of free base.

Carbonation reduces the latency and increases the duration of block by decreasing intraneuronal pH:

$$pKa - pH = \log \frac{\text{ionized drug}}{\text{unionized drug}}$$

## Phamacokinetics and dynamics

*Uptake of drugs into CSF*
- Via dura
- Via arachnoid granulations and radicular arteries
- Diffusion into epidural fat
- Nerve trunks in paravertebral space.

Increased epidural blood flow in pregnancy increases the rate of epidural absorption. Increased lipid solubility also causes increased fat absorption, preventing an overall increase in CSF delivery.

Uptake of epidural morphine is sufficient to cause analgesia through a systemic route of action.

*Spread of epidural LA.* Spreads in a cephalad and caudad direction from the site of injection. In the thoracic region, the spread is symmetrical, in the lumbar area it is mostly cephalad, and in the caudal area it is mostly cephalad.

*Epidural dosage for a healthy adult*
- 10–12 ml to block to $T_{10}$
- 20–25 ml to block to $T_4$.

Increase these doses by 0.1 ml/segment for each 2 inches over 5 feet in height. Decrease these doses by 30% in the third trimester (venous distension reduces volume of the epidural space, progesterone increases nerve sensitivity to LA), 50% if advanced arteriosclerosis, and 30–50% for thoracic epidurals.

## Advantages of continuous epidural infusions

- Safer if migration of catheter into subarachnoid space
- Less motor block than with top-ups
- Better analgesia – avoids peaks and troughs
- Better cardiovascular stability

- Lower total dose of local anaesthetic required
- Avoids top-ups
- Fewer side-effects, e.g. less nausea, vomiting and pruritus with opioids.

### Bupivacaine

Increased cardiotoxicity of bupivacaine due to:

- increased progesterone in pregnancy
- acidosis, e.g. pregnancy
- β-blockers
- calcium-channel blockers.

## SPINAL BLOCK

The degree of sympathetic block is greater and the onset of hypotension faster with spinal compared with epidural blockade.

Sympathetic block tends to be 2–3 segments above the level of sensory block, unlike epidurals where sensory and sympathetic blocks are usually at the same level.

## EPIDURAL AND SPINAL OPIOIDS

Introduced by Yaksh and Rudy in 1976.

Neuraxial opioids decrease LA requirements, thereby reducing motor blockade and improving pain relief. Compared with parenteral administration, opioids increase the duration of block and may decrease serious morbidity and mortality in high-risk surgical patients, probably through improving postoperative pulmonary function. Epidural opioids also speed the onset of block.

Lipophilicity determines onset, speed and duration of analgesia. Increasing lipophilicity results in greater systemic action of opioids. Epidural fentanyl (intermediate solubility) is reported to be no more effective than parenteral administration.

### Lipid solubility

The relative lipid solubility of certain drugs is as follows: morphine < pethidine < alfentanyl < diamorphine < fentanyl < buprenorphine. There is an inverse relationship between lipid solubility and potency.

Low lipophilicity of morphine results in drug migrating rostrally in the CSF to cause delayed respiratory depression. Lipid-soluble drugs penetrate the dorsal horn faster with quicker onset of action. Early respiratory depression occurs via systemic absorption from vertebral veins and via azygous veins to superior vena cava. Systemic administration of NSAIDs may decrease opioid requirements and enhance analgesia.

# COMPLICATIONS OF SPINAL/EPIDURAL ANAESTHESIA

## Safety

Mechanisms of toxicity include vasoconstriction, vascular injury and alteration in blood flow to the spinal cord; also injection of incorrect solution, bacterial contamination and chronic inflammation from catheters.

2-Chloroprocaine and hypertonic saline both cause spinal cord damage. Phenol contamination of intrathecal LA (described by Wooley & Roe in 1954).

## Cardiac arrest

More common with spinal (0.06%) than with epidural (0.01%) anaesthesia. In some cases, associated with intraoperative sedation (fentanyl, thiopentone, diazepam). Cardiac arrest is often preceded by cyanosis, suggesting hypoventilation, hypotension and bradycardia.

## Hypotension

Due to loss of tone in resistance and capacitance vessels, causing decreased venous return, vasodilatation and decreased cardiac output.

Block below sympathetic outflow tract ($T_1$–$L_2$) has no effect on BP. Hypotension is worse if cardioaccelerator fibres ($T_2$–$T_4$) are blocked, which removes the ability to compensate for other circulatory changes. Crystalloid preload has a variable effect on preventing hypotension following spinal anaesthesia. Fluids alone have been shown to be unable to maintain BP in 50% of patients, and ephedrine in 17%, but metaraminol maintained BP in all patients following spinal anaesthesia. If there is any delay in performing the regional block, much of the fluid preload is redistributed to the extracellular compartment, reducing any benefit of preloading. Fluids should therefore only be given after establishment of the block as the block evolves. Vagal overactivity may cause severe hypotension in some patients.

Hypotension following a regional block during pregnancy may be treated safely with small doses of ephedrine (3–6 mg) or phenylephrine (80–100 $\mu$g). The use of pure $\alpha$-agonists at higher doses may be associated with reduced placental flow, despite an increased MAP. Hypotension following a combined spinal/extradural technique is less marked by rapid establishment of a low spinal block followed by careful extradural extension into higher segments. Ephedrine causes nausea more frequently when given as a bolus (36%), compared with an infusion (5%).

## Respiratory system

Respiratory impairment will occur if the block is too high. Impairment of force of cough and bronchoconstriction. Brainstem depression of respiratory centre due to direct effect of LA.

## Total spinal blockade

Characterized by rapid onset of hypotension, respiratory arrest and loss of consciousness. May not be revealed by test dose. Requires immediate intubation, i.v. fluids and vasopressors.

## Backache

Significant increase in long-term backache if epidural given during labour (18.2% vs. 10.2%), for instrumental delivery or emergency LSCS (19.2%). No increased risk if epidural used for elective LSCS.

Day-case spinals are associated with 37% headache and 55% backache; therefore avoid use for day cases. Quinke > Sprogt > Whitacre at 1 day but no difference by 1 week.

## Headache

Postdural puncture headache is caused by loss of CSF through dural tear with loss of CSF cushion and traction on pain-sensitive intracranial structures. Described by Bier in 1989 who suffered a severe postdural headache after an experiment on himself resulted in a dural tap. Traction above the tentorium is transmitted via the trigeminal nerve to the frontal region; traction below the tentorium is transmitted by the vagus to the occiput and neck. Incidence is not affected by posture following spinal. Incidence following spinal is reduced with small-gauge pencil-point needles: Quinke > Sprogt > Whitacre at 1 day but little difference between needles at 1 week. Epidural catheters introduced into the CSF following dural tap reduce incidence of headache, perhaps by a fibroblast reaction sealing the tear.

Dura usually seals spontaneously within 1 week, but in persisting cases may cause intracerebral haemorrhage, subdural haemorrhage and cranial nerve palsies. Bed rest and hydration may improve symptoms. Epidural saline infusion, i.v. caffeine and abdominal binders are also reported to reduce symptoms.

Perform an autologous blood patch at 1–3 days if symptoms do not resolve. Largest study from USA (American Society for Obstetric Anesthesia and Perinatology) showed 182 of 185 women completely and permanently cured of symptoms using an average of 10 ml of blood injected 4 days after the dural tear. Symptoms are often relieved immediately. MRI scanning shows that the clot has an initial mass effect, with anterior displacement and compression of the dura and nerve roots over a mean of 4.6 vertebral segments, mostly cephalad. Clot resolution occurs by 7 h to leave a thick mature clot over the dorsal dura. A small amount of blood may enter the CSF (which accelerates its clotting). Spread of blood back into subcutaneous fat may cause backache following blood patch. No residual adhesions are formed in the epidural space.

### Neural damage

More common if associated with paraesthesia during puncture or local anaesthetic injection.

Direct trauma to the spinal cord may result if the needle is inserted above $L_1$. Causes severe lancinating pain in the dermatomes below the level of insertion.

Transverse myelitis is also documented.

### Spinal haematoma

Rare but significant morbidity (irreversible neurological injury and paraplegia). Estimated as 1:150 000 for epidural block and 1:220 000 for spinal block. Risk factors include coagulopathies (antiplatelet or oral anti-coagulant drugs, chronic alcohol abuse, chronic renal failure), anatomical abnormalities (7%), technical difficulties (25%), bloody tap (25%), multiple punctures (20%) and insertion of an epidural catheter (50%).

A recent USA series of 43 cases had a mean age of 74 years and 75% were female. Cases occurred up to 12 days after low-molecular-weight heparin (LMWH) was started, with diagnosis being made a median of 24 h after onset of symptoms. Usually presenting as lower limb weakness or numbness and *not* severe radicular back pain as is traditionally taught. Requires immediate surgical decompression to avoid permanent neurological damage.

More case reports of spinal haematoma with LMWH than with unfractionated heparin. May be due to fibrinolytic activity of LMWH and greater inhibition of platelet binding to fibrinogen and endothelium. Combination of LMWH and NSAID may further increase risk.

### Other complications

*Spinal abscess.* Onset of fever and back pain over 1–3 days. CSF leucocytosis.

*Horner's syndrome.* Sympathetic blockade presumed due to tracking of LA.

*Shivering.* Reduced by warming i.v. solutions and adding fentanyl to the LA.

*Urinary retention.* Attributed to loss of bladder sensation but still occurs if sensation intact.

*Gastrointestinal.* Nausea and vomiting due to a central effect of LA. Dopaminergic stimulation by opioids. Loss of sympathetic inhibition results in small bowel contraction and expression of gut contents through a bowel perforation.

*Foreign body.* Breakage of catheter. Shearing of catheter if withdrawn back through the needle.

*Prolonged labour.* Most studies show an increased risk of instrumental delivery of LSCS.

## SIDE-EFFECTS OF CENTRAL OPIOIDS

### Respiratory depression

0.09% incidence with extradural morphine, and 0.36% following spinal morphine. Can occur up to 24 h, especially with water-soluble opioids.

Worse in the presence of other respiratory depressants, patient supine, rapid injection (intrathecal), elderly, respiratory disease and increased intra-abdominal pressure.

### Pruritus

- Intrathecal – 46%
- Epidural – 8.5%.

Especially common with morphine. Less common if bupivacaine is mixed with opioid.

Can be reduced with naloxone (5–10 $\mu$g/kg per h), propofol (10 mg), droperidol (2.5 mg) or ondansetron (8 mg).

### Nausea and vomiting

Much more common with intrathecal opioids than with epidural opioids. Occurs in 20% of patients given epidural morphine.

Scopolamine patch decreases incidence in labour.

### References

Auroy Y, Narchi P, Messiah A, Litt L, Rouvier B, Samii K 1997 Serious complications related to regional anaesthesia. Anesthesiology 87: 479–486

Carrie L E S 1993 Postdural puncture headache and extradural blood patch. Editorial. British Journal of Anaesthesia 71: 179–180

Carson D F, Serpell M G 1995 Clinical characteristics of commonly used spinal needles. Anaesthesia 50: 523–525

Checketts M R, Wildsmith J A W 1999 Central nerve block and thromboprophylaxis – is there a problem? British Journal of Anaesthesia 82: 164–167

Critchley L A H 1996 Hypotension, subarachnoid block and the elderly patient. Anaesthesia 51: 1139–1143

Hodgson P S, Neal J M, Pollock J E, Liu S S 1999 The neurotoxicity of drugs given intrathecally (spinal). Anesthesia and Analgesia 88: 797–809

Horlocker T T, Wedel D J 1998 Spinal and epidural blockade and perioperative low molecular weight heparin: smooth sailing on the Titanic. Anesthesia and Analgesia 86: 1153–1156

Mulroy M F, Norris M C, Liu S S 1997 Safety steps for epidural injection of local anaesthetics: review of the literature and recommendations. Anesthesia and Analgesia 85: 1346–1356

Rao T L, El-Etr A A 1981 Anticoagulation following placement of epidural and subarachnoid catheters: an evaluation of neurologic sequelae. Anesthesiology 55(6): 618–620

Vakharia S B, Thomas P S, Rosebaum A E, Wasenko J J, Fellows D G 1997 Magnetic resonance imaging of cerebrospinal fluid leak and tamponade effect of blood patch in postdural puncture headache. Anesthesia and Analgesia 84: 585–590

Yeager M P, Glass D D, Neff R K, Brinck-Johnsen T 1987 Epidural anesthesia and analgesia in high-risk surgical patients. Anesthesiology 66: 729–736

# 11. Pharmacology

## OXYGEN

Discovered by Joseph Priestley in 1777. Manufactured by:

- fractional distillation of liquid air
- passing air over an artificial zeolite, which entraps $N_2$, leaving a gas containing greater than 90% $O_2$.

Critical temperature: 119°C
Critical pressure: 50 bar
Boiling point: −182.5°C

Vacuum insulated evaporator (VIE) stores $O_2$ at −180°C at a pressure of ≈10 bar. One litre of liquid oxygen evaporates to give 842 l $O_2$ at standard temperature and pressure (STP). Contents of a VIE are measured by weighing scales on which the VIE sits.

## NITROUS OXIDE

Sweet-smelling, non-irritant colourless gas. First prepared by Joseph Priestley in 1772. First used as an anaesthetic agent in 1845 by Horace Wells. Now manufactured by heating ammonium nitrate with products washed through water and caustic soda to remove NO and $NO_2$:

$$NH_4NO_3 \xrightarrow{240°C} 2H_2O + N_2O$$

Critical temperature: 36.5°C
Critical pressure: 71.7 bar
Boiling point: −89°C
Blood:gas solubility: 0.42
MAC: 105%

Exists in cylinder as a liquid so pressure in cylinder does not reflect contents. Measure contents by weight

Filling ratio: temperate, 0.75; tropics, 0.67

### Entonox

- 500 l cylinders – store at > 10°C for 2 h or, alternatively, place in water at 37°C for 5 min and invert three times before use
- 2000 and 5000 l cylinders – store at 10–45°C for 24 h in horizontal position. Do not store < 0°C for > 10 min after delivery.

Only Entonox cylinders contain a dip tube. If Entonox laminates, lower level of fluid contains ≈ 80% $N_2O$ and 20% $O_2$, which is delivered to patient via a dip tube. The mixture gradually becomes richer in $O_2$. If gas was withdrawn from the top of the cylinder, it would initially contain 20% $N_2O$ and 80% $O_2$, but as this mixture was withdrawn, the remaining liquid would become very low in $O_2$ and a hypoxic mixture would eventually be delivered to the patient.

Analgesia is due to release of endogenous opioids and direct effect at opioid receptors.

### Side-effects

- Diffusion hypoxia
- Diffusion into air-filled cavities (35 times more soluble in blood than $N_2$)
- Diffusion out of gas-filled pockets at end of surgery, e.g. retinal detachment
- SNS stimulant, but if SNS already stimulated, e.g. LVF, $N_2O$ causes hypotension, particularly in the presence of opioids
- Reduced bowel motility
- Limits $F_iO_2$
- Increases intracranial pressure
- Nausea and vomiting
- Irreversibly inactivates cob(I)alamin, the active form of vitamin $B_{12}$, essential for methionine-synthase activity in the brain. Recurrent exposure to nitrous oxide has been documented to cause vitamin $B_{12}$ deficiency (subacute combined degeneration of the cord, megaloblastic anaemia, spastic paraparesis, encephalopathy). Cobalamin-deficient patients are particularly susceptible (deficient $B_{12}$ consumption, $B_{12}$ malabsorption)
- High-dose (> 70%) nitrous oxide is teratogenic in rats. There is concern over effects in humans
- Increased spontaneous abortion rate in female staff exposed to waste gas. Dental assistants exposed to more than 5 h/week of unscavenged $N_2O$ take longer to become pregnant than those exposed to lesser amounts

## XENON

Proposed as a replacement for nitrous oxide. The only inert gas with anaesthetic properties at ambient pressure, having a MAC of 71% and the lowest blood/gas partition coefficient of any anaesthetic gas, making induction and recovery very rapid. Minimal haemodynamic effects. Prepared from air where it is present in a concentration of 0.000 009%, making it very expensive (£10/l).

## CARBON DIOXIDE

Colourless, pungent gas. Prepared by:

- by-product of beer fermentation
- waste gas from burning fuel
- by-product of $H_2$ manufacture.

Critical temperature: −31°C
Critical pressure: 73.8 bar
Filling ratio: temperate, 0.75; tropics, 0.67

### References

Dingley J, Ivanova-Stoilova T M, Grundler S, Wall T 1999 Xenon: recent developments. Anaesthesia 54: 335–346

Langton J A 1994 Gases used in anaesthesia. In: Nimmo W S, Rowbotham D J, Smith G (eds) Anaesthesia, 2nd edn. Blackwell Scientific Publications, Oxford

Lee P, Smith I, Piesowicz A, Brenton D 1999 Spastic paraparesis after anaesthesia. Lancet 353: 554

Shaw A D S, Morgan M 1998 Nitrous oxide: time to stop laughing? Anaesthesia 53: 213–215

Smith W D A 1972 A history of nitrous oxide and oxygen anaesthesia. British Journal of Anaesthesia 44: 212–215

## DRUG INTERACTIONS

- *Pharmacokinetics* determine the relationship between dose administered and concentration delivered to site of action, i.e. effect of body on drug.
- *Pharmacodynamics* determine the relationship between concentration of drug at site of action and intensity of effect produced, i.e. effect of drug on body.

## MONOAMINE OXIDASE INHIBITORS (MAOIs)

MAO-A is found in CNS, and MAO-B in liver, lungs and kidneys. Most new MAOIs are selective for type A and are reversible within 48 h.
  Actions:

- Decrease sympathetic tone with decreased ability to respond to stress
- Postural hypotension
- Decrease plasma cholinesterase and thereby prolong action of suxamethonium
- Synergistic with insulin to cause hypoglycaemia
- No serious interaction with common agents except pethidine. Reaction with pethidine (via norpethidine) causes pyrexia, hypertension, CNS excitation and coma. Unlikely to occur with other opioids
- Indirect sympathomimetics are contraindicated because they cause excess noradrenaline release.

## TRICYCLICS

- Inhibit reuptake of noradrenaline at nerve terminals, potentiating action of adrenaline, noradrenaline and other catecholamines.
- Anticholinergic side-effects potentiate anticholinergic effect of other drugs, e.g. atropine, glycopyrrolate
- Quinidine-like membrane-stabilizing effects with prolonged PR interval, widened QRS complex and risk of VF.

Therefore tricyclics result in an increased risk of arrhythmias and hypotension.

## SELECTIVE SEROTONIN REUPTAKE INHIBITORS (fluoxetine (Prozac), sertraline, paroxetine)

Second-generation antidepressants replacing tricyclics. Selectively inhibit presynaptic 5HT reuptake, causing an increase in serotonin at the synaptic cleft.

- Common side-effects include nausea, diarrhoea, headache, insomnia and syndrome of inappropriate ADH secretion (particularly in the elderly)
- Overdose is usually associated with few symptoms unless combined with MAOIs or tricyclics when a serotonin syndrome may occur, characterized by coma, hyperreflexia, autonomic instability (fever, diarrhoea, tachycardia, labile BP), DIC, myoglobinaemia, renal failure and death
- $P_{450}$ inhibition causes interaction with haloperidol, tricyclics, theophylline, phenytoin, carbamazepine and warfarin.

### Anaesthetic implications

Exclude hyponatraemia and clotting abnormalities preoperatively.

Inhibition of midazolam metabolism prolongs its action. Seratomimetic drugs (pethidine, pentazocine, dextromethorphan) may cause a serotonin syndrome. May antagonize the $\mu$ opioid receptor to cause reduced effects of opioids.

## ANTICONVULSANTS

- Barbiturates and phenytoin induce $P_{450}$ hepatic enzymes with increased dose requirements of anaesthetic drugs
- Also cause resistance to non-depolarizers (except atracurium) possibly via effect on ACh receptors
- No significant reaction of benzodiazepines with anaesthetic drugs.

## ANGIOTENSIN-CONVERTING ENZYME (ACE) INHIBITORS

May improve perioperative CVS stability but are associated with peri- and postoperative hypotension. Consider stopping drug 24 h before surgery.

## H$_2$ ANTAGONISTS

*Ranitidine.* Causes sinus bradycardia and AV block, especially following i.v. administration.

*Cimetidine.* Inhibits hepatic cytochrome $P_{450}$, increasing levels and thus toxicity of lignocaine, nifedipine and propanolol (Table 11.1). Potentiation of action of warfarin and theophyllines. Cimetidine competes with creatinine for renal excretion.

**Table 11.1** Drugs affecting hepatic enzymes

| Hepatic enzyme induction | Hepatic enzyme inhibition |
| --- | --- |
| Alcohol | Cimetidine |
| Barbiturates | Erythromycin |
| Phenytoin | Ciprofloxacin |
| Carbamazepine | |
| Sodium valproate | |

## DROPERIDOL

Butyrophenone; used for neuroleptic anaesthesia and as an antiemetic. Causes:

- mental detachment
- catatonia
- dopaminergic antagonism (acts at chemoreceptor trigger zone)
- $\alpha$-adrenergic antagonism, causing hypotension. Exacerbates hypotensive effects of anaesthetic agents

- amphetamine antagonism
- gamma-aminobutyric acid (GABA) antagonism.

Large doses cause extrapyramidal movements. Gives some protection against catecholamine-induced arrhythmias. Reduces oxygen uptake. Has minimal effects on CVS, respiratory or liver function.

## LEUCOTRIENE ANTAGONISTS (montelukast, zafirlukast)

Leucotriene receptor antagonists block receptors in bronchial smooth muscle and are therefore of use in treating asthma:

- Zafirlukast – inhibits cytochrome $P_{450}$ enzyme
- Montelukast – metabolized by cytochrome $P_{450}$ enzyme.

### References

Fee J P H, McCaughey W 1994 Preoperative preparation, premedication and concurrent drug therapy. In: Nimmo W S, Rowbotham D J, Smith G (eds) Anaesthesia, 2nd edn. Blackwell Scientific Publications, Oxford, p 677–703
Kam P C A, Chang G W M 1997 Selective serotonin reuptake inhibitors. Anaesthesia 52: 982–988
Licker M, Morel D R 1998 Inhibitors of the renin angiotensin system: implications for the anaesthesiologist. Current Opinion in Anaesthesiology 11: 321–326
Vuyk J 1997 Drug interactions in anaesthesia. Current Opinion in Anaesthesiology 10: 267–270

## ECSTASY

Ecstasy (3,4-methylenedioxymethamphetamine, MDMA) is an amphetamine derivate with similar properties to sister drugs 'Eve' (3,4-methylene-dioxyethamphetamine) and 'Ice' (3,4-methylenedioxyamphetamine). First produced in 1914 as an appetite suppressant but not used again until the 1970s when it was reintroduced for psychotherapy to give energy and euphoria.

Acute effects include empathy, heightened alertness, acute psychosis trismus and tachycardia. Positive effects tend to decrease with regular use, while negative effects increase. Hangover lasts 4–5 days and is associated with depression and impaired memory.

MDMA causes the release of 5HT, one of the neurotransmitters implicated in control of mood. In primates, it causes irreversible loss of serotonergic nerve fibres. 5HT is a neurotransmitter triggering the thermoregulatory centre in the hypothalamus to increase body temperature.

Main problems in the management of these patients are:

- Acute side-effects related to hyperpyrexia causing a syndrome similar to malignant hyperthermia with rhabdomyolysis, DIC and multiple organ failure. Mortality relates to the extent and duration of hyperthermia. Rapid cooling and use of dantrolene if core temperature > 40°C have been recommended.
- Drinking of large amounts of water at 'raves' to prevent dehydration causes dilutional hyponatraemia and cerebral oedema. This may also be associated with the syndrome of inappropriate production of antidiuretic hormone.
- Acute liver failure may occur due to either a reaction to MDMA itself or a reaction to a contaminant.

**References**

Hall A P 1997 'Ecstasy' and the anaesthetist. British Journal of Anaesthesia 79: 697–698

# INTRAVENOUS INDUCTION AGENTS

## THIOPENTONE

Prepared as 6% anhydrous sodium carbonate in nitrogen to prevent thiopentone forming acid with the $CO_2$ present in air. pH of 2.5% solution = 10.8.

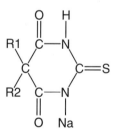

Highly lipid-soluble and rapidly distributed into the tissues. Pharmacokinetics are those of a three compartment model. Undergoes first-order kinetics.

80% protein bound; $t_{1/2}$ = 12 h. Induction dose 4–5 mg/kg. Oxidized by liver to inactive metabolites with renal excretion. Serious allergic reactions are rare but severe.

## Physiological effects

- ↓ myocardial contractility and peripheral vasodilation

- ↑ bronchial muscle tone and laryngeal spasm
- ↓ ICP, ↓ CNS flow, ↓ CNS metabolism
- ↓ IOP
- ↓ SNS > PNS.

### Accidental intra-arterial thiopentone injection

- Immediate pain and blanching
- Arterial obstruction due to vascular spasm and obstruction by thiopentone crystals.

#### Treatment
- Leave needle in place
- Irrigate with saline. Commence anticoagulation with heparin and then warfarin for 2 weeks
- Give 10 ml of 1% procaine to buffer thiopentone and act as LA
- Consider papaverine 40 mg, phenoxybenzamine 0.5 mg or urokinase
- Sympathetic block, e.g. brachial plexus block
- Keep limb warm, elevate and continue with the GA to dilate vessels.

## PROPOFOL (di-isopropylphenol)

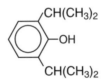

Emulsified in soya bean oil and egg phosphatide (formerly Cremphor EL).
$t_{1/2}$ = 4 h. Induction dose 2–3 mg/kg. Highly lipid-soluble.
Metabolized by liver and extrahepatic sites (?lung). Hepatic excretion.
Delay in loss of eyelash reflex. Short duration of action makes drug suitable for day-case anaesthesia and ITU sedation.

### Physiological effects

- Hypotension due to vasodilation more than myocardial depression
- Tachycardia. Resets baroreceptors to allow ↓ BP
- Bronchial muscle tone unchanged. Less laryngospasm than other induction agents.

## METHOHEXITONE

Prepared in 6% anhydrous sodium carbonate. pH of 1% solution = 11.1.
$t_{1/2}$ = 4 h. Induction dose 1–1.5 mg/kg. Metabolized to 4-OH methohexitone

(inactive). Causes involuntary muscle movement (including hiccough). Pain on injection.

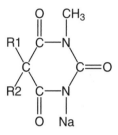

Less cardiovascular depression than with thiopentone. Epileptiform EEG, therefore good for electroconvulsive therapy. Rapid recovery, therefore good for day-case surgery.

## ETOMIDATE

Carboxylated imidazole; pH 3.3. Dissolved in propylene glycol.

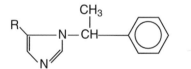

$t_{1/2}$ = 1.2 h; 75% protein bound. Induction dose 0.3 mg/kg.

Inhibits 17$\alpha$- and 11$\beta$-hydroxylase, impairing adrenal function. Broken down by esterase hydrolysis in plasma and liver. Renal excretion.

Most haemodynamically stable of all i.v. induction agents. Causes post-operative nausea and vomiting. Venous thrombosis. Worst agent for pain on injection. Dose-related myoclonus.

## KETAMINE

Phencyclidine derivative; pH 4.0.

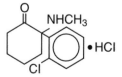

$t_{1/2}$ = 2.5 h; 12% protein bound. Racemic mixture; S form is 3–5 times more potent than R form. S form causes hallucinations.

Liver breakdown by demethylation and hydroxylation to form norketamine (active). Metabolism slowed in the presence of halothane and benzodiazepines.

Renal excretion. Contraindicated with ischaemic heart disease, hypertension and in psychiatric patients.

### Physiological effects

- ↑ CNS metabolic rate
- ↑ BP, ↑ HR, ↑ CO (possibly secondary to ↑ $Ca^{2+}$ flux modulated by cAMP)
- Salivation. Bronchial smooth muscle dilation
- Dissociative analgesia possibly via NMDA receptors.

## MIDAZOLAM

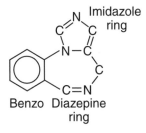

Benzo Diazepine ring

Addition of a fused imidazole ring to the benzodiazepine structure. Prepared as a solution at pH 3.5 with an open ring structure making the drug water-soluble. After injection, the change in pH closes the ring to form a highly lipophilic compound.

$t_{1/2}$ = 2.5 h; 94% protein bound. Hydroxylated by the liver to active metabolites. Renal excretion.

Hypnotic, anxiolytic, amnesic and anticonvulsant. Induction dose of 0.15–0.3 mg/kg. Relatively slow induction. Hypotension due to vasodilation and negative inotropic effect. Causes apnoea on induction in 10–20% of patients. Minimal effect on ICP.

Reversed with the benzodiazepine antagonist, flumazenil.

### References

Hirota K, Lambert D G 1996 Ketamine: its mechanism(s) of action and unusual clinical uses. British Journal of Anaesthesia 77: 441–444

Mather L E, Edwards S R 1998 Chirality in anaesthesia – ropivacaine, ketamine and thiopentone. Current Opinion in Anaesthesiology 11: 383–390

Ostwald P, Doenicke A W 1998 Etomidate revisited. Current Opinion in Anaesthesiology 11: 391–398

White M, Kenny G N C 1994 Intravenous anaesthetic agents. In: Nimmo W S, Rowbotham D J, Smith G (eds) Anaesthesia, 2nd edn. Blackwell Scientific Publications, Oxford

# LOCAL ANAESTHETICS

## PHARMACOLOGY AND PHYSIOLOGY

Local anaesthetics are weak bases. The proportion of drug existing in an ionized form is dependent upon the pH of the solution. The non-ionized form diffuses into the axoplasm where it becomes charged and binds with sodium channels.

$$pH - pKa = \log \frac{\text{ionized } [BH^+]}{\text{unionized } [B]}$$

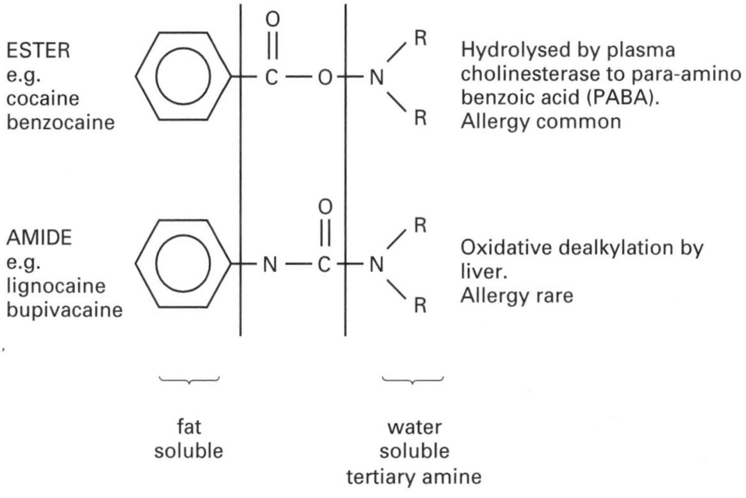

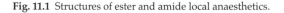

**ESTER**
e.g.
cocaine
benzocaine

Hydrolysed by plasma cholinesterase to para-amino benzoic acid (PABA). Allergy common

**AMIDE**
e.g.
lignocaine
bupivacaine

Oxidative dealkylation by liver. Allergy rare

fat soluble

water soluble tertiary amine

**Fig. 11.1** Structures of ester and amide local anaesthetics.

### Frequency-dependent block

Open sodium channels are more susceptible to local anaesthetic binding than those in a closed state. Thus, the higher the frequency of stimulation, the more intense the block. Nerves that carry high-frequency impulses, e.g. sensory nerves, are more susceptible to block than those carrying low-frequency impulses, e.g. motor nerves. This frequency-dependent block may explain why cardiac toxicity of local anaesthetics is more pronounced at faster heart rates.

### Differential nerve block

Three successive nodes of Ranvier must be blocked by local anaesthetic to block nerve conduction. Thicker nerves have more widely spaced nodes and therefore take longer to be blocked. Thus small-diameter A$\delta$ and C pain fibres are blocked earlier than large A$\alpha$ motor fibres. If muscle relaxation in addition to analgesia is required (e.g. to reduce a dislocation), a higher dose of local anaesthetic is required.

### pH effects

Local anaesthetics are usually prepared as the salt to provide solubility and stability. Most local anaesthetics dissolved in water have a pKa of $\approx 8$. At a physiological pH of 7.4, more cation will be present than base. Addition of bicarbonate increases the proportion of drug present in the unionized form and increases the speed of onset. Local anaesthetics with low pKa have an increased speed of onset. Potency $\propto \uparrow$ pKa.

Inflamed tissues have a low pH, so LA exists mostly in the ionized form and thus little drug reaches the sodium channels.

### Vasoconstriction/dilation

All local anaesthetics cause vasoconstriction at very low doses, but vasodilate at higher doses. Cocaine causes vasoconstriction by inhibiting noradrenaline uptake.

### Convulsions

Appear to be triggered by the limbic system to cause seizures electrographically resembling temporal lobe epilepsy: dysphoria, metallic taste in the mouth, circumoral numbness, slurred speech, dizziness, fine twitching of the small muscles of the face and hands, drowsiness, generalized convulsion. Highest blood levels seen after intercostal block, interpleural block and topical anaesthesia of upper airway. Lowest levels seen with spinal anaesthesia.

### Cardiotoxicity

Unlike other local anaesthetics, bupivacaine toxicity usually manifests as myocardial depression rather than neurological symptoms. Highly protein bound to myocardial tissue. VF arrest is best treated with early administration of bretylium. Animal studies suggest noradrenaline may be more effective than adrenaline during cardiopulmonary resuscitation.

## SPECIFIC DRUGS

**EMLA cream** (Eutectic mixture of local anaesthetic)

Eutectic means having a low melting point, below that of either compound separately. Mixture of 2.5% lignocaine and 2.5% prilocaine. In addition to its use for venepuncture, has also been used for split-skin grafts, removal of anal warts and postherpetic neuralgia. Large doses can cause methaemoglobinaemia. Depresses local immune response when applied topically to open wounds.

### Amethocaine gel

4% amethocaine gel has a much more rapid onset than EMLA and is a vasodilator, but local histamine release may cause itching. It is rapidly absorbed from mucous membranes and should never be applied to inflamed, traumatized or highly vascular surfaces. Should not be left on for more than 45 min because of risk of methaemoglobinaemia.

### Tetracaine gel

New topical agent. Applied for at least 45 min before cannulation. Anaesthesia lasts for 4–6 h after removal. Has vasodilatory effects which may improve ease of cannulation.

### Prilocaine

Prilocaine is metabolized to toluidine which reduces Hb to methaemoglobin. A dose greater than 600 mg prilocaine risks methaemoglobinaemia (reduction of > 1.5 mg/dl Hb). Treat with 1 mg/kg methylene blue i.v.

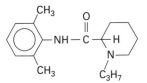

Ropivacaine

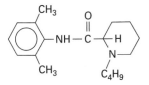

Bupivacaine

**Fig. 11.2** Ropivacaine and bupivacaine.

### Ropivacaine

An amide anaesthetic structurally similar to bupivacaine, with similar potency and duration as bupivacaine but less cardiotoxicity (Fig. 11.2). This may be because it is manufactured in the S (–) form, whereas bupivacaine exists in the racemic (RS) form. The sensory block is similar to that provided by bupivacaine but the motor block is slower in onset, less intense and shorter in duration. It is an effective vasoconstrictor (bupivacaine vasodilates) and has no detrimental effect on placental blood flow. Cardiotoxicity and CNS symptoms occur at higher doses compared with bupivacaine.

## MAXIMUM RECOMMENDED DOSES

Table 11.2  Maximum recommended doses of some common local anaesthetics

|  | Plain | With adrenaline |
|---|---|---|
| Lignocaine | 3 mg/kg | 7 mg/kg |
| Bupivacaine | 2 mg/kg | 2 mg/kg |
| Prilocaine | 5 mg/kg | 8 mg/kg |
| Cocaine | 2 mg/kg | |
| Amethocaine | 1.5 mg/kg | |

### References

McClure J H 1996 Ropivacaine. British Journal of Anaesthesia 76: 300–307
Neal M J 1992 Medical pharmacology at a glance. Blackwell Scientific Publications, Oxford
O'Sullivan G 1998 What's new in local anaesthetics for obstetric anaesthesia? Current Opinion in Anaesthesiology 11: 259–263
Tucker G T 1994 Local anaesthetic drugs: mode of action and pharmacokinetics. In: Nimmo W S, Rowbotham D J, Smith G (eds) Anaestheisa, 2nd edn. Blackwell Scientific Publications, Oxford

## NEUROMUSCULAR BLOCKADE

## NEUROMUSCULAR BLOCKING DRUGS

*Tubocurarine* (dTC). Long-acting non-depolarizing quaternary ammonium compound. First neuromuscular blocker to be used clinically by Griffiths and Johnson in Montreal in 1942. Prepared from the plant *Chondrodendron tomentosum*; 50% protein bound. Hypotension secondary to histamine release and also SNS > PNS blockade, causing bradycardia. Minimal metabolism. Excreted in bile and urine.

*Gallamine.* Blocks vagus and acts as $\beta_1$-agonist to cause tachycardia and hypertension. Crosses placenta, so contraindicated in obstetrics. 85% renal excretion; therefore avoid in renal failure.

## Benzylisoquinoliniums

*Doxacurium.* Long-acting non-depolarizing drug with no cardiovascular side-effects; 25% recovery of twitch height in 2–3 h. Excreted by the kidney unchanged, with minor pathway via the liver. Therefore prolonged action in hepatic and renal failure.

*Mivacurium.* Short-acting non-depolarizing drug. Consists of three stereoisomers, two with short elimination half-lives of 1.8–1.9 min, the third with an elimination half-life of 53 min but only one-tenth as potent. Hydrolysed by plasma cholinesterases to inactive metabolites. Duration of action prolonged by same factors that affect suxamethonium, e.g. atypical enzymes. Weak ability to release histamine.

*Atracurium.* Intermediate-acting non-depolarizing drug. Minimal cardiovascular effects. Amount of histamine release is proportional to the rate of injection. Spontaneous degradation by ester hydrolysis and Hofmann degradation. Breakdown product of laudanosine is known to cause cerebral irritation which may accumulate to significant levels when using prolonged infusions, e.g. ITU.

*Cisatracurium.* Purified form (1R-cis, 1R'-cis isomer) of one of the 10 stereoisomers of atracurium, accounting for about 15% of the racemic mixture. Intermediate-acting non-depolarizing drug. It is more potent and has a slightly longer duration of action than atracurium. It provides greater cardiovascular stability because it lacks histamine-releasing effects. Mostly broken down by Hofmann degradation to form laudanosine, with a small amount removed by the liver and kidney. Plasma esterases do not appear to hydrolyse cisatracurium directly. Hepatic or renal impairment have little pharmacokinetic effect.

## Steroid derivatives

*Pancuronium.* Long-acting non-depolarizing drug; 80% protein bound. Deacetylated by liver to three inactive metabolites: 75% excreted in urine, 25% via bile. Indirect SNS effects (via release of noradrenaline from nerve endings) to cause ↑ CO, ↑ HR and ↑ BP. Potentiated by its additional vagal blockade. Minimal histamine release.

*Vecuronium.* Intermediate-acting non-depolarizing drug. No cardiovascular side-effects. Safe in liver failure. No histamine release. 60% eliminated in bile, half of which is broken down to the 3 OH-metabolite.

*Pipecuronium.* Long-acting non-depolarizing drug with no cardiovascular side-effects. Excreted by the kidney unchanged with minor pathway via the liver. Therefore prolonged in hepatic and renal failure. No histamine release.

*Rocuronium.* Intermediate-acting non-depolarizing drug. Neuromuscular blocking drugs of low potency are thought to have a faster onset of action because of the higher concentration gradient between plasma and post-synaptic nicotinic receptor (Bowman 1988). Similar kinetics to vecuronium but with faster biphasic onset (80% of block within 60 s followed by remainder over 2–3 min). Vagolytic action may cause 10–12% increase in HR. Does not cause histamine release. Not metabolized, and excreted unchanged in urine and bile. Prolonged action in liver failure but not in renal failure. Rocuronium 1.0 mg/kg can be used as an alternative to suxamethonium 1.0 mg/kg for rapid sequence induction provided there is no anticipated difficulty in intubation. The clinical duration of this dose of rocuronium is, however, 60 minutes.

Table 11.3 Short-acting non-depolarizing neuromuscular blocking drugs

| Drug | ED$_{95}$ (mg/kg) | Intubation (mg/kg) | Onset (s) | 95% recovery (min) |
|---|---|---|---|---|
| Vecuronium | 0.05 | 0.10–0.20 | 90–150 | 60–120 |
| Atracurium | 0.25 | 0.40–0.60 | 90–150 | 60–90 |
| Cisatracurium | 0.05 | 0.15 | 100–160 | 50–70 |
| Rocuronium | 0.30 | 0.60–1.00 | 60–90 | 60–120 |
| Mivacurium | 0.08 | 0.20–0.25 | 90–150 | 20–40 |

Table 11.4 Long-acting non-depolarizing neuromuscular blocking drugs

| Drug | ED$_{95}$ (mg/kg) | Intubation (mg/kg) | t$_{1/2}$ β (min) |
|---|---|---|---|
| Pancuronium | 0.06 | 0.10 | ≈ 100 |
| Pipecuronium | 0.05 | 0.10 | ≈ 100 |
| Doxacurium | 0.03 | 0.05 | ≈ 100 |

## PRIMING

Priming accelerates onset of block by ≈ 30 s. Use dose of 20% ED$_{95}$, pre-oxygenate and keep priming interval < 2 min. Also accelerate onset of block by using large (2–3 times ED$_{95}$) single doses of non-depolarizer, e.g. increasing dose of vecuronium from 0.1 to 0.4 mg/kg speeds onset from 3.5 to 1.5 minutes.

# SUXAMETHONIUM

$$(CH_3)_3N^+ - CH_2 - O - \overset{\displaystyle O}{\overset{\|}{C}} - CH_2$$
$$(CH_3)_3N^+ - CH_2 - O - \underset{\displaystyle O}{\overset{\|}{C}} - CH_2$$

Stimulates all sympathetic and parasympathetic ganglia, cholinergic autonomic receptors, muscarinic receptors in the sinus node of the heart and nicotine receptors. In low doses, causes negative inotropic and chronotropic effects, attenuated by atropine.

Side-effects include:

- masseter muscle rigidity and malignant hyperthermia
- increased intraocular pressure
- increased intragastric pressure but increased lower oesophageal sphincter pressure
- increased intracerebral pressure
- myalgia and muscle damage
- anaphylactic reactions
- hyperkalaemia – raises plasma $K^+$ by 0.5–0.8 mmol, particularly in burns and renal failure
- bradycardia, particularly with second doses in neonates
- dual block.

Metabolized by plasma cholinesterase ($t_{1/2}$ = 2–4 min). Decreased plasma cholinesterase with congenital and acquired conditions.

*Congenital.* Several genes control the structure of plasma cholinesterase (Table 11.5). Normal homozygote genetic structure is $E1^U$, $E1^U$. Common abnormal variants are:

- atypical gene – $E1^a$
- fluoride gene – $E1^f$
- silent gene   – $E1^s$.

**Table 11.5** Common genotypes of plasma cholinesterase

|            | Incidence | DN | FN | Response to suxamethonium |
|------------|-----------|----|----|---------------------------|
| $E1^U$, $E1^U$ | 96%     | 80 | 61 | Normal                    |
| $E1^U$, $E1^a$ | 4%      | 62 | 50 | Slightly prolonged        |
| $E1^U$, $E1^f$ | 1:200   | 74 | 52 | Slightly prolonged        |
| $E1^a$, $E1^a$ | 1:2000  | 21 | 19 | Prolonged                 |
| $E1^a$, $E1^f$ | 1:20 000 | 53 | 33 | Moderately prolonged      |

Commonest abnormality is the heterozygous state for the atypical gene ($E1^U, E1^a$) present in 4% of the Caucasian population. This results in prolongation of neuromuscular blockade for ≈ 30 min. Heterozygous forms of the other abnormal genes result in prolongation of neuromuscular blockade for > 3 h.

In vitro, dibucaine prevents normal plasma cholinesterase breaking down benzoylcholine. Normal benzoylcholine breakdown produces a colour change, the percentage inhibition of which is related to the dibucaine number (DN). A dibucaine number > 77 is present in normal homozygotes; lower numbers suggest impaired plasma cholinesterase activity. Use of fluoride instead of dibucaine allows detection of the abnormal fluoride gene, by measuring the fluoride number (FN).

### Acquired
- Liver disease, chronic renal failure, MI
- Pregnancy, oral contraceptive pill
- Haemodialysis, plasmapheresis, cardiopulmonary bypass
- Hypothyroidism
- Ester local anaesthetics
- Anaesthetic drugs metabolized by cholinesterase – etomidate, neostigmine, phenothiazines
- Propanolol
- Burns.

*Decrease suxamethonium fasciculations with* gallamine, benzodiazepines, lignocaine, calcium, magnesium or thiopentone.

*Suxamethonium-induced hyperkalaemia due to:*
- upregulation of extrajunctional ACh receptors, which leak $K^+$ in response to suxamethonium
- whole muscle cell membrane behaving as motor end-plate.

## RAPACURONIUM

Non-depolarizing analogue of vecuronium undergoing phase III trials, with similar pharmacokinetic properties to suxamethonium. Aminosteroid with even lower potency than rocuronium, resulting in faster onset time (time of maximum depression of TOF twitch) (Table 11.6).

**Table 11.6** A comparison of the pharmacokinetic properties of suxamethonium and rapacuronium

|  | Rapacuronium 1.5 mg/kg | Suxamethonium 1.0 mg/kg |
|---|---|---|
| Max. depression of first twitch of TOF | 83 s | 67 s |
| Duration of block (25% recovery first twitch) | 11 min | 3 min |

Vagolytic effect results in transient 23% increase in heart rate. Calcium-channel blockade causes vasodilation and transient fall in blood pressure. Possible histamine release may explain relatively high (11% vs. 4% suxamethonium) incidence of bronchospasm. These side-effects may limit clinical introduction/use of this drug.

## AUTONOMIC EFFECTS OF NEUROMUSCULAR BLOCKERS

### Autonomic ganglia

- Suxamethonium – stimulates
- dTC – blocks.

### Cardiac muscarinic receptors

- Suxamethonium – stimulates
- Gallamine – strong block
- Pancuronium – moderate block
- Rocuronium – weak block
- Vecuronium – clinically insignificant block.

## ONSET OF NEUROMUSCULAR BLOCKADE

Relative sensitivity of muscles to neuromuscular blockade is as follows: muscles of upper airway > peripheral muscle and intercostal muscles > diaphragm. Therefore, optimal intubating conditions develop earlier than a similar depth of block in the hand. Sufficient relaxation for intubation is usually present well before complete loss of the TO4 in the adductor pollicis.

A normal tidal volume requires just 15% of maximum diaphragm strength, so adequate respiratory effort can still occur whilst limbs are still paralysed. Forearm/hand muscles are of comparable sensitivity to intercostals and may explain why ventilatory weakness is still present until the adductor pollicis muscle has recovered completely. Any weakness detectable in peripheral muscles is likely to be associated with difficulty in maintaining an airway.

Neonatal diaphragmatic paralysis occurs at the same time as peripheral muscle groups, making peripheral neuromuscular monitoring a good indicator of respiratory muscle reversal.

## REVERSAL OF NEUROMUSCULAR BLOCKADE

Sustained head lift, tongue protrusion, hand grip, coughing and vital capacity of > 10 ml/kg require patient cooperation and are only crude measures.

Inspiratory effort > –25 cmH$_2$O is required before spontaneous respiration becomes adequate (equates with 15 ml/kg vital capacity). Adequate gag/swallowing correlates with $> -40$ cmH$_2$O. Five-second head lift equates to $-55$ cmH$_2$O inspiratory pressure.

In neonates and infants, hip flexion to $> 90°$ equates with a maximum inspiratory force of $-30$ cmH$_2$O, which is adequate for spontaneous respiration.

Although anticholinesterases appear to accelerate the reversal of mivacurium, there is a theoretical possibility that inhibition of plasma cholinesterase may retard the hydrolysis of mivacurium and thereby prolong neuromuscular blockade.

Use of intermediate rather than long-acting neuromuscular blockers reduces the risk of postoperative incomplete reversal.

## NEUROMUSCULAR BLOCKADE BY OTHER DRUGS

- Aminoglycosides – pre-junctional block
- Tetracyclines – post-junctional block
- Calcium-channel blockers – interfere with pre-junctional Ca$^{2+}$ flux
- Magnesium – potentiates block
- Metoclopramide – prolongs action of suxamethonium by 50%.

## MONITORING

Monitor to assess degree of relaxation, help adjust dosage, assess development of phase II block, provide early recognition of patients with abnormal cholinesterases, and to assess cause of apnoea.

Stimulate peripheral nerve and assess visually, by feeling the strength of contraction or mechanically (mechanomyography, electromyography). Ulnar nerve in forearm is motor only to adductor pollicis in hand, which is easily accessible. Facial nerve stimulation is a better indicator than ulnar nerve to predict when intubation is possible.

### Patterns of nerve stimulation

All stimulation should be supramaximal. Achieved by increasing the intensity of the stimulus until twitch height increases no further.

- *Single twitch.* A 2 ms stimulus is applied every few seconds and subsequent contractions monitored. Insensitive since $> 75\%$ of postsynaptic receptors must be blocked before there is any diminution in twitch height.
- *Train of four* (Ali et al 1970). A 2 Hz stimulus is applied no more often than every 10 s. Compare first ($T_1$) and last twitch ($T_4$). TO4 ratio ($T_1$:$T_4$) indicates degree of neuromuscular blockade:

  - $T_4$ disappears at 75% depression of $T_1$ (1st, 2nd and 3rd twitches present)
  - $T_3$ disappears at 80% depression of $T_1$ (1st and 2nd twitches present)
  - $T_2$ disappears at 90% depression of $T_1$ (1st twitch only)
  - $T_1$ disappears at 100% depression of $T_1$ (no twitches).

A TO4 count of 0–1 is needed for adequate intubating conditions, but a count of three twitches provides adequate relaxation for most surgery. A TO4 ratio > 0.70, or $T_1:T_0$ > 0.75, corresponds to adequate clinical recovery, but normal pharyngeal function requires a ratio > 0.90.

Neuromuscular reversal can be given when $T_2$ has reappeared, i.e. when $T_1$ is about 20% of its control height.

- **Tetanic stimulation.** Supramaximal stimulation of 50 Hz for 5 s. With non-depolarizing block, peak height is reduced and fades. Release of acetylcholine is reduced (possibly presynaptic effect) and postsynaptic receptors are blocked, limiting sustained contraction.
- **Post-tetanic count.** A 1 Hz stimulus is applied 5–10 s after tetanic stimulus. May result in response (post-tetanic potentiation), even if none is seen with original TO4. Due to increased synthesis and mobilization of acetylcholine following tetanus. Appearance of post-tetanic count precedes return of TO4 by 30–40 minutes.
- **Double-burst stimulation** (Engbaek et al 1989). Three 0.2 ms bursts of 50 Hz tetanus, each burst separated by 20 ms and repeated after 750 ms. Similar to TO4, but tactile evaluation is more sensitive because fade of the two resultant contractions is more marked.

## DIFFERENCES BETWEEN DEPOLARIZING AND NON-DEPOLARIZING BLOCKS

Table 11.7  Depolarizing versus non-depolarizing block

| Depolarizing block | Non-depolarizing block |
|---|---|
| Reduced twitch height | Reduced twitch height |
| No fade of TO4/tetanus | Fade of TO4/tetanus |
| No post-tetanic potentiation | Post-tetanic potentiation |

### References

Ali H H, Utting J E, Gray T C 1970 Stimulus frequency in the detection of neuromuscular block in humans. British Journal of Anaesthesia 42: 967–968

Davis L, Britten J J, Morgan M 1997 Cholinesterase. Its significance in anaesthetic practice. Anaesthesia 52: 244–260

Donati F, Bevan D R 1992 Not all muscles are the same. Editorial. British Journal of Anaesthesia 68: 235–236

Engbaek J, Viby-Mogensen J 1999 Can rocuronium replace succinylcholine in a rapid-sequence induction of anaesthesia? Acta Anaesthesiologica Scandinavica 43: 1–3

Engbaek J, Ostergaard D, Viby-Mogensen J 1989 Double-burst stimulation (DBS); a new pattern of nerve stimulation to identify residual neuromuscular block. British Journal of Anaesthesia 62: 247–248

Goulden M R, Hunter J M 1999 Rapacuronium (Org 9487): do we have a replacement for succinylcholine? British Journal of Anaesthesia 82: 489–492

Hilmi I, Ginsburg R. Mivacurium 1994 In: Kaufman L, Ginsburg R (eds) Anaesthesia review II. Churchill Livingstone, London

McCourt K C, Salmela L, Mirakhur R K et al 1998 Comparison of rocuronium and
    suxamethonium for use during rapid sequence induction of anaesthesia.
    Anaesthesia 53: 867–871
Meistelman C, McLoughlin C 1993 Suxamethonium – current controversies. Current
    Anaesthesia and Critical Care 4: 53–58
Norman J 1999 Assessing paralysis. British Journal of Anaesthesia 82: 321–322

## OPIOIDS AND OTHER ANALGESICS

### FENTANYL (anilino-piperidine)

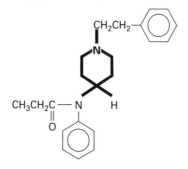

Fentanyl was the first of the potent anilino-piperidine opioids, being 200 times
as potent as morphine with a high therapeutic index. Its high lipid
solubility causes accumulation of the drug in lipophilic tissues, particularly
the lungs on first pass, with a resultant prolongation in elimination half-life
(150–400 min). 84% is protein bound to albumin and $\alpha$- and $\beta$-globulins;
80% undergoes N-dealkylation by liver metabolism to inactive norfentanyl,
so has prolonged duration of action with liver disease. Little change in drug
kinetics in patients with renal disease.

### ALFENTANIL (anilino-piperidine)

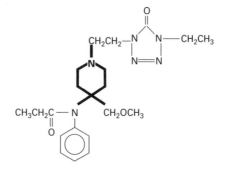

Alfentanil has 20% of the potency of fentanyl. Less lipid-soluble than fentanyl, with 90% bound to $\alpha_1$-acid glycoprotein. It is shorter acting and 80% is biotransformed by liver metabolism, so has prolonged duration of action with liver disease. Little change in drug kinetics in patients with renal disease.

## SUFENTANIL (anilino-piperidine)

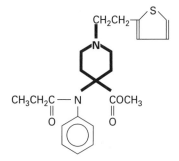

Shorter acting than fentanyl with an elimination half-life of 140–200 min. 80% is biotransformed by liver metabolism, so has prolonged duration of action with liver disease. Little change in drug kinetics in patients with renal disease except in uraemic patients.

## REMIFENTANIL (anilino-piperidine)

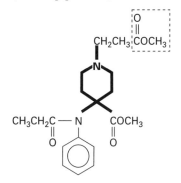

Remifentanil is an ultra-short-acting synthetic opioid with $\mu$-specific opioid activity. Vials of remifentanil contain glycine which is an inhibitory neurotransmitter, making it unsuitable for subarachnoid and extradural injection. 70% bound to $\alpha_1$-acid glycoprotein. It has cardiovascular and side-effect profiles similar to fentanyl. Not associated with histamine release. The ester linkage (shown by the dotted line) makes remifentanil susceptible to rapid hydrolysis by tissue and blood non-specific esterases (distinct from pseudocholinesterase) and it therefore has a rapid clearance (elimination $t_{1/2}$ = 5 min) independent of renal and hepatic function. The major metabolite is a pure $\mu$-opioid agonist excreted by the kidney, but with a potency 1/4600 of the parent compound. Placental transfer occurs rapidly, but metabolism and redistribution prevent adverse neonatal effects. Prolonged duration of action with liver disease. Little change in drug kinetics in patients with renal disease.

Less nausea and vomiting than with other longer-acting opioids. As with other opioids, muscle rigidity at high dose may occur. When assessed by the effect on reduction in MAC, the relative potencies of sufentanil, fentanyl, remifentanil and alfentanil are 1:10:10:80.

## PETHIDINE

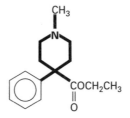

Greater (>70%) protein binding (mostly $\alpha_1$-acid glycoprotein) than morphine. Metabolized by N-demethylation to the active metabolite, norpethidine and inactive pethidinic acid and norpethidinic acid. Accumulation of norpethidine in renal impairment may prolong the action of pethidine and cause tremor, agitation and seizures. Despite significant pulmonary clearance, 80% is biotransformed by liver metabolism, so liver disease is associated with increased elimination half-life.

Said to be the opioid of choice for biliary colic because its atropine-like effect will counteract the opioid action on smooth muscle. Topical atropine, however, does not relax a contracted gall bladder and there no is evidence that pethidine is any better than equianalgesic doses of other opioids.

## MORPHINE

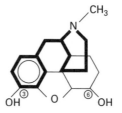

Metabolized to morphine 3-glucuronide (M3G) and the active metabolite morphine 6-glucuronide (M6G). 10% of morphine conjugation occurs in extrahepatic and GI tissues; 80% biotransformed by liver metabolism, but kinetics of morphine remain unaltered until end-stage liver disease. Renal failure is associated with accumulation of M3G and M6G and prolonged action.

## DIAMORPHINE

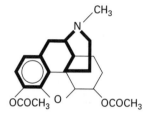

3,6-diacetylmorphine (heroin). Hydrolysed in liver and blood to 6-monoacetyl morphine, a potent opioid.

## CODEINE

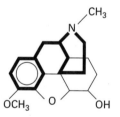

3-methoxy morphine. Approximately 10–20% of the potency of morphine. Methyl ether group reduces metabolism so increasing oral bioavailability. Undergoes extensive hepatic metabolism, mostly to inactive conjugated compounds but 10–20% metabolized to morphine.

## TRAMADOL

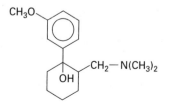

A phenylpiperidine derivative with a structure similar to pethidine and elimination $t_{1/2}$ of 5–7 h. Same analgesic potency as pethidine. Analgesic effects through:

- moderate affinity at $\mu$ receptors and weak activity at $\kappa$ receptors
- enhancing the function of the spinal descending inhibitory pathways and blocking spinal nociceptive pathways by inhibition of reuptake of both 5HT and norepinephrine at synapses.
- presynaptic stimulation of 5HT release.

As it enhances monoaminergic transmission, it is contraindicated in patients taking MAOIs. Does not cause significant respiratory depression or histamine release. Exists as a chiral mixture with (+) form acting at $\mu$ receptors and (–) form causing monoamine reuptake inhibition. Has 10–20% of the potency of morphine but causes less respiratory depression and less depression.

20% bound to plasma protein with an elimination $t_{1/2}$ of 5 h. Demethylation by the liver ($P_{450}$) accounts for 86% of the metabolism. The O-desmethyl-tramadol metabolite is active with a $t_{1/2}$ of 9 h. Most metabolites are excreted in the urine. Hepatic and renal impairment causes significant prolongation of action.

For moderate/severe pain, 3 mg/kg is an effective initial dose. Associated with common but mild side-effects of headache, nausea, vomiting and dizziness. Reduced side-effects with oral slow-release preparations.

Committee on Safety of Medicines (CSM) has received 27 reports of convulsions possibly associated with tramadol, although many of the patients were known epileptics. Some reports have shown interaction with coumarin anticoagulants to prolong the INR and there have also been reports of drug abuse.

**References**

Budd K, Langford R 1999 Tramadol revisited. British Journal of Anaesthesia 82: 493–496

Sear J W 1998 Recent advances and developments in the clinical use of i.v. opioids during the preoperative period. British Journal of Anaesthesia 81: 38–50

Smith M A, Morgan M 1997 Remifentanil. Anaesthesia 52: 291–293

Thompson J P, Rowbotham D J 1996 Remifentanil – an opioid for the 21st century. British Journal of Anaesthesia 76: 341

## VOLATILE AGENTS

**Table 11.8** Physical properties of volatile agents

|  | Halothane | Enflurane | Isoflurane | Sevoflurane | Desflurane |
|---|---|---|---|---|---|
| Blood:gas solubility | 2.3 | 1.9 | 1.4 | 0.6 | 0.42 |
| MAC | 0.75 | 1.68 | 1.15 | 2 | 7 |
| Boiling point (°C) | 50 | 56 | 48 | 58 | 24 |
| Saturated vapour pressure (kPa) | 32 | 24 | 32 | 21 | 88 |
| % metabolism | 20 | 2 | 0.2 | 2 | 0.02 |

## HALOTHANE

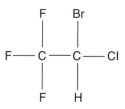

Instability in light is improved by addition of 0.01% thymol. Arrhythmogenicity associated with alkane structure. Maximum recommended safe dose of adrenaline is 0.1 mg/10 min. Least irritant of all the volatiles for gas induction.

### Halothane hepatitis

The National Halothane Study (USA 1966) studied 750 000 anaesthetics. Spectrum of damage from minor derangement of LFTs to fulminant hepatic failure (FHF). There were seven cases of unexplained FHF (1:35 000 halothane exposures). Hepatitis was associated with more than one exposure to halothane, recent exposure to halothane, family history of halothane hepatotoxicity, obesity, female sex and drug allergies. Eosinophilia and autoantibodies were common.

There are two patterns of hepatitis:

- *mild* – usually subclinical with transient derangement in LFTs
- *fulminant hepatic failure* – defined by Neuberger & Williams (1988) as 'the appearance of liver damage within 28 days of halothane exposure in a person in whom other known causes of liver disease had been excluded'.

75% of patients with halothane hepatitis have antibodies reacting to

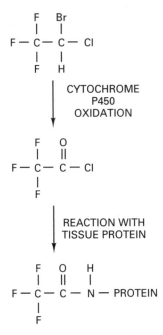

**Fig. 11.3** Proposed mechanism of formation of trifluoroacetyl halide antigen.

halothane-altered antigens. Route of metabolism of halothane depends upon $O_2$ tension in liver. At high $O_2$ tension, an oxidative route generates trifluoroacetyl halide (TFAH) (Fig. 11.3), which covalently binds to liver proteins, forming haptens. Halothane-directed antibodies detectable by ELISA test have been identified that are directed against TFAH antigens. Present in 70% of cases of halothane-induced FHF. The significance of the more minor reductive route at low $O_2$ tension is debated. It may be associated with direct liver damage with release of fluoride. National database of FHF patients set up at St. Mary's Hospital, London (Prof. R.M. Jones) to whom these patients should be reported.

**GUIDELINES FOR HALOTHANE EXPOSURE** Committee on Safety of Medicines 1997

Halothane is well known to be associated with hepatotoxicity, particularly if patients are re-exposed. This risk decreases as the time between halothane exposure increases, but a risk persists regardless of the time since last exposure.

The Committee on Safety of Medicines (CSM) received reports of 15 cases of halothane-induced acute liver failure requiring liver transplants between 1985 and 1995. Ten patients had at least one previous halothane exposure of which four were in the preceding month, and six had had previous adverse reactions to halothane.

The CSM recommend that halothane be avoided if there has been a previous exposure within 3 months, previous adverse reaction to halothane, family history of adverse reaction to halothane or pre-existing liver disease, unless there are overriding clinical needs.

## ENFLURANE

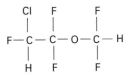

Causes paroxysmal epileptiform EEG spike wave activity at > 3%. Fluoride ions may approach toxic levels in prolonged or high-dose anaesthesia. May generate significant amounts of carbon monoxide in the presence of dry baralyme or soda lime (see 'Circle systems', p. 344).

### Enflurane hepatitis

There are several reports of FHF. Patients tend to be older, have more rapid onset of symptoms and have postoperative pyrexia. Degree of hepatotoxicity is unsure.

## ISOFLURANE

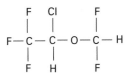

### Isoflurane hepatitis

Limited number of reports of hepatotoxicity. Patients tend to be younger. May generate significant amounts of carbon monoxide in the presence of dry baralyme or soda lime (see 'Circle systems', p. 344).

## DESFLURANE

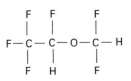

Differs from isoflurane only by substitution of a fluorine for a chlorine atom. Change from partial chlorination causes ↓ potency, ↑ volatility, ↓ solubility, ↑ stability and ↑SVP. The strength of the carbon–fluorine bond increases stability with 0.02% metabolism and stability in soda lime. Requires heated vaporizer because of high SVP.

Has similar CVS effects to isoflurane (↑HR, ↓SVR). Not arrhythmogenic, even with adrenaline. Coronary artery vasodilator (no evidence for coronary steal). Respiratory depression equivalent to isoflurane. Irritant to upper respiratory tract, therefore not suitable for gas induction. EEG effects similar to isoflurane with dose-related depression. No renal/hepatic toxicity reported.

May generate significant amounts of carbon monoxide in the presence of dry baralyme or soda lime (see 'Circle systems', p. 344).

## SEVOFLURANE

Has similar CVS effects to isoflurane but less tachycardia and coronary vasodilation (no evidence for coronary steal). Less myocardial depression than halothane. Not arrhythmogenic, even with adrenaline. No more irritant than halothane to upper respiratory tract. Greater respiratory depression than halothane but faster elimination results in less postoperative respiratory depression. EEG effects similar to isoflurane, with dose-related depression. Decomposed by soda lime to compounds A and B (see Fig. 11.4; 'Circle systems', p. 344); 2% metabolized. Levels of fluoride ions > 50 $\mu$mol/l (thought to be the threshold for nephrotoxicity) and post-anaesthetic albuminuria have been reported, but there is no evidence of significant post-anaesthetic renal impairment. However, consider avoiding in patients with renal failure. Also reported to cause small post-anaesthetic increase in serum ALT, suggesting mild transient hepatic injury.

Use of sevoflurane is associated with more rapid recovery than either propofol or isoflurane.

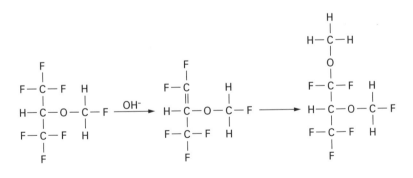

Fig. 11.4 Decomposition of sevoflurane (by soda lime) to compounds A and B.

# References

Committee on Safety of Medicines 1997 Guidelines for halothane exposure. Current Problems 23: 7

Elliot R H, Strunin L 1993 Hepatotoxicity of volatile anaesthetics. Review. British Journal of Anaesthesia 70: 339–348

Jones R 1995 The new inhalational agents: desflurane and sevoflurane. What is the clinical role of 3rd generation fluorinated anaesthetics and how do they compare with 2nd generation agents? Acta Anaesthesiologica Scandinavica 39(suppl.): 130–131

Langbein T, Sonntag H, Trapp D et al 1999 Volatile anaesthetics and the atmosphere: atmospheric lifetimes and atmospheric effects of halothane, enflurane, isoflurane, desflurane and sevoflurane. British Journal of Anaesthesia 82: 66–73

Neuberger J, Williams R 1988 Halothane hepatitis. Digestive Diseases 6: 52–54

Robinson B J, Uhrich T D, Ebert T J 1999 A review of recovery from sevoflurane anaesthesia: comparisons with isoflurane and propofol including meta-analysis. Acta Anaesthesiologica Scandinavica 43: 185–190

Smith I, Nathanson M, White P F 1996 Sevoflurane – a long-awaited volatile anaesthetic. British Journal of Anaesthesia 76: 435–445

Young C J, Apfelbaum J L 1998 A comparative review of the newer inhalational anaesthetics. CNS Drugs 10: 287–310

# 12. Equipment

## GASES

### Cylinders

Gas cylinders are manufactured from chromium molybdenum steel as a seamless tube.

*Colours.* Conform to International Standards Organisation (Table 12.1).

**Table 12.1** Gas cylinder colours

|  | Body | Shoulder |
| --- | --- | --- |
| Oxygen | Black | White |
| Nitrous oxide | French blue | French blue |
| Air | Grey | Black/white |
| Carbon dioxide | Grey | Grey |
| Helium | Brown | Brown |
| Cyclopropane | Orange | Orange |
| Entonox | French blue | French blue/white |
| Nitric oxide | Pink | Pink |

*Marks on cylinders.* Test pressure, dates of test, chemical formula of gas and tare weight (i.e. weight when empty).

### Gas pressures

- $N_2O$      – 51.6 bar (liquid). No reduction in cylinder pressure until 75% empty
- $CO_2$      – 44 bar (liquid)
- Cyclopropane – 4 bar (liquid)
- $O_2$      – 137 bar
- Entonox      – 137 bar.

Filling ratio = weight of gas in cylinder/weight of water cylinder would hold. For $CO_2$ and $N_2O$, filling ratio = 0.75 in temperate climates and 0.67 in tropics.

## VACUUM

Vacuum required to give 0.53 kPa pressure below atmospheric pressure, producing 40 l/min suction of air.

## ANAESTHETIC MACHINE SAFETY FEATURES

- Copper reinforced gas hoses to prevent kinking, with specific colours for each gas. Non-interchangeable Schraeder valves at wall with different threads to connect to the anaesthetic machine
- One-way valves at yokes to prevent leaks
- Pin index system for cylinders
- Pressure-reducing valves (from 137 to 4 bar)
- Sintered bronze filters proximal to rotameters to prevent ingress of dust
- Oxygen flow knob on rotameter more proud than others with serrated surface
- Oxygen enters fresh gas flow from rotameter last
- Rotameters have a stop to prevent bobbin disappearing from site at high gas flows
- Gold/tin coating on surface of rotameter to prevent static electricity causing bobbin to stick
- Flow restrictors sited proximal to rotameters to protect them from sudden surges in pressure and distal to rotameters to protect them from back pressure
- Interlocking vaporizers
- Oxygen failure alarm
- Emergency $O_2$ flush without locking valve (> 35 l/min)
- Air entrainment if oxygen delivery fails
- Blow-off valve at 43 kPa to protect back bar
- Blow-off valve in patient circuit at 5 kPa.

**CHECKLIST FOR ANAESTHETIC APPARATUS 2** Association of Anaesthetists of Great Britain and Ireland 1997

Recommended check is based on the use of an oxygen analyser which will detect misfilling of oxygen cylinders, contamination of oxygen reservoirs and crossed-over pipelines.

Full checklist is the responsibility of the anaesthetist and should be performed prior to each operating session.

1. **Check that the anaesthetic machine is connected to the electricity supply (if appropriate) and switched on**

- Take note of any information or labelling on the anaesthetic machine referring to the current status of the machine. Particular attention should be paid to recent servicing. Servicing labels should be fixed in the service logbook.

2. **Check that an oxygen analyser is present on the anaesthetic machine**
   - Ensure that the analyser is switched on, checked and calibrated
   - The oxygen sensor should be placed where it can monitor the composition of the gases leaving the common gas outlet.

3. **Identify and take note of the gases which are being supplied by the pipeline, confirming with a 'tug test' that each pipeline is correctly inserted into the appropriate gas supply terminal**

Note. Carbon dioxide cylinders should not be present on the anaesthetic machine unless requested by the anaesthetist. A blanking plug should be fitted to any empty cylinder yoke.

   - Check that the anaesthetic machine is connected to a supply of oxygen and that an adequate supply of oxygen is available from a reserve oxygen cylinder
   - Check that adequate supplies of other gases (nitrous oxide, air) are available and connected as appropriate
   - Check that all pipeline pressure gauges in use on the anaesthetic machine indicate 400 kPa.

4. **Check the operation of flow meters**
   - Ensure that each flow control valve operates smoothly and that the bobbin moves freely throughout its range
   - Check the operation of the emergency oxygen bypass control.

5. **Check the vaporizers**
   - Ensure that each vaporizer is adequately filled but not overfilled
   - Ensure vaporizer is seated correctly on the back bar and not tilted
   - Check the vaporizer for leaks (with the vaporizer off) by temporarily occluding the common gas outlet
   - When checks have been completed, turn the vaporizer(s) off
   - A leak test should be performed immediately after changing any vaporizer.

6. **Check the breathing system to be employed**
   - The system should be visually inspected for correct configuration. All connections should be secured by 'push and twist'
   - A pressure leak test should be performed on the breathing circuit by occluding the patient port and compressing the reservoir bag

- The correct operation of unidirectional valves should be carefully checked.

**7. Check that the ventilator is configured appropriately for its intended use**
- Ensure that the ventilator tubing is correctly configured and securely attached
- Set the controls for use and ensure that an adequate pressure is generated during the inspiratory phase
- Check that the pressure relief valve functions
- Check that the disconnect alarm functions correctly
- Ensure that an alternative means to ventilate the patient's lungs is available

**8. Check that the anaesthetic gas scavenging system is switched on and is functioning correctly**

- Ensure that the tubing is attached to the appropriate expiratory port(s) of the breathing system or ventilator.

**9. Check that all ancillary equipment which may be needed is present and working**
- This includes laryngoscopes, intubation aids, intubation forceps, bougies etc. and appropriately sized face masks, airways, tracheal tubes and connectors
- Check that the suction apparatus is functioning and that all connections are secure
- Check that the patient can be tilted head-down on the trolley, operating table or bed.

**10. Ensure that the appropriate monitoring equipment is present, switched on and calibrated ready for use**

- Set all default alarms as appropriate. (It may be necessary to place monitors in the stand-by mode to avoid unnecessary alarms before being connected to the patient.)

## VAPORIZERS

Because desflurane has such a high saturated vapour pressure (88 kPa), standard vaporizers are unsuitable for its storage and delivery. Use of a conventional vaporizer would require very high fresh gas flows to achieve 1 MAC equivalent of desflurane. The low boiling point of desflurane (24°C) also makes a conventional vaporizer unsuitable. The Tech 6 desflurane vaporizer (Fig. 12.1) uses a servo-controlled electronic system which heats the vaporizer chamber to a constant 39°C (higher than the boiling point) at a pressure of 1500 mmHg. The desflurane is delivered into the fresh gas flow (FGF) at equal pressures through a pressure-regulating valve which increases

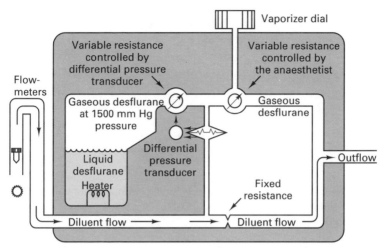

**Fig. 12.1** Desflurane vaporizer. (Reproduced with permission from New Generation Vaporizers, Pharmacia.)

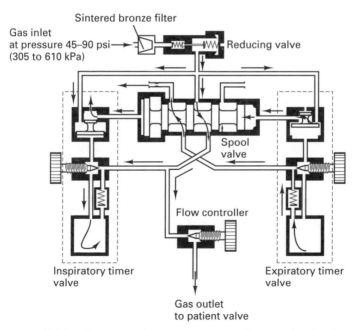

**Fig. 12.2** Nuffield Penlon 200 ventilator – inspiratory mode. (Reproduced with permission from Davey et al 1992.)

desflurane delivery as the FGF increases. Unlike conventional ventilators, use of the Tech 6 vaporizer at high altitude requires manual adjustment to increase desflurane concentrations.

## VENTILATORS

### Nuffield 200 series ventilator

This is a time-cycled pressure generator. It has variable expiratory and inspiratory timers and a variable inspiratory flow rate control (Fig. 12.2).

*Paediatric Newton valve.* Capable of delivering tidal volume between 10 and 300 ml at flow rates of 0.5–18 l/min. At small tidal volumes, pressure-controlled ventilation is preferable to volume-controlled ventilation because the final volume delivered is dependent upon circuit leaks, circuit compliance and fresh gas flow rates.

### References

Andrews J J, Johnston R V 1993 The new Tech 6 desflurane vaporizer. Anesthesia and Analgesia 76: 1338–1341

Association of Anaesthetists of Great Britain and Ireland 1997 Checklist for anaesthetic apparatus 2. AAGBI, London

Cartwright D P, Freeman M F 1999 Vaporisers. Anaesthesia 54: 519–520

Gardner M C, Adams A P 1996 Anaesthetic vaporizers: design and function. Current Anaesthesia and Critical Care 7: 315–321

Davey A, Moyle J T B, Ward C S (eds) 1992 Ward's anaesthetic equipment, 3rd edn. WB Saunders, London

Howell R S C 1989 Medical gases (1) – manufacture and uses. In: Kaufman L (ed) Anaesthesia review 7. Churchill Livingstone, Edinburgh, p 87–104

Howell R S C 1990 Medical gases (2) – distribution. In: Kaufman L (ed) Anaesthesia review 8. Churchill Livingstone, Edinburgh, p 195–210

Moyle J T B, Davey A 1998 Automatic ventilators. In: Ward C (ed) Ward's anaesthetic equipment, 4th edn. WB Saunders, London

## BREATHING CIRCUITS

## MAPLESON'S CLASSIFICATION OF BREATHING SYSTEMS

For all adult circuits, a 110 cm hose holds a volume of 550 ml. T-piece reservoir should equal the tidal volume (more reservoir volume causes increased resistance and rebreathing).

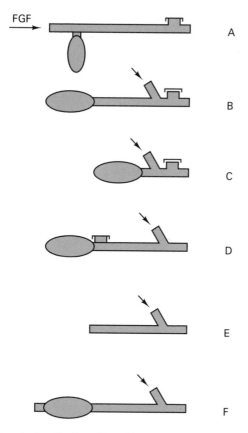

**Fig. 12.3** Mapleson's classification of breathing systems.

**Table 12.2** Breathing circuit flow rates

| Mapleson classification | Spontaneous ventilation | IPPV |
|---|---|---|
| A | 70 ml/kg per min | 2.5 × MV |
| B | 2.5 × MV | 2.5 × MV |
| C | 2.5 × MV | 2.5 × MV |
| D | 2.5 × MV | 70 ml/kg per min |
| E | | |
|   Adult | 2.5 × MV | 2.5 × MV |
|   < 20 kg | 3 (1000 + 100 ml/kg) | 1000 + 100 ml/kg (minimum flow = 3 l) |
|   *or* | 3 (5 × frequency × kg) | 5 × frequency × kg |
| Lack (coaxial A) | 50 ml/kg per min | |
| Bain (coaxial D) | | 70 ml/kg per min |

## PAEDIATRIC CIRCUITS

Deadspace and resistance are most important during spontaneous respiration. Circuit resistance is higher with smaller circuits ($\propto 1/r^4$). Use of low flows with T-piece or Bain circuit results in carbon dioxide being rebreathed only at the latter part of inspiration, which may not affect alveolar ventilation. Rebreathed gas has the advantage of being warm and humidified.

### References

Jones M J 1994 Breathing systems and vaporizers. In: Nimmo W S, Rowbotham D J, Smith G (eds) Anaesthesia, 2nd edn. Blackwell Scientific Publications, Oxford, p 486–505

Moyle J T B, Davey A 1998 Breathing systems and their components. In: Ward C (ed) Ward's anaesthetic equipment, 4th edn. WB Saunders, London

## CIRCLE SYSTEMS

Rebreathing was introduced by Snow in 1850. Circle systems were pioneered by Sword in 1926.

## ANAESTHETIC CIRCUITS

- *Open circuit* – respiratory tract open to the atmosphere and no rebreathing, e.g. open drop mask for ether
- *Semi-open circuit* – anaesthetic gases carried by fresh gas but may be diluted with room air
- *Semi-closed circuit* – anaesthetic gases carried by fresh gas and no dilution with room air, e.g. Mapleson D
- *Closed circuit* – respiratory tract closed to the atmosphere on both inspiration and expiration.

### Advantages of closed-circuit anaesthesia

- Conservation of heat
- Maintenance of humidity of inspired gases
- Additional monitoring of oxygen consumption, circuit leaks and tidal volume
- Oxygen reservoir if failure of supply
- Decreased pollution
- Less volatile agent used, with cost saving.

### Disadvantages of closed-circuit anaesthesia

- Cost of circle system and soda lime

- Complexity of system
- Unsuitable for short operations when equilibration does not have time to occur
- Possible to deliver hypoxic mixtures of gases or mixtures with little volatile, leading to awareness
- Slow changes in depth of anaesthesia
- Accumulation of anaesthetic metabolites.

## CARBON DIOXIDE ABSORBER

Soda lime contains:

- 94% $Ca(OH)_2$
- 5% NaOH
- 1% KOH
- trace of silicates (prevent powdering)
- 15% water (more efficient $CO_2$ absorption and less absorption of anaesthetic gases)
- pH indicator, e.g. Clayton Yellow turning from pink to white when exhausted.

Size 4–8 mesh (i.e. granules $\frac{1}{4}-\frac{1}{8}$ inch in diameter); 50% volume of canister is granules, 50% is air. Pack tightly to avoid channelling.

### Reaction of soda lime

$$2NaOH + CO_2 \rightarrow Na_2CO_3 + H_2O + heat$$
$$Na_2CO_3 + Ca(OH)_2 \rightarrow CaCO_3 + 2NaOH$$

Trichloroethylene is decomposed by soda lime to phosgene (toxic). Sevoflurane is decomposed by soda lime and baralyme to compounds A, B, C, D and methanol. Concentrations of compound A in circle systems producing renal injury can approach those found in clinical practice. The effect of dryness is complex, with fresh dry absorbent destroying compound A as it is made but causing greater production of compound A if exposed to sevoflurane in excess of about 1 h. Greater degradation with baralyme than with soda lime. If soda lime becomes excessively dry (< 5% water), use of sevoflurane risks formation of formic acid, causing airway irritation.

Temperature within canister may exceed 60°C. Canister should at least equal tidal volume. Therefore, minimum 500 g soda lime becomes exhausted after about 2 h; 100 g soda lime can theoretically absorb 25 l of $CO_2$, but this figure is reduced by channelling and uneven absorption. Large cylinders contain 2 kg soda lime which can be inverted once the upper chamber becomes exhausted. 'Regeneration' of soda lime on standing occurs due to migration of hydroxyl ions to the surface of granules.

## CIRCLE LAYOUT

There are 64 different possible combinations of layout. The most efficient has been found to be that shown in Figure 12.4.

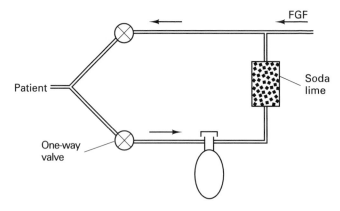

**Fig. 12.4** Layout for optimal circle system.

## EQUILIBRATION OF CIRCLE GASES

The wash-in and wash-out curves for changes in vapour concentration within a closed circuit are exponential. Assuming net gas uptake is minimal:

$$\text{Time constant (Tc) for circle} = \frac{\text{volume of circle system}}{\text{FGF}}$$

- 1 Tc = 63% equilibration of FGF with circle gases
- 2 Tc = 86% equilibration of FGF with circle gases
- 3 Tc = 95% equilibration of FGF with circle gases.

For example, in a circuit of volume 4 l with FGF = 8 l/min, Tc = 0.5 min. Therefore, 95% of any change in the percentage of volatile selected will be reflected in the circuit within 1.5 min (Tc × 3). However, at low FGF, e.g. 1 l/min, Tc = 2 min and therefore 95% equilibration will not be achieved until 12 min. Hence, increase flow rather than volatile to deepen anaesthesia.

At low flow rates of $O_2$ and $N_2O$ into a circle system, the uptake of $N_2O$ exceeds that of $O_2$, and the [$O_2$] in the circle exceeds that set by the rotameters. After 30 min equilibration, uptake of $N_2O$ is less than that of $O_2$, and the [$N_2O$] in the circle exceeds that set by the rotameters. After the start of an anaesthetic, 15 ml/kg $N_2$ will be released from tissues, lowering [$N_2O$]. This effect is lessened with denitrogenation prior to closing the circuit.

Thus it is difficult to predict exact concentrations of gases, so use of anaesthetic gas monitoring is mandatory to prevent hypoxic mixtures or mixtures that are deficient in volatile, resulting in awareness. Monitor *expired* gases, which are a better reflection of alveolar gas concentrations than inspired gases.

## PRINCIPLES OF CLOSED CIRCUIT VOLATILE ADMINISTRATION

$$V_{O_2} \, (ml/min) = kg^{0.75} \times 10$$

Direct administration of volatiles into the circuit was pioneered by Lowe.

Uptake of volatile $\propto 1/\sqrt{time}$, so the same dose of volatile is taken up between each square of time after induction, i.e. 1, 4, 9, 16, etc. min. Thus one dose is taken up by 1 min after induction, two doses by 4 min after induction, three doses by 9 min after induction etc. This does not take into account the amount of volatile needed to prime the circuit or any uptake by soda lime or rubber in the circuit. Therefore, extra priming dose needs to be given within the first 9 min.

Aim for $ED_{95}$ of volatile within circuit, i.e. $\approx 1.3$ MAC. Thus, at any time after induction, volatile anaesthetic uptake is as follows:

$$Q_{AN} = (1.3 - \% \, N_2O/100) \times MAC \times \lambda_{B/G} \times time^{-0.5}$$

where:
$Q_{AN}$ = uptake of anaesthetic
$\lambda_{B/G}$ = blood/gas solubility of volatile.

## VAPORIZER OUTSIDE CIRCLE (VOC)

At high FGFs, the volatile concentration inspired by the patient will approach that leaving the vaporizer (Fig. 12.5).

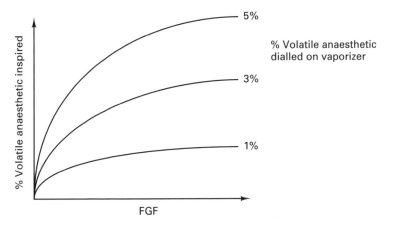

**Fig. 12.5** Effect of fresh gas flow (FGF) on the percentage of volatile inspired for vaporizers outside the circle.

## VAPORIZER INSIDE CIRCLE (VIC)

At low FGFs, the volatile concentration inspired by the patient will be much higher than that leaving the vaporizer (Fig. 12.6).

Draw-over vaporizers for VIC must not have wicks, because water vapour from saturated gases condenses on them to cause inaccurate volatile delivery. Need draw-over vaporizer with low internal resistance if using spontaneous respiration, e.g. Goldman vaporizer. Plenum vaporizers have too high an internal resistance.

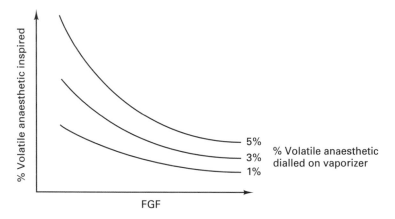

**Fig. 12.6**  Effect of fresh gas flow (FGF) on the percentage of volatile inspired for vaporizers inside the circle.

## CIRCLE SYSTEMS AND CARBOXYHAEMOGLOBINAEMIA

In 1995, reports were received from the USA of patients developing significant carboxyhaemoglobinaemia during anaesthesia. This phenomenon was only observed while using halogenated volatile agents (enflurane, isoflurane, desflurane) in association with circle systems. Cases usually occurred on Monday mornings when oxygen had been left flowing through the circuit over the weekend.

Further investigation found that barium hydroxide (baralyme) in the canister was generating significant amounts of carbon monoxide, particularly at low water content as it dried out. Dry baralyme or soda lime (e.g. gas flowing through an anaesthesia circuit over a weekend period) results in excessive carbon monoxide formation which may reach fatal levels (35 000 ppm CO documented with desflurane; safe limit is 35 ppm for 1 h).

In the UK, barium hydroxide is not available and soda lime only dries significantly (< 2% water) in circuits where the FGF is placed upstream from the absorbent canister – an arrangement not found in circle systems in the UK. No cases of carboxyhaemoglobinaemia have been reported in the UK and it is thought unlikely that the problems seen in the USA will occur in the UK.

### References

Baxter P J, Garton K, Kharasch E D 1998 Mechanistic aspects of carbon monoxide formation from volatile anesthetics. Anesthesiology 89: 929–941

Committee on Safety of Medicines 1997 Circle systems and volatile agents. Current Problems 23: 7

Fang Z X, Kandel L, Laster M J, Ionescu P, Eger E I 1996 Factors affecting production of compound A from the interaction of sevoflurane with baralyme and soda lime. Anesthesia and Analgesia 82: 775–781

Jones M J 1994 Breathing systems and vaporizers. In: Nimmo W S, Rowbotham D J, Smith G (eds) Anaesthesia, 2nd edn. Blackwell Scientific Publications, Oxford, p 486–505

White D C 1992 Closed and low flow system anaesthesia. Current Anaesthesia and Critical Care 3: 98–107

## MONITORING

Inadequate monitoring or observation causes 8.2% of all anaesthetic fatalities; 90% of 'monitor-detectable' incidents would be picked up with the correct use of pulse oximetry or capnography.

**RECOMMENDATIONS FOR STANDARDS OF MONITORING DURING ANAESTHESIA AND RECOVERY** Association of Anaesthetists of Great Britain and Ireland 1994. Adapted from Harvard minimum monitoring standards (1986) and revised from 1988 Association guidelines

- Anaesthetist should be present continuously and make an adequate record of the procedure
- Monitoring should be commenced prior to induction and continued until the patient is awake
- Anaesthetic machine function should be monitored with an oxygen analyser, $CO_2$ and circuit pressure monitoring devices
- Patient should be monitored by clinical observations (colour, respiratory movement, auscultation etc.), continuous monitoring devices (ECG, pulse oximeter, capnography) and intermittent monitoring devices (BP, neuromuscular function)
- Adequate monitoring is needed even with brief anaesthetics, during the transport of patients, and with sedation that might cause cardiovascular or respiratory complications.

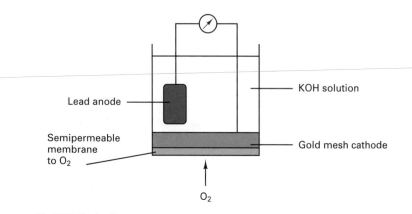

**Fig. 12.7** Fuel cell.

## INSPIRED OXYGEN CONCENTRATION

### Fuel cell

In a fuel cell (Fig. 12.7) the current is proportional to the partial pressure of oxygen:

$$Pb + 2OH^- \rightarrow PbO + H_2O + 2e^-$$

### Clarke electrode

In a Clarke electrode (Fig. 12.8) the current is proportional to the partial pressure of oxygen. This type of electrode is usually used in blood gas machines.

$$2H_2O + O_2 + 4e^- \rightarrow 4OH^-$$

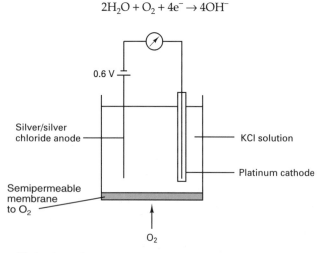

**Fig. 12.8** Clarke electrode.

## Paramagnetic analysis

Based on the fact that oxygen is paramagnetic and attracted towards magnetic fields. Most other gases are diamagnetic and repelled from magnetic fields.

*Dumbbells analyser.* Consists of nitrogen-filled dumbbells with each ball resting within a magnetic field. Any oxygen in the sample gas is attracted into the magnetic field and displaces the nitrogen dumbbells out of the magnetic field. As the dumbbells swing, a mirror attached to them displaces a light beam onto photocells.

*Datex analyser.* The sample gas is separated from the reference gas by a thin diaphragm attached to a pressure transducer. An alternating current applied to the gases causes pressure oscillations across the diaphragm, which is displaced in proportion to the oxygen concentration in the sample gas.

## PULSE OXIMETER

### Mechanism

Light is transmitted through tissue at two alternating wavelengths:

- red at 660 nm.
- near infrared at 940 nm (not visible).

*Beer's law,* used to calculate the absorption (Fig. 12.9), states

$$I_t = I_o \, e^{-dce}$$

where:
$I_t$ = intensity of reflected light
$I_o$ = intensity of incident light
$d$ = distance light is transmitted through liquid
$c$ = concentration of solute
$e$ = extinction coefficient of solute.

The pulse oximeter measures the variation in absorption caused by the arterial pulse, cancelling out the effects of other tissues, venous blood and background light (Fig. 12.10). It is accurate to within 2%, but falls to ± 5% with saturations below 80%.

### Factors affecting accuracy

- Smoking – overestimates the saturation by the % of HbCO present (≈ 3% in urban dwellers, 15% in heavy smokers)
- Methaemoglobin – saturation tends towards 85%
- Cardiac dyes – cause underestimation
- HbF and hyperbilirubinaemia have no effect on accuracy of readings
- Extraneous light, motion artefact and diathermy all interfere with absorption
- Atrial fibrillation and vasoconstriction result in a poor pulse volume, which causes errors in measurement.

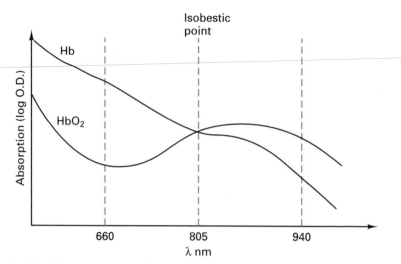

**Fig. 12.9** Absorption spectra of haemoglobin and oxyhaemoglobin.

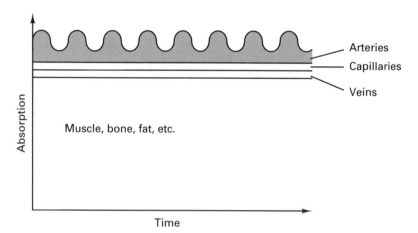

**Fig. 12.10** Composition of the absorption spectra. (Reproduced with permission from Davey et al 1992.)

## CAPNOGRAPHY

Uses spectrophotometry to measure absorption of $CO_2$ in sample chamber (Beer's law) and compares results with known $CO_2$ concentration in a reference chamber (Fig. 12.11).

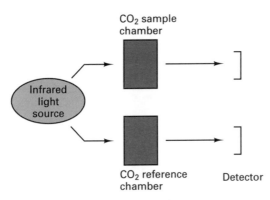

**Fig. 12.11** Infrared analyser for carbon dioxide.

### Arrangement of sampling chamber

The sampling chamber can have one of two arrangements:

1. Attached close to endotracheal tube to measure absorption directly through fresh and expired gases. Avoids delays in sampling time but necessitates a heavy, bulky detector attached to the endotracheal tube.
2. Sampling tube attached close to endotracheal tube which continuously samples gases at 150 ml/min. Avoids bulky attachment but several seconds delay in measuring expired $CO_2$. If used with a circle system, sampled gas must be returned to the circuit to prevent emptying of the circle gases.

### Factors affecting accuracy

- Length and size of sampling tubing and rate of sampling
- $N_2O$ has similar absorption to $CO_2$ and therefore requires compensation in calculations
- High respiratory rate, e.g. children, can underestimate $P_{ET}CO_2$ if sampling rate is too slow
- PEEP and CPAP can cause overestimation of readings
- $P_{ET}CO_2$ is usually 0.3–0.6 kPa below $P_aCO_2$, but with severe COAD it may be > 2 kPa.

### Patterns of capnography displays

*IPPV.* During ventilation with a Bain circuit, $P_{ET}CO_2$ does not return to zero during inspiration because FGF is less than the minute volume. During inspiration, the trace is distorted by the mixing of expired and fresh gas.

*Severe COAD* causes a prolonged sloping expiratory phase because of the wide spread in V/Q̇ values. Alveoli emptying last have the least ventilation, the lowest V/Q̇ and thus the highest $P_{ET}CO_2$.

*Pulmonary embolus* causes a flat expiratory plateau lower than the true $P_{ET}CO_2$ because of dilution of expiratory gases with air from non-perfused alveoli.

*Shunting,* e.g. secretions blocking alveoli, causes a rise in $P_{ET}CO_2$, but the difference is only small since the AV difference is only $\approx 0.6$ kPa.

## Clinical uses

- Detection of oesophageal intubation
- Disconnection/apnoea alarm
- Estimation of $P_aCO_2$. $P_{ET}CO_2$ is 0.3–0.6 kPa less than $P_aCO_2$, with the least difference at large tidal volumes. $P_{ET}CO_2$ has been measured at higher values than $P_aCO_2$, possibly due to time-dependent mismatching of ventilation and perfusion occurring in normal lungs at large tidal volumes
- Monitoring IPPV and hyperventilation
- $\downarrow P_{ET}CO_2$ with pulmonary embolus, $\downarrow$ cardiac output, hyperventilation, hypothermia or hypovolaemia
- $\uparrow P_{ET}CO_2$ with hypoventilation, pyrexia or malignant hyperthermia
- Detection of rebreathing
- Monitors early return of spontaneous respiratory effort
- Detects soda lime exhaustion.

## VOLATILE AGENT MONITORING

### Drager Narcotest halothane indicator

Uses a rubber band under tension attached to a pointer. Halothane is absorbed by rubber, causing change in elasticity and thus length of the rubber band. Only measures to 3%.

### Infrared absorption spectroscopy

Asymmetric, polyatomic molecules absorb infrared radiation, e.g. $CO_2$, $N_2O$. $H_2$ and $O_2$ do not. Similar arrangement as the capnograph $CO_2$ detector. Volatile agents have overlapping absorption spectra (Fig. 12.12) and therefore the gas being measured must be specified.

### Peizoelectric crystal

Quartz crystal coated in oil. Volatile agent absorbed into oil which changes the weight and thus the frequency of oscillation of the crystal.

### Raman scattering

Argon laser beam is shone through the sample gas. It emerges at a different wavelength, the change being dependent upon the type of volatile agent.

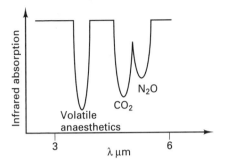

**Fig. 12.12** Infrared absorption spectrum.

# NON-INVASIVE BLOOD PRESSURE

## Mercury manometer

*Korotkoff sounds:*

I   – first appearance of pulse
II  – reduced intensity of pulsation
III – increased intensity of pulsation
IV – reduced intensity of pulsation
V  – loss of all sound ≡ diastole.

## Finapres

Utilizes the technique of Penaz. Digital cuff is servo-controlled so that its pressure is equal to the blood pressure in that digit. The pressure waveform of the cuff is calibrated with the systolic, diastolic and mean blood pressures from a conventional cuff and displayed continuously on an oscilloscope. Less accurate with peripheral vasoconstriction and susceptible to movement artefact.

## Arterial tonometry

Microtransducers compress a large artery, e.g. brachial, and continuously monitor the arterial blood pressure. Calibrated by standard BP cuff. Not yet available commercially.

## Pulse wave detection velocity

Two photometric sensors at different sites, e.g. forehead and finger, compare rate of propagation of the arterial pulse, which is related to blood pressure. Viscoelasticity decreases with age and may affect accuracy in the elderly. Calibrated by standard BP cuff. Not yet available commercially.

## CENTRAL VENOUS PRESSURE

IPPV increases intrathoracic pressure and overestimates mean CVP. Spontaneous respiration decreases intrathoracic pressure and underestimates mean CVP. Measure the peak pressure of the 'a' wave during the end-expiratory pause.

Right atrial pressure is a reasonable indicator of left atrial pressure with normal myocardial and pulmonary function.

### References

Association of Anaesthetists of Great Britain and Ireland 1994 Recommendations for standards of monitoring during anaesthesia and recovery: report of a Working Party (revised edition). AAGBI, London

Hanning C D, Alexander-Williams J M 1995 Pulse oximetry: a practical review. British Journal of Anaesthesia 311: 367–370

Lennmarken C, Vegfors M 1998 Advances in pulse oximetry. Current Opinion in Anaesthesiology 11: 639–644

Moyle J T B 1994 Pulse oximetry. Principles and practice series. BMJ Publishing Group, London

O'Flaherty D 1994 Capnography. Principles and practice series. BMJ Publishing Group, London

Runciman W B, Ludbrook G L 1994 Monitoring. In: Nimmo W S, Rowbotham D J, Smith G (eds) Anaesthesia, 2nd edn. Blackwell Scientific Publications, Oxford, p 704–739

Ward C (ed) 1998 Ward's anaesthetic equipment, 4th edn. WB Saunders, London

## PHYSICS

## GAS LAWS

*Henry's law.* Amount of gas dissolved ∝ partial pressure of the gas.

*Fick's law.* Rate of diffusion across a membrane ∝ concentration gradient.

*Graham's law.* Rate of diffusion ∝ 1 / molecular weight.

*Charles' law.* The volume of a gas changes in proportion to the change in temperature.

*Boyle's law.* The volume of a gas is inversely proportional to pressure.

*Gay-Lussac's law.* At constant volume, the absolute pressure of a given mass of gas varies directly with the absolute temperature.

*Adiabatic change.* A change in pressure, volume or temperature without changes in energy of gas (i.e. heat is lost or added).

## AVOGADRO'S HYPOTHESIS

Equal volumes of 'ideal' gases at the same temperature and pressure contain the same number of molecules. (Avogadro's number = $6.022 \times 10^{23}$ molecules occupying 22.4 l at STP.)

## PRESSURE

*Dalton's law of partial pressures.* The pressure exerted by a mixture of gases is equal to the sum of the pressures which each gas would exert on its own.

*Vapour pressure.* A vapour is saturated when it is in equilibrium with its own liquid, i.e. as many molecules leave the surface as rejoin it. When vapour pressure equals atmospheric pressure, the liquid boils.

## SOLUBILITY

*Ostwald solubility coefficient.* The amount of gas that dissolves in unit volume of liquid under the stated temperature and pressure.

*Bunsen solubility coefficient.* The amount of gas that dissolves in unit volume of liquid at standard temperature (273 K) and pressure (101.3 kPa).

## TEMPERATURE

*Critical temperature.* Temperature above which a gas cannot be liquefied.

*Critical pressure.* Pressure above which a gas at its critical temperature cannot be liquefied.

*Pseudocritical temperature.* Temperature at which a mixture of gases separate out into their separate components, e.g. $N_2O$ and $O_2$ in Entonox at $-5.5°C$.

*Specific heat capacity.* Amount of heat required to increase the temperature of a substance by $1°C/kg$.

## GAS FLOW

*Hagen–Poiseuille equation.* For laminar flow:

$$\dot{Q} = \frac{P \times \pi \times r^4}{8 \times \eta \times L}$$

where P= pressure, r = tube radius, L = tube length, $\eta$ = viscosity.

Liquid tends to flow smoothly in straight and uniform tubes. Abrupt changes in diameter or direction of flow cause turbulent flow, which is dependent upon density ($\rho$) rather than viscosity.

For turbulent flow:

$$\dot{Q} \propto \frac{\rho}{r^5}$$

When Reynold's number (R) exceeds 2000, flow becomes turbulent:

$$R = \frac{v \times \rho \times r}{\eta}$$

*Bernoulli effect.* Fall of pressure at a constriction in a tube. Increased gas/fluid velocity results in increased kinetic energy with a reduction in potential energy and thus a decrease in pressure.

Venturi devices use the Bernoulli effect for suction, e.g. Venturi oxygen mask.

*Coanda effect.* Streaming of gas at a division in tubing along only one of the divisions. Used as logic valve in some ventilators.

*Poynting effect.* A mixture of gases (e.g. Entonox) remains in a gaseous state, even though one component ($N_2O$) would normally be liquid at high storage pressures.

## HUMIDIFICATION

*Absolute humidity* is the mass of water vapour present in a given volume of air.

*Relative humidity* is the ratio of the mass of water vapour to the mass of water vapour when fully saturated, expressed as a percentage.

### Saturation

- Fully saturated air – 44 g/m$^3$
- Upper trachea – 34 g/m$^3$

   > 20 $\mu$m drops condense on breathing circuit
   5 $\mu$m drops settle on trachea
   1 $\mu$m drops reach alveoli.

### Measurements

- Hair hygrometer
- Regnault's hygrometer – measures dew point
- Electrical resistance
- Mass spectrometer.

### Methods of humidification

- *Heat and moisture exchanger* – also acts as bacterial filter. Can achieve levels of humidity in trachea of 20–25 g/m$^3$. Cheap.
- *Bubble humidifier* – fresh gas is bubbled through water. More efficient if bubbles are small, increasing their surface area. Heated water also improves efficiency by supplying energy for latent heat of vaporization. Bacterial multiplication is prevented by heating water to high temperatures, $\approx$ 60°C. This risks scalding of patient, so a thermistor is needed near the ETT. Can achieve levels of humidity of 40 g/m$^3$.
- *Venturi effect* – humidifies gas to 60 g/m$^3$.

- *Water dropped onto heated wire.*
- *Ultrasonic* – can achieve levels of humidity > 90 g/m$^3$.
- *Spinning plate* – can achieve levels of humidity > 90 g/m$^3$.

## ELECTRICITY

*Macroshock.* Skin-to-skin contact:
- 1 mA     – tingle
- 15 mA    – let-go threshold
- 50 mA    – respiratory arrest
- 100 mA   – VF.

*Microshock.* Direct myocardial contact. Current $\geq$ 100 $\mu$A. Less effect at higher frequency, e.g. diathermy at 20 kHz.

### Classification of electrical equipment

- *Class 1 equipment* – earthed metal casing
- *Class 2 equipment* – outer casing protected by double insulation with no exposed metal work; therefore an earth wire is not required
- *Class BF* – surface contact with patient. Maximum patient leak = 100 $\mu$A
- *Class CF* – may contact the heart directly. Maximum patient leak = 10 $\mu$A.

### References

Moyle J T B, Davey A 1998 Physical principles. In: Ward C (ed) Ward's anaesthetic equipment, 4th edn. WB Saunders, London
Parbrook G D, Davis P D, Parbrook E O 1995 Basic physics and measurement in anaesthesia. Butterworth-Heinemann Ltd, Oxford

# 13. Reports

## GUIDELINES FOR THE MANAGEMENT OF A MALIGNANT HYPERTHERMIA CRISIS 1998

See 'Malignant hyperthermia' (p. 114).

## IMMEDIATE POSTANAESTHETIC RECOVERY 1993

### Basic recovery facilities

Patient should normally be placed in the left lateral position and transferred on a tipping trolley to the recovery room. This should be fully staffed, available at all times and be able to give continuous individual nursing care to each patient. Handover should include pre-existing diseases, airway and cardiovascular problems, postoperative orders and analgesia.

Observations should include $O_2$ administration and saturation, respiratory rate, heart rate, blood pressure, level of consciousness, pain and i.v. infusions.

Patients should not be discharged to the ward until they can maintain their own airway and have protective reflexes, cardiovascular and respiratory stability, adequate analgesia and are normothermic.

Day-case patients on discharge should be accompanied by a responsible adult, be given written advice on analgesia and hospital contact number, and be warned against drinking alcohol and operating machinery for at least 24 hours.

### Recovery room

Effective emergency call system, defibrillator and anaesthetic machine must be available in the recovery room. Room must be well lit with waste gas scavenging and temperature of 21–22°C. Children should be segregated from adults.

Each bay should contain an $O_2$ source, breathing circuit (e.g. Mapleson C), pulse oximeter, ECG, suction and BP measuring equipment.

Each recovery trolley should contain an $O_2$ cylinder, be capable of tipping head-down, have suction equipment and have padded cot sides.

### Training of recovery staff

Minimum standards of training for recovery room staff.

## DAY CASE SURGERY 1994

See 'Day case anaesthesia' (p. 153).

## THE ANAESTHESIA TEAM 1998

### Recommendations

- A team-based approach to anaesthesia offers many advantages for the provision of a high-quality anaesthesia service.
- Pre-admission screening is a vital early component of pre-anaesthetic assessment. It reduces cancellations and promotes effective usage. It does not replace the need for the anaesthetist's preoperative visit.
- Anaesthetists must have dedicated, skilled assistance wherever anaesthesia is administered.
- Recovery areas must have trained staff available throughout all operating hours and until the last patient meets all the criteria for discharge.
- All acute hospitals providing in-patient surgical services must have an acute pain team led by a consultant anaesthetist.

## RECOMMENDATIONS FOR THE TRANSFER OF PATIENTS WITH ACUTE HEAD INJURIES TO NEUROSURGICAL UNITS 1996

See 'Neuroanaesthesia' (p. 74).

## GUIDELINES FOR OBSTETRIC ANAESTHESIA SERVICES 1998

See 'Obstetrics' (p. 254).

## MANAGEMENT OF ANAESTHESIA FOR JEHOVAH'S WITNESSES 1999

See 'Blood' (p. 144).

# OTHER GUIDELINES

## GUIDELINES FOR AUTOLOGOUS BLOOD TRANSFUSION British Committee for Standards in Haematology Blood Transfusion Task Force 1997

See 'Blood' (p. 142).

## INTERNATIONAL TASKFORCE ON PATIENT SAFETY 1993

Anaesthetist should be present for each anaesthetic.
Anaesthetist remains responsible during recovery period.
*Highly desirable monitoring:*

- low pressure/oxygen failure alarm
- oxygen analyser
- oximeter
- capnograph
- ECG.

*Mandatory:*

- BP and pulse every 5 min.

UK recommendations include ECG displayed from induction.

## REPORT OF THE JOINT WORKING PARTY ON ANAESTHESIA IN OPHTHALMIC SURGERY Royal College of Anaesthetists and College of Ophthalmologists 1993

See 'Anaesthesia for ophthalmic surgery' (p. 92).

## SEDATION AND ANAESTHESIA IN RADIOLOGY Royal College of Radiologists and Royal College of Anaesthetists 1992

### Sedation
Defined as 'a technique in which the use of drugs produces a state of depression of the central nervous system enabling treatment to be carried out, but during which, verbal contact with the patient is maintained throughout the period of sedation. The drugs and techniques used should carry a margin of safety wide enough to render unintended loss of consciousness unlikely'.

### Anaesthesia
Defined as 'any technique in which drugs produce loss of consciousness, as defined by failure to respond to verbal command'.

Patients must be carefully screened before the radiological procedure to identify those at increased risk.

Sedation is the responsibility of the radiologist and requires a nurse or technician to monitor the patient during the procedure.

Anaesthesia should only be administered by anaesthetists with the help of an operating department assistant. Full monitoring (non-invasive BP, oximetry, ECG), oxygen, suction, tipping trolley etc. should be available. A suitable recovery area is necessary. Adequate resuscitation facilities must be available.

Staff of all grades and specialities should be able to perform at least basic life support. They should all receive training in the detection of adverse reactions both to contrast media and to sedative drugs.

Cadaveric organs for transplantation. **A CODE OF PRACTICE FOR THE DIAGNOSIS OF BRAIN STEM DEATH** Department of Health 1998

See 'Organ donation and transplantation' (p. 179).

**GUIDELINES FOR PREOPERATIVE CHEST X-RAYS** Royal College of Radiologists 1995

Guidelines recommend that preoperative chest X-rays (CXRs) are not indicated routinely. They may be necessary in patients with known malignancy or possible tuberculosis. Anaesthetists may also request CXRs for dyspnoeic patients and those with known cardiac disease. Many patients with cardiorespiratory disease have a recent CXR available and a repeat CXR may not be needed.

**INFECTIVE ENDOCARDITIS PROPHYLAXIS** Endocarditis Working Party of the British Society for Antimicrobial Chemotherapy 1997 (As summarized in the *British National Formulary* 1999)

See 'Anaesthesia and cardiac disease' (p. 11).

**STANDARDS AND GUIDELINES FOR GENERAL ANAESTHESIA FOR DENTISTRY** Royal College of Anaesthetists 1999

See 'Dental anaesthesia' (p. 79).

### References

Association of Anaesthetists of Great Britain and Ireland 1990 Checklist for anaesthetic machines. AAGBI, London

Association of Anaesthetists of Great Britain and Ireland 1992 HIV and other blood borne viruses – guidance for anaesthetists. AAGBI, London

Association of Anaesthetists of Great Britain and Ireland 1993 Immediate postanaesthetic recovery. AAGBI, London

Association of Anaesthetists of Great Britain and Ireland 1994 Recommendations for standards of monitoring during anaesthesia and recovery: report of a working party (revised edition). AAGBI, London

Association of Anaesthetists of Great Britain and Ireland 1994 Day case surgery. AAGBI, London

Association of Anaesthetists of Great Britain and Ireland 1995 Suspected anaphylactic reactions associated with anaesthesia (revised edition). AAGBI, London

Association of Anaesthetists of Great Britain and Ireland 1996 A report received by Council of the Association of Anaesthetists on blood borne viruses and anaesthesia – an update. AAGBI, London

Association of Anaesthetists of Great Britain and Ireland 1997 Checklist for anaesthetic apparatus 2. AAGBI, London

Association of Anaesthetists of Great Britain and Ireland 1998 Guidelines for the management of a malignant hyperthermia crisis. AAGBI, London

Association of Anaesthetists of Great Britain and Ireland 1998 The anaesthesia team. AAGBI, London

Association of Anaesthetists of Great Britain and Ireland 1999 Management of anaesthesia for Jehovah's Witnesses. AAGBI, London

Association of Anaesthetists of Great Britain and Ireland and the Obstetric Anaesthetists Association 1998 Guidelines for obstetric anaesthesia services. AAGBI and OAA, London

British Committee for Standards in Haematology Blood Transfusion Task Force: Autologous Transfusion Working Party (Napier J A, Bruce M, Chapman J et al) 1997 Guidelines for autologous transfusion. II. Perioperative haemodilution and cell salvage. British Journal of Anaesthesia 78: 768–771

British National Formulary 1999 Infective endocarditis prophylaxis. British National Formulary 37(5.1)

Department of Health 1998 A code of practice for the diagnosis of brain stem death including guidelines for the identification and management of potential organ and tissue donors. HMSO, London

Neuroanaesthesia Society of Great Britain and Ireland and the Association of Anaesthetists of Great Britain and Ireland 1996 Recommendations for the transfer of patients with acute head injuries to neurosurgical units. NSGBI/AAGBI, London

Royal College of Anaesthetists 1992 Sedation and anaesthesia in radiology. Report of a Joint Working Party. RCA, London

Royal College of Anaesthetists and College of Ophthalmologists 1993 Report of the Joint Working Party on Anaesthesia in Ophthalmic Surgery. RCA and CO, London

Royal College of Anaesthetists 1999 Standards and guidelines for general anaesthesia and dentistry. RCA, London

Royal College of Radiologists 1995 Making the best use of a department of clinical radiology Guidelines for doctors, 3rd edn. RCR, London

## NATIONAL CONFIDENTIAL ENQUIRIES INTO PERIOPERATIVE DEATHS (NCEPOD)

CEPOD was established in 1988 to review surgical and anaesthetic practice in the UK. The first report covered three areas, but it has been a national report (NCEPOD) since 1989. It involves all NHS and most private hospitals. The reports are anonymous and confidential and are peer-reviewed by consultants representing the medical colleges.

### CEPOD 1987

Covered three areas (i.e. not national): N.E. Thames Health Authority (HA), Northern HA and South Western HA.

### Recommendations

- Need for national assessment of clinical practice.
- No SHO/registrar should undertake any emergency case without consultation with their consultant/SR.
- Resources should be concentrated on a single site.
- Neurological and neonatal surgery should be performed in specialist units.
- Patients must be adequately resuscitated preoperatively if possible.
- Moribund patients should be allowed to die with dignity.

## NCEPOD 1989 – Children

Involved all hospitals, i.e. first national CEPOD. Covered deaths in children ≤ 10 years occurring within 30 days of surgery, of which there were 115 non-cardiac deaths and 160 cardiac deaths.

### Recommendations

- Anaesthetists should not undertake occasional paediatric anaesthesia.
- No trainee should anaesthetize a child without discussion with the consultant.
- Neonates should be transferred to a paediatric centre.

## NCEPOD 1990 – Deaths

Random sample of 20% of adult postoperative deaths. 19 000 deaths, mostly within 5 days of surgery. 59% of anaesthetists were working without assistance.

### Recommendations

- All essential services should be on one site.
- Surgeon and anaesthetist should be in agreement about need for surgery.
- Proper pain relief needs a high-dependency unit.
- Provision of daytime emergency theatre is needed to prevent delays.
- All grades of anaesthetist should be involved in audit and continuing education.

## NCEPOD 1991/2 – Specific procedures

Reviewed 15 specific surgical procedures from all specialities.

### Recommendations

- Surgical and anaesthetic skills should be more matched to the condition of the patient.

- 42% of deaths after total hip replacement were found to have a pulmonary embolus. Therefore a local policy on prophylaxis must be determined and followed.
- Some patients with GI obstruction had no NG tube, resulting in aspiration.
- Stresses importance of fluid balance in the elderly.
- Patients about to die should not be subjected to surgery.
- Capnography and ventilator disconnect alarms are underused.

## NCEPOD 1992/3

Reviewed 19 816 deaths in patients aged 6–70 years.

### Recommendations

- Trainees with less than 3 years' training should not anaesthetize without appropriate supervision.
- Practitioners should recognize their limitations and not hesitate to consult a more experienced colleague.
- The skills of the anaesthetist and surgeon should be appropriate for the physiological and pathological status of the patient.
- Appropriately trained staff must accompany all patients with life-threatening conditions during transfer between and within hospitals.
- The medical profession must develop and enforce standards of practice for the management of many common acute conditions (e.g. head injury, aortic aneurysm, GI bleeding).

## NCEPOD 1993/4 – Postoperative deaths

Reviewed one death per consultant surgeon or gynaecologist.

### Recommendations

- Surgical operations should not be started in hospitals without appropriate critical care services.
- Anaesthetist must have appropriately skilled and dedicated non-medical assistants.
- Consultation between surgeons and anaesthetists needs to be more frequent in order to promote a team approach.
- The use of protocols in the management of certain clinical conditions needs to be increased.

## NCEPOD 1994/5 – Postoperative deaths

Reviewed 1818 deaths within 3 days of surgery.

### Recommendations

- High-dependency and ICU beds are still inadequate and resources need to be increased to correct deficiencies.
- Communication between specialists and between grades needs to be more frequent and more effective.
- Patients > 90 years of age, those with aortic stenosis, those who need radical pelvic surgery and those in for emergency vascular operations require individual attention by consultant anaesthetists and consultant surgeons.
- Clinical records and data collection need to be improved.

## NCEPOD 1995/6 – Out-of-hours operating

Reviewed 53 162 'out-of-hours' cases performed over a period equal to 1 week's work for each participating hospital.

### Key points

- Decision-making – too many decisions were taken by juniors; the decision to operate should be made by consultants
- Preoperative management – guidance from experienced staff was needed, including preoperative ICU admission if necessary
- Management of intravenous fluids – was sometimes poor
- Records and charts – were often poorly kept.

### Recommendations

- All hospitals admitting emergency surgical patients must be of sufficient size to provide 24-hour operating rooms. There should also be sufficient medical staff to perform these functions.
- These provisions should be continuous throughout the year: trauma and acute surgical emergencies do not recognize weekends or public holidays.
- Patients expect to be treated and managed by trained and competent staff. Patients assume trainees to be taught appropriately and supervised as necessary. Consultants should acknowledge these facts and react accordingly.

## NCEPOD 1996/7 – Specific surgical procedures

Reviewed 2541 deaths following specific surgical operations.

### Recommendations

*Obstructed airway in head and neck surgery.* Management should be planned between surgical and anaesthetic staff. Awake fibreoptic intubation and tracheostomy using LA should be considered amongst the options. A fibreoptic intubating laryngoscope should be readily available for use in all surgical hospitals.

*Anaesthesia for carotid endarterectomy.* Invasive arterial pressure monitoring should be routine and perioperative BP control needs to be excellent.

*Oesophageal surgery.* Preoperative resuscitation was often inadequate. One-lung ventilation should be performed by anaesthetists with appropriate experience in the technique. Attention to postoperative respiratory care is essential to achieve a good outcome.

*CVP monitoring during anaesthesia and surgery.* May be indicated for patients with acute or chronic medical conditions. CVP is a core anaesthetic skill that needs regular practice.

*Non-steroidal anti-inflammatory drugs.* Must be used with caution in patients with renal impairment, hypertension and cardiac failure, GI ulceration and asthma.

*Other recommendations.* Morbidity/mortality meetings should take place in all anaesthetic departments. Surgeons need to recognize the limits of surgical procedures; a decision to operate may not be in the best interests of the patient.

## NCEPOD 1997/8 – Deaths at the extremes of age

Reviewed 19 643 deaths occurring within 30 days of surgery in children (≤ 15 yrs) and elderly (≥ 90 yrs).

### Recommendations – Paediatric surgery

- Anaesthetic and surgical trainees need to know when they must inform their consultants before undertaking any paediatric procedures.
- The death of any child within 30 days of surgery should be subjected to peer review.
- The concentration of paediatric surgical services would increase expertise and reduce occasional practice.

### Recommendations – Surgery for the elderly

- Fluid management is often poor and should be accorded the same status as drug prescription. Multidisciplinary reviews to develop good working practices are required.
- A team of senior physicians, surgeons and anaesthetists need to be closely involved with these patients who have poor physical status and high intraoperative risk.
- Pain management must be provided by those with appropriate specialized experience.
- The decision to operate must be accompanied by a decision to provide appropriate post-operative care.

- No elderly patient requiring an urgent operation, once fit for surgery, should wait more than 24 hours.

## NCEPOD 1998/9 – One in ten sample of death (to be published Nov. 2000)

Will allow comparison with the 1992 NCEPOD report which considered one in five deaths. Will be available on NCEPOD website (www.ncepod.org.uk).

### References

Buck N, Devlin H B, Lunn J N 1987 The Report of a Confidential Enquiry into Perioperative Deaths. Nuffield Provincial Hospitals Trust and the King Edward's Hospital Fund for London, London

Callum K G, Gray A J G, Hoile R W, Ingram G S, Martin I C, Sherry K M 1999 Extremes of Age: The Report of the National Confidential Enquiry into Perioperative Deaths 1999. NCEPOD, London

Campling E A, Devlin H B, Lunn J N 1990 The Report of the National Confidential Enquiry into Perioperative Deaths 1989. NCEPOD, London

Campling E A, Devlin H B, Hoile R W, Lunn J N 1992 The Report of the National Confidential Enquiry into Perioperative Deaths 1990. NCEPOD, London

Campling E A, Devlin H B, Hoile R W, Lunn J N 1993 The Report of the National Confidential Enquiry into Perioperative Deaths 1991/2. NCEPOD, London

Campling E A, Devlin H B, Hoile R W, Lunn J N 1995 The Report of the National Confidential Enquiry into Perioperative Deaths 1992/3. NCEPOD, London

Campling E A, Devlin H B, Hoile R W, Ingram G S, Lunn J N 1997 The Report of the National Confidential Enquiry into Perioperative Deaths 1995/6. NCEPOD, London

Gallimore S C, Hoile R W, Ingram G S, Sherry K M 1997 The Report of the National Confidential Enquiry into Perioperative Deaths 1994/5. NCEPOD, London

Gray A J G, Hoile R W, Ingram G S, Sherry K M 1998 The Report of the National Confidential Enquiry into Perioperative Deaths 1996/7. NCEPOD, London

Lunn J N, Devlin H B, Hoile R W 1996 The Report of the National Confidential Enquiry into Perioperative Deaths 1993/4. NCEPOD, London

## REPORTS ON CONFIDENTIAL ENQUIRIES INTO MATERNAL DEATHS IN THE UNITED KINGDOM

England and Wales reports published every 3 years from 1952 to 1984. Changed to combined triannual UK reports from 1984.

### Definitions of maternal deaths

*Maternal deaths.* Deaths of women while pregnant or within 42 days of termination of pregnancy, from any cause related to or aggravated by the pregnancy or its management, but not accidental or incidental causes.

*Direct.* Deaths resulting from obstetric complications of the pregnant state, from interventions, omissions, incorrect treatment, or from a chain of events resulting from any of the above.

*Indirect.* Deaths resulting from previous existing disease, or disease that developed during pregnancy and which was not due to direct obstetric causes, but which was aggravated by the physiological effects of pregnancy.

**Table 13.1** Maternal deaths directly associated with anaesthesia, United Kingdom 1985–96

|         | Number of deaths directly associated with anaesthesia | Rate per million maternities | % of maternal deaths |
|---------|-------------------------------------------------------|------------------------------|----------------------|
| 1985–87 | 6                                                     | 2.6                          | 4.3                  |
| 1988–90 | 4                                                     | 1.7                          | 2.7                  |
| 1991–93 | 8                                                     | 3.5                          | 6.5                  |
| 1994–96 | 1                                                     | 0.5                          | 0.8                  |

## REPORTS ON CONFIDENTIAL ENQUIRIES IN MATERNAL DEATHS IN THE UNITED KINGDOM 1991–93 (published 1996)

There were 128 direct maternal deaths in 1991–93 (Fig. 13.1).

### Deaths associated with anaesthesia

14 deaths were associated with anaesthesia, of which 8 were directly

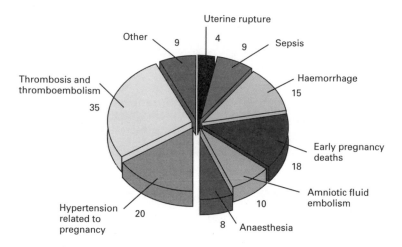

**Fig. 13.1** Causes of direct maternal deaths 1991–93.

attributable to anaesthesia. Of these direct deaths, 7 were associated with substandard anaesthetic care. Hypoxia and airway obstruction were responsible for 5 deaths, acute respiratory distress syndrome for 2 deaths, and 'failure of tissue perfusion' for 1 death. Anaesthesia contributed to a further 6 deaths (indirect deaths).

All direct deaths following caesarian section were associated with general rather than regional anaesthesia.

Lack of consultant involvement, inadequate diagnosis and assessment of severity of illness, aspiration of stomach contents, hypovolaemic shock and lack of availability of intensive care facilities were the main factors associated with mortality. It was particularly noted that monitoring (especially pulse oximetry) and recording of physiological variables were substandard in many cases, as was good record-keeping.

## Recommendations

- Recognition of the need for intensive care for any serious complication is essential. Any patient requiring mechanical ventilation should be transferred to an intensive care unit. High dependency units may be appropriate for patients who are at risk of developing organ failure or those with single-organ (non-pulmonary) organ failure.
- Patients with haemolysis, elevated liver enzymes and low platelets (HELLP) syndrome should be expected to show serious morbidity, particularly renal failure, disseminated intravascular coagulopathy and pulmonary oedema. Early recognition and referral to at least a high-dependency care unit may improve outcome.
- The quality of medical record-keeping must be improved.
- The anaesthetist must be involved with management of the 'at risk' patient at an early stage and provide liaison with high dependency and intensive care. Intensive and high-dependency care facilities should be readily available on the same hospital site for obstetric patients.
- Development of clinical guidelines and local protocols should be encouraged.

### SUMMARY OF THE REVISED GUIDELINES FOR THE MANAGEMENT OF MASSIVE OBSTETRIC HAEMORRHAGE
Report on Confidential Enquiries into Maternal Deaths in the United Kingdom 1994

- Summon all the extra staff required, particularly the duty anaesthetic registrar.
- Inform haematology and blood transfusion.
- Take blood for cross-matching and coagulation studies. Order a minimum of 6 units, only using group O Rh D-negative blood if transfusion must be given immediately. Use of packed cells requires

additional colloid (gelatins or hydroxyethylstarch solutions, not dextrans) once > 40% blood volume is lost.

- Insert at least two 14G intravenous cannulae. CVP measurement should be continuously displayed and invasive BP is extremely useful.
- Perform regular Hb, platelet and coagulation studies. Restoring normovolaemia is a priority. Consider FFP, cryoprecipitate and platelets.
- Pressure bags ensure rapid fluid administration. Blood filters are rarely necessary and slow down infusion rates. Administer all fluids, and in particular blood, through a blood warmer.
- Additional calcium is only necessary if there is evidence of $Ca^{2+}$ deficiency. Use 10% calcium chloride in preference to gluconate.
- Regular monitoring of pulse, BP, CVP, blood gases and urinary output. Consider early transfer to an intensive care unit.

## SUMMARY OF GUIDELINES FOR THE TREATMENT OF OBSTETRIC HAEMORRHAGE IN WOMEN WHO REFUSE BLOOD TRANSFUSION Report on Confidential Enquiries into Maternal Deaths in the United Kingdom 1996

- Mostly Jehovah's Witnesses, of which there are 125 000 in the UK.
- Massive obstetric haemorrhage may occur rapidly, and in patients who may refuse blood transfusion the management of massive haemorrhage should be considered in advance.
- Patients who refuse blood transfusions should be managed in a unit which has facilities for prompt management of haemorrhage, including hysterectomy.
- Hb and ferritin should be monitored closely during pregnancy and haematinics used throughout pregnancy to maximize iron stores. Donation of blood for subsequent autotransfusion is inappropriate, because the amount of blood required to treat massive obstetric haemorrhage is far in excess of the amount that could be donated during pregnancy.
- Extra vigilance is required in managing these patients, to detect early bleeding and clotting abnormalities. Prompt and early intervention is necessary, particularly with regard to surgery.
- The consultant anaesthetist and haematologist should be informed as soon as abnormal bleeding has been detected.
- Dextrans should be avoided for fluid replacement because of their possible effects on haemostasis. Intravenous crystalloid and plasma expanders such as Haemaccel should be used. Intravenous vitamin K should be given if bleeding is severe. Desmopressin,

methylprednisolone and fibrinolytic inhibitors such as aprotinin and tranexamic acid should be considered.
- The use of hyperbaric oxygen therapy has enabled survival with a haemoglobin concentration of 2.6 g/dl, although it is recognized that it is unrealistic to book women only where this facility is available.
- If the patient refuses to accept blood or blood products, her wishes must be respected. Any adult patient (over 18 years old) who has the necessary mental capacity to do so is entitled to refuse treatment, even if the refusal is likely to result in death.
- If the woman survives the acute episode, erythropoietin, parenteral iron therapy and adequate protein for haemoglobin synthesis should be given.

## REPORTS ON CONFIDENTIAL ENQUIRIES INTO MATERNAL DEATHS IN THE UNITED KINGDOM 1994–96
(published 1998)

There were 134 direct maternal deaths in 1994–96 (Fig. 13.2).

### Deaths associated with anaesthesia

Only 1 death was directly attributable to anaesthesia, involving hypotension and cardiac arrest following a combined spinal and epidural anaesthesia which caused extensive sympathetic block.

There were 20 additional deaths in which anaesthesia was associated with death, although only 12 involved substandard care. Lack of consultant

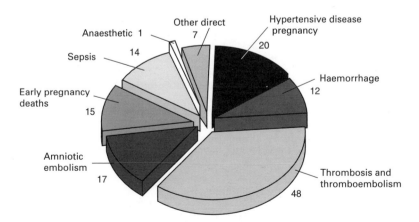

**Fig. 13.2** Causes of direct maternal deaths 1994–96.

availability, failure of communication and wise decision-making, failure of trainee doctors to recognize severity of illness, delay in providing adequate resuscitation, delay in obtaining blood products, delay or inadequate access to intensive or high-dependency units and split site working were the main factors associated with mortality in these 20 cases.

A large increase in deaths associated with thromboembolism, from 13 to 21 per million maternities, was noted. There were also increases in deaths from amniotic fluid embolism, sepsis and pregnancy-induced hypertension. In addition to a decrease in deaths from anaesthesia, there was also a decrease in deaths resulting from haemorrhage.

### Recommendations

- Each unit should draw up guidelines for the management of pre-eclampsia and eclampsia, obstetric haemorrhage, the use of thromboprophylaxis, the use of antibiotics for caesarian section, management of patients who decline blood products and the management of ectopic pregnancy. Implementation of these guidelines should be subject to regular audit.
- A single senior clinician should have overall responsibility for the management of pre-eclampsia/eclampsia, and in particular for fluid balance. These patients should be transferred to a more specialized centre at an appropriate stage.
- Women in haemorrhagic shock following rupture of an ectopic pregnancy should be transferred promptly to theatre. This must not be delayed by attempts to restore a normal circulating blood volume.
- Women must be assessed for the risk of thromboembolism and given prophylactic heparin if appropriate.

### References

Department of Health 1991 Report on Confidential Enquiries into Maternal Deaths in the United Kingdom 1985–87. HMSO, London

Department of Health 1994 Report on Confidential Enquiries into Maternal Deaths in the United Kingdom 1988–90. HMSO, London

Department of Health 1996 Report on Confidential Enquiries into Maternal Deaths in the United Kingdom 1991–93. HMSO, London

Department of Health 1998 Report on Confidential Enquiries into Maternal Deaths in the United Kingdom 1994–96. HMSO, London

May A E 1994 The Confidential Enquiry into Maternal Deaths 1988–1990. Editorial. British Journal of Anaesthesia 73: 129–131

# Appendix

## INTRODUCTION

The purpose of this examination is to assess trainees who have completed a minimum of 12 months of recognized training. It is expected, however, that most trainees will have completed 18 months of training before attempting the Primary FRCA examination. The topics outlined in the Primary FRCA examination syllabus indicate areas in which knowledge should be demonstrated.

It is accepted that a candidate's depth of knowledge will vary from subject to subject depending upon its relevance to the basic science and clinical practice of anaesthesia undertaken in the first year or 18 months of training.

This examination is designed to test:

- the candidates' understanding of the fundamentals of clinical anaesthetic practice including equipment and resuscitation
- the candidates' knowledge of the fundamental principles of Anatomy, Physiology, Pharmacology, Physics, Clinical Measurement and Statistics as is appropriate for the discipline of anaesthesia
- the candidates' clinical skills and attitudes appropriate to the above level of training

## ANAESTHESIA AND RESUSCITATION

*Candidates should be able to demonstrate a good understanding of the fundamentals of clinical anaesthetic practice, with an ability to discern when more senior assistance will be required.*

### Anaesthetic equipment and safety

Physical principles underlying the function of the anaesthetic machine, pressure regulators, flowmeters, vaporizers, breathing systems. Absorption of carbon dioxide

Principles of lung ventilators, disconnection monitors

Manufacture and storage of oxygen, nitrous oxide, carbon dioxide, compressed air

Pipeline and suction systems, gas cylinders

Humidification devices

Minimum monitoring requirements

Environmental control of the operating theatre including scavenging systems for waste anaesthetic gases and vapours

Pre-use checks of anaesthetic machine, breathing systems and monitoring apparatus

Anaesthetic records and critical incidents

Function and use of related anaesthetic and resuscitation equipment including that used for regional anaesthesia. Airways, tracheal tubes, tracheostomy tubes, laryngeal masks, oxygen therapy equipment, self-inflating bags, spinal and epidural needles, intravenous cannulae and transfusion devices

Sterilization and cleaning of equipment

**Preoperative assessment**

Implications for anaesthesia of commoner medical conditions. In particular, respiratory diseases (e.g. asthma, chronic obstructive airway disease), cardiac disease (e.g. angina pectoris, valvular disease, myocardial infarction, pacemakers, arrhythmias), vascular disease (e.g. hypertension), sickle cell disease and anaemias, rheumatoid arthritis, renal dysfunction and insufficiency, plasma electrolyte disturbance (e.g. hyper- and hypokalemia), diabetes mellitus, liver disease

Implications for anaesthesia of commoner surgical conditions, trauma, intestinal obstruction and acute abdominal emergencies

ASA classification and other pre-anaesthetic scoring systems such as Glasgow coma scale

Interpretation of relevant preoperative investigations, plasma electrolytes, haematology, disturbances of acid/base status, ECG, X-rays, pulmonary function tests and clotting abnormalities

Preoperative assessment of a patient of any age (excluding neonates) for elective or emergency surgery

Restriction of food and fluid by mouth, cessation of smoking, correction of dehydration

Assessment of difficulty of tracheal intubation

Precautions in the management of the infective patient (e.g. hepatitis B positive or HIV positive)

Anaesthetic implications of current drug therapy such as beta blockers, anti-hypertensive drugs, tricyclic antidepressant agents and monoamine-oxidase inhibitors, insulin, anti-diabetic drugs, anticoagulants, contraceptives

Assessment of postoperative analgesic needs

**Premedication**

Rationale for premedicant drugs. Choice of drugs, advantages and disadvantages

**Induction**

Intravenous and inhalational induction of anaesthesia; advantages and disadvantages, techniques

Recognition and management of anaphylactic and anaphylactoid reactions including follow up and patient information

Indications for tracheal intubation

Management of difficult intubation and failed intubation

Recognition of correct placement of tracheal tube, oesophageal and endobronchial intubation, complications

Causes of regurgitation and vomiting during induction, prevention and management

Technique of cricoid pressure. Pulmonary aspiration

Induction of anaesthesia in special circumstances, head injury, full stomach, upper airway obstruction

**Intraoperative**

*Ability to deal with emergencies before, during and after anaesthesia and the ability to stabilize a patient's condition until senior assistance can be obtained.*

Techniques of maintenance of anaesthesia. To provide adequate analgesia using opioids and other analgesic drugs. To prevent awareness. Management of appropriate intermittent positive pressure ventilation. Airway control. Intraoperative fluid therapy. Minimal monitoring

Diagnosis and management of important critical incidents during anaesthesia including: cyanosis, hypertension, hypotension, cardiac arrhythmias, bronchospasm, respiratory obstruction, increased peak inspiratory pressure, hyper- and hypocarbia, failed intubation, failed reversal

Management of massive haemorrhage, volume expansion, blood transfusion (hazards including incompatibility reaction), gas embolism, malignant hyperthermia

Correct intraoperative positioning on theatre table – complications, prone position

Diagnosis and treatment of pneumothorax


## Postoperative

Causes and treatment of failure to breathe at end of operation, suxamethonium apnoea – management

Care of the unconscious patient

Recovery room diagnosis and treatment of inadequate pulmonary ventilation, cyanosis, hypo- and hypertension, shivering, stridor. Oxygen therapy, indications and techniques

Methods of pain management. Assessment of pain and analgesic techniques

Prevention, diagnosis and treatment of postoperative pulmonary atelectasis, deep vein thrombosis and pulmonary embolus

Postoperative fluid therapy

Causes and treatment of postoperative nausea and vomiting

Minor and major adverse sequelae to anaesthesia and their management


## Anaesthesia in special circumstances

Principles of obstetric anaesthesia

Principles of the care of children (excluding neonates and infants) undergoing anaesthesia for straightforward surgical procedures, including ENT, eye and dental operations

Principles of general anaesthesia for simple ophthalmic procedures and a penetrating eye injury

Patients with a pacemaker

Advantages and problems associated with day surgery, appropriate anaesthetic techniques

Principles of neurosurgical anaesthesia as applied to the management of the head-injured patient

Problems of anaesthesia in the obese patient

Repeat anaesthesia – hepatic injury

Implications for the anaesthetist of viral hepatitis and HIV infections

Laparoscopic and minimally invasive procedures

Management of patients requiring transfer

## Regional anaesthesia

Indications, technique and management of the complications of spinal and epidural (including caudal approach) analgesia. Techniques including intravenous regional anaesthesia, brachial plexus block, femoral nerve block, inguinal field block, ankle block and dorsal nerve of the penis block

Local anaesthesia for awake tracheal intubation

## Resuscitation

*Immediate care and resuscitation in patients of all ages. The guidelines promulgated by the European Resuscitation Council and the Resuscitation Council [UK] will be followed. The syllabus will include:*

Patient assessment

The principles and practice of life support

The principles and practice of recognition and management of life-threatening arrhythmias including defibrillation and drug therapy

The techniques of venous access and the intraosseous route

Management of the airway and ventilation in the emergency including care of cervical spine

Specific problems in paediatric resuscitation

Ethical aspects of resuscitation

## Trauma

Pathophysiology of trauma and hypovolaemia

Assessment, immediate care and management of trauma patients of all ages

Performance and interpretation of the primary and secondary survey

Immediate specific treatment of life-threatening illness or injury, with special reference to thoracic and abdominal trauma

Care of cervical spine injury

Emergency airway management and oxygen therapy

Cannulation of major vessels for resuscitation and monitoring

Management of hypovolaemic shock

Chest drain insertion and management

Pain management in trauma victims

## ANATOMY

*Candidates should be able to demonstrate a good understanding of human anatomy relevant to the practice of anaesthesia.*

### Respiratory system

Mouth, nose, pharynx, larynx, trachea, main bronchi, segmental bronchi, structure of bronchial tree

Pleura, mediastinum

Lungs, lobes, bronchopulmonary segments. Structure of lungs

Innervation of respiratory tract, blood supply and lymphatic drainage

Diaphragm, muscles of respiration, innervation

### Cardiovascular system

Heart, chambers, conducting system, blood and nerve supply. Pericardium

Great vessels, main peripheral arteries and veins

Fetal circulation

### Nervous system

Brain and spinal cord, structure of spinal cord, age variation, spinal meninges, subdural and extradural space, contents of extradural space, CSF

Spinal nerves, dermatomes

Cervical plexus, brachial plexus, nerves of arm

Intercostal nerves

Lumbar plexus, nerves of abdominal wall

Sacral and coccygeal plexuses, nerves of leg

Autonomic nervous system, sympathetic innervation, sympathetic chain, ganglia and plexuses

Stellate ganglion

Parasympathetic innervation. Coeliac plexus

Cranial nerves. Trigeminal ganglion

**Vertebral column**

Cervical, thoracic and lumbar vertebrae

Sacrum, sacral hiatus

Ligaments of vertebral column

**Areas of special interest**

Base of skull

The thoracic inlet and 1st rib

Intercostal spaces including paravertebral space

Abdominal wall (including the inguinal region)

Antecubital fossa

Large veins of neck

Large veins of leg

Diaphragm

Anatomy of tracheostomy, cricothyrotomy

Eye and orbit

Axilla

## PHYSIOLOGY AND BIOCHEMISTRY

*Candidates should have a good general understanding of human physiology, and recognize the need to apply physiological principles and knowledge to the clinical practice of anaesthesia.*

**General**

Organization of the human body and control of internal environment

Differences between neonates, infants, children, adults and the elderly

Function of cells; genes and their expression

Cell membrane characteristics; receptors

Protective mechanisms of the body

## Biochemistry

Acid–base balance and buffers

Ions, e.g. $Na^+$, $K^+$, $Ca^{++}$, $Cl^-$, $HCO3^-$

## Body fluids and their functions and constituents

Capillary dynamics and interstitial fluid

Osmolarity: osmolality, partition of fluids across membranes

Lymphatic system

Special fluids especially cerebrospinal fluid and ocular fluids. Also pleural, pericardial and peritoneal fluids

## Haematology and Immunology

Red blood cells: haemoglobin and its variants. Blood groups

Haemostasis and coagulation

White blood cells

The inflammatory response

Immunity and allergy

## Muscle

Action potential generation and its transmission

Neuromuscular junction and transmission

Muscle types

Skeletal muscle contraction

Smooth muscle contraction

Motor unit

## Heart/Circulation

Cardiac muscle contraction

The cardiac cycle: pressure and volume relationships

Regulation of cardiac function; general and cellular

Control of cardiac output

Rhythmicity of the heart

Electrocardiogram and arrhythmias

Neurological and humoral control of systemic blood pressures, blood volume and blood flow (at rest and during physiological disturbances, e.g. exercise, haemorrhage and Valsalva manoeuvre)

Peripheral circulation: capillaries, vascular endothelium and arteriolar smooth muscle, tissue

Characteristics of special circulations including: pulmonary, coronary, cerebral, renal, portal and fetal

**Renal tract**

Blood flow and glomerular filtration and plasma clearance

Tubular function and urine formation

Regulation of fluid and electrolyte balance

Regulation of acid–base balance

Micturition

**Respiration**

Gaseous exchange: $O_2$ and $CO_2$ transport, hypoxia and hyper- and hypocapnia, hyper- and hypobaric pressures

Pulmonary ventilation: volumes, flows, dead space. Effect of IPPV on lungs

Mechanics of respiration: ventilation/perfusion abnormalities

Regulation of respiration

Non-respiratory functions of the lungs

**Nervous system**

Functions of nerve cells and synaptic mechanisms

The brain: functional divisions – cortex, midbrain, medulla, limbic system, brain stem and cerebellum

Intracranial pressure: cerebrospinous fluid, blood flow

Maintenance of posture

Autonomic nervous system

Neurological reflexes

Motor function: spinal and peripheral

Senses: receptors, nociception, special senses

Pain: afferent nociceptive pathways, dorsal horn, peripheral and central mechanisms, neuromodulatory systems, supraspinal mechanisms, visceral pain, neuropathic pain, influence of therapy on nociceptive mechanisms

Spinal cord: anatomy and blood supply, effects of spinal cord section

## Liver

Functional anatomy and blood supply

Metabolic functions

## Gastrointestinal

Gastric function; secretions, nausea and vomiting

Gut motility, sphincters and reflex control

Digestive functions

## Metabolism

Nutrients: carbohydrates, fats, proteins, vitamins and minerals

Metabolic pathways, energy production and enzymes; metabolic rate

Hormonal control of metabolism: regulation of plasma glucose, response to trauma

Physiological alterations in starvation, obesity, exercise and the stress response

Body temperature and its regulation

## Endocrinology

Mechanisms of hormonal control: feedback mechanisms, effect on membrane and intracellular receptors

Hypothalamic and pituitary function

Adrenocortical hormones

Adrenal medulla

Pancreas

Thyroid and parathyroid hormones and calcium homeostasis

## Pregnancy

Physiological changes associated with normal pregnancy

Functions of the placenta: dynamics of placental transfer

Fetus: changes at birth

## PHARMACOLOGY

Candidates should have a good understanding of general pharmacological principles, together with knowledge of drugs likely to be encountered in (a) basic anaesthetic practice and (b) current treatment of patients presenting for anaesthesia.

### GENERAL PHARMACOLOGY

#### Applied chemistry

Types of intermolecular bonds

Laws of diffusion. Diffusion of molecules through membranes

Solubility and partition coefficients

Ionization of drugs

Drug isomerism

Protein binding

#### Mode of action of drugs

Receptors: Dynamics of drug:receptor interaction. Graphical representations of receptor binding. Agonists, antagonists, agonist/antagonists, partial agonists, inverse agonists. Efficacy and potency. Receptor function and regulation. Tolerance

Metabolic pathways; enzymes; drug:enzyme interactions; Michaelis Menten equation

Ion channels: Types of ion channels. Relation to receptors. Gating mechanisms. Types of drug action

Signal transduction: cell membrane/receptors/ion channels to intracellular molecular targets, second messengers

Membranes: Action of gases and vapours

Other mechanisms: Osmotic effects. pH effects. Adsorption and chelation. Oxidation and reduction

Mechanisms of drug interactions: Inhibition and promotion of drug uptake. Competitive protein binding. Receptor interactions. Enzyme inducers and inhibitors. Addition, subtraction and synergism

Effects of metabolites and other degradation products.

Methodology of clinical trials

**Pharmacokinetics**

Drug uptake from the gastrointestinal tract

Presystemic metabolism: bioavailability

Drug uptake from the skin. Transdermal administration systems

Drug uptake by tissues: Muscle, subcutaneous, CSF, extradural space. Factors determining the distribution of drugs: perfusion, molecular size, solubility, protein binding. Significance of drug uptake by the lung

The influence of drug formulation on disposition

Body compartments

Distribution of drugs to organs and tissues: Influence of specialized membranes. Tissue binding and solubility. Materno–fetal distribution. Distribution in CSF and extradural space

Modes of drug elimination: Direct excretion

Metabolism in organs of excretion: phases I & II

Non-organ breakdown of drugs

Pharmacokinetic analysis: Concept of a pharmacokinetic compartment. Apparent volume of distribution. Clearance. Clearance concepts applied to whole body and individual organs

Relation to the Fick principle

Simple compartmental models

Physiological models based on perfusion and partition coefficients

Pharmacokinetic variation: influence of body size, sex, age, disease, pregnancy, anaesthesia, trauma, surgery, smoking, alcohol and other drugs

Pharmacodynamics: concentration-effect relationships. Hysteresis

Pharmacogenetics. Familial variation in drug response

Adverse reactions to drugs: hypersensitivity, allergy, anaphylaxis, anaphylactoid reactions

## SYSTEMATIC PHARMACOLOGY

Anaesthetic gases and vapours

Hypnotics, sedatives and intravenous anaesthetic agents

Opioids and other analgesics

Non-steroidal anti-inflammatory drugs

Neuromuscular blocking agents

Drugs acting on the autonomic nervous system: cholinergic and adrenergic agonists and antagonists

Drugs acting on the heart

Antihypertensives

Anticonvulsants

Diuretics

Antibiotics

Corticosteroids and other hormone preparations

Antacids. Drugs influencing gastric secretion and motility

Antiemetic agents

Local anaesthetic agents

Plasma volume expanders

Antihistamines

Antidepressants

Anticoagulants

## PHYSICS AND CLINICAL MEASUREMENT

*Trainees should understand the physical principles upon which methods of clinical measurement are based. Knowledge of clinical measurement techniques should be limited to principles and basic method.*

Mathematical concepts: sinusoids, exponentials and parabolas. Exponential functions and logarithms

Basic measurement concepts: linearity, drift, hysteresis, signal:noise ratio, dynamic response

SI units. Fundamental and derived units

Simple mechanics: Mass, Force, Work and Power

Heat: simple calorimetry. Conduction, convection, radiation. Mechanical equivalent of heat: laws of thermodynamics

Physics of gases. Absolute and relative pressure. The gas laws. Triple point: critical temperature. Density and viscosity of gases. Laminar and turbulent flow. The Bernoulli principle

Freezing point, melting point. Latent heat. Vapour pressure. Colligative properties; osmometry

Basic concepts of electricity and magnetism. Capacitance, inductance and impedance Amplifiers. Band width, filters.

Amplification of biological potentials: ECG, EMG, EEG. Sources of electrical interference

Processing, storage and display of physiological measurements. Bridge circuits

Basic principles of lasers

Principles of cardiac pacemakers and defibrillators

Electrical hazards: causes and prevention. Electrocution, fires and explosions. Diathermy and its safe use

Principles of pressure transducers.

Resonance and damping, frequency response

Measurement of pressure. Direct and indirect methods of blood pressure measurement. Pulmonary artery pressure

Measurement of volume and flow in gases and liquids. The pneumotachograph and other respirometers. Peak flow measurement. Spirometry. Cardiac output

Measurement of temperature and humidity

Measurement of gas concentrations, especially oxygen, carbon dioxide, nitrogen, nitrous oxide, volatile anaesthetic agents

Measurement of pH, $pCO_2$, $pO_2$

Simple tests of pulmonary function

Capnography

Pulse oximetry

Measurement of neuromuscular blockade

Measurement of pain

## BASIC STATISTICS

*Candidates will be required to demonstrate understanding of basic statistical concepts, but will not be expected to have practical experience of statistical methods. Emphasis will be placed on methods by which data may be summarized and presented, and on the selection of statistical measures for different data types. Candidates will be expected to understand the statistical background to measurement error and statistical uncertainty.*

## Descriptive statistics

Categories of data. Statistical distributions (Gaussian, $c_2$, binomial) and their parameters. Non-parametric measures of location and variability. Graphical presentation of data

## Deductive and inferential statistics

Simple probability theory. Confidence intervals. Linear regression. Linear correlation

The null hypothesis. Type I and type II errors. Probability of error occurrence, and the power of a test to detect a significant difference, Bland-Altman plot. Choice of simple statistical tests for different data types

## SKILLS DIRECTORY

### Clinical assessment

*History:*

Respiratory symptoms

Cardiovascular symptoms

Airway/intubation difficulties

Relevant neurological history: head injury; headache; raised intracranial pressure; space-occupying lesion; 'fits and faints'

Assessment and management of acute pain

Musculo-skeletal problems

Mental state: apprehension; depression; psychosis; mania; mental handicap

Gastro-intestinal problems

Obstetric considerations

Renal problems

Hepatic problems

Endocrine problems: thyroid; pituitary; adrenal; diabetes mellitus

Skin problems

Congenital disorders

Hereditary disorders

Haemoglobinopathies

Coagulopathies

Anaesthetic history: personal; familial

Medication: current; past

Allergies

Drug reactions

Drug interactions

Social problems: smoking; alcohol; recreational drugs; 'high risk' groups; domestic/social circumstances

### Physical examination:

Nutritional state: obesity; cachexia; dehydration; skin

Respiratory system: cyanosis/clubbing; dyspnoea/orthopnoea; chest deformities; chest movement; operation scars; chest observation/palpation/percussion/auscultation

Cardiovascular system: cyanosis/oedema; pulse; anatomy of veins and arteries; jugular venous pressure; arterial blood pressure; heart size/sounds/murmurs

Teeth/airway/intubation assessment: dental problems; jaw opening/thyro-mental distance/Mallampati criteria/Wilson risk factors/mobility of cervical spine/neck masses

Neurological signs: coma/charts/scores; raised intracranial pressure/papilloedema; cranial nerves; wasting/muscle power; reflexes; loss of mobility; sensory testing; pain scores

Anaemia

Jaundice

Abdomen: masses; bowel sounds; free fluid

Musculo-skeletal problems (relevant to positioning)

Vascular access – suitability of sites

Cricoid pressure

Cricothyrotomy/tracheostomy anatomy

Pleural drain sites

Epidurals/spinals/caudals

Local nerve blocks for brachial plexus, femoral nerve and dorsal nerve of penis

## Data interpretation

### *Clinical:*

Respiratory function: peak flow, vital capacity, vitalograph and spirometry measurements

Exercise tolerance

Electrocardiographs

Interpreting charts

Fluid balance

Central venous pressure measurement

### *Radiological:*

Chest radiographs

Neck and thoracic inlet films

Abdominal fluid levels/air/masses

Skull films

Other imaging investigations (simple data only)

### *Laboratory tests:*

Haematology

Coagulation

Haemoglobin electrophoresis

Thyroid function

Urea and electrolytes

pH and blood gases

Renal function

Liver function

Adrenal function

## Communication

Consent for:

- general anaesthesia (discuss risks)
- epidural/caudal/spinal/regional/local blocks (discuss risks)
- Explanation of need for preoperative:

- hepatitis screening

- HIV testing

- sickle cell status

Explanation of analgesic methods:

- oral/sublingual/rectal/subcutaneous/i.m./i.v./nasal/transdermal drugs

- inhalational analgesia

- patient controlled analgesia

- epidural/regional techniques/local blocks

- possible side-effects and complications

Discussion of preoperative medication choices

Explanation of postoperative expectations and care

Instructions to nurses:

- preoperative preparation

- premedication

- postoperative care

- postoperative analgesia

Checking patient into anaesthetic room/operating theatre

Instructions for supervision of anaesthetic recovery/discharge from recovery area

Explanation to patients/relatives of problems/complications:

- suxamethonium apnoea/difficult intubation

- anaphylaxis/malignant hyperthermia

- post-spinal headache

**Technical skills**

*Clinical:*

Resuscitation: basic life support; mouth to mouth/nose ventilation; intubation and pulmonary ventilation; cricothyrotomy/mini-tracheotomy; external chest compression; arrhythmia recognition and management (drugs/defibrillators/pacemakers); vascular access; fluid balance assessment/management

Venous access

Central venous pressure monitoring

Arterial pressure monitoring

Pleural drain insertion

Emergency pericardiocentesis

Lumbar puncture/spinal anaesthesia

Epidural anatomy and cannulation: management of associated hypotension; other relevant protocols

Caudal block

Nerve blocks

Intravenous regional analgesia

*Equipment:*

Anaesthetic machine checks

Checking pipelines

Changing and checking cylinders

Connecting up breathing systems

Breathing system checks

Setting up/checking/monitoring lung ventilators

Setting up/checking alarm limits for monitoring equipment

Data collection from monitors

Checking resuscitation equipment

Connecting up resuscitation equipment

Defibrillator settings

Recovery room equipment

What is missing?

What is misconnected?

What is wrongly set up?

What hazards are there?

Composing equipment checklists: resuscitation equipment; epidural/spinal packs; paediatric intubation set; difficult intubation kit; failed intubation management; CVP monitoring; arterial pressure monitoring

## SYLLABUS FOR THE FINAL FRCA EXAMINATION

### INTRODUCTION

The purpose of this examination is to assess trainees who have obtained the Primary FRCA examination and completed a minimum of 30 months' recognized training. The candidates will be expected to have a knowledge of medicine and surgery appropriate to the practice of anaesthesia, intensive care medicine and pain management.

This examination is designed to test the candidate's knowledge and ability to apply that knowledge in the broad fields of anaesthesia, intensive care medicine and pain management covered during training for this examination.

A knowledge of the **principles** of the specialized areas of post-fellowship training is required, but not the details of practice.

### ANAESTHESIA

*Trainees will be expected to demonstrate knowledge consistent with post-Primary FRCA examination training under the following headings:*

Anaesthetic equipment

Preoperative assessment

Pre-medication

Pre-, peri- and postoperative management of anaesthesia

Anaesthesia for patients with co-existing disease including diabetes and cardiovascular disorders

Anaesthesia for particular disciplines – obstetric, ENT, dental/maxillofacial, orthopaedic, trauma, vascular, ophthalmic, paediatric, day stay, neuroradiology (anaesthesia and sedation)

Regional anaesthesia

Audit and quality control

Ethics, relevant legislation and the duty of care

#### Obstetrics

Physiological changes of pregnancy

Anaesthesia in early pregnancy

Antenatal assessment of the pregnant woman

Medical diseases complicating pregnancy

Pain relief in labour

Anaesthesia for operative obstetrics

Emergencies in obstetrics

Maternal morbidity and mortality

Neonatal resuscitation

## ENT

Preoperative assessment, particularly prediction of a difficult intubation. Management of patients of all ages to include patients with: stridor; intubation difficulties; sleep apnoea; concomitant diseases

Local techniques and surface analgesia

Acute ENT emergencies (e.g. bleeding tonsils, croup, epiglottitis, foreign bodies)

Laryngoscopy and bronchoscopy

Knowledge of special tubes, gags and equipment for microlaryngoscopy, bronchoscopy, laser surgery (e.g. venturi devices, ventilating bronchoscope and fibreoptic bronchoscopy)

Middle ear surgery including hypotensive techniques

Major head and neck surgery

Emergency airway management including tracheostomy

Postoperative management

## Dental/Maxillofacial

Preoperative assessment

Day case/inpatient requirements

Resuscitation facilities

Dental chair anaesthesia

Paediatric anaesthesia

Sedative, anaesthetic and analgesic techniques for dental extractions

Assessment and management of the difficult airway including fibreoptic intubation

Anaesthesia for maxillofacial surgery including the perioperative management of the fractured jaw and other major facial injuries

Postoperative management for all patients undergoing dental or maxillofacial procedures

## Orthopaedic

Preoperative assessment with particular reference to the problems of children, the elderly and the patient with rheumatoid arthritis

Emergency anaesthesia for fractures

Routine anaesthesia for joint replacement surgery, arthroscopy, fractured bones, dislocations and tendon repair

Procedures under tourniquet

Anaesthesia for spinal surgery

Regional blocks

Perioperative analgesia

Prevention, diagnosis and management of fat emboli, deep vein thromboses and pulmonary emboli

## Trauma

Management of head injury, spinal injury and multiple trauma with major blood loss

Major incident management, triage and anaesthesia in situations outside the hospital

Transfer of the traumatized patient

Management of the burned patient

## Vascular

Resuscitation and management of major vascular accidents

Management of the patient with atherosclerotic disease

Management of the patient for major vascular surgery

Postoperative management

Postoperative analgesia

Anaesthesia for non-cardiac surgery in patients with cardiac disease

## Ophthalmic

Preoperative assessment with particular reference to patients with underlying disease

Strabismus, cataract and detached retina surgery

Penetrating eye injury

Control of intraocular pressure

Anatomy relevant to local anaesthetic blocks

Peribulbar and retrobulbar techniques of local anaesthesia

Postoperative care

## Paediatric

Preoperative assessment and psychological preparation for surgery

Anaesthetic management of children for major elective and emergency surgery

The anaesthetic implications of major congenital anomalies including congenital heart disease

Management of recovery

Management of postoperative pain in children

Management of acute airway obstruction including croup and epiglottitis

## Day stay

Selection criteria and preoperative evaluation

Instructions to patients

Regional analgesia

General anaesthesia

Appropriate drugs

Recovery assessment

Postoperative analgesia

## Diagnostic imaging – anaesthesia and sedation

Preanaesthetic preparation

Techniques appropriate for adults and children for CT scanning and MR imaging

Post-investigation care

## Regional

Basic sciences applied to regional anaesthesia: anatomy, physiology and pharmacology

Principles and practice of spinal and extradural anaesthesia, intravenous regional anaesthesia and nerve blocks

Recognition and management of adverse effects

*In addition, candidates will be assessed on their understanding of principles in the following areas:*

## Cardiac anaesthesia

Preoperative assessment and management of patients with cardiac disease

Anaesthesia for cardiovascular imaging

Pacemakers

Non-invasive and invasive vascular and non-vascular monitoring appropriate to the cardiovascular system

Anaesthesia for cardiac surgery

Principles of cardiopulmonary bypass and cardiac surgery

Postoperative management

## Thoracic anaesthesia

Preoperative lung function tests

Local and general anaesthesia for bronchoscopy to include techniques of ventilation

Familiarity with fibreoptic bronchoscopic techniques for airway management and diagnostic procedures

Techniques of one-lung anaesthesia to include single and double lumen endobronchial tubes

Principles of thoracic anaesthesia to include management of pneumothorax

Principles of underwater seals on chest drains

Tracheostomy and other techniques of emergency airway management

## Neurosurgical anaesthesia

Preoperative assessment and management of patients with neurological disease

Anaesthesia for imaging relevant to the CNS

Principles of anaesthesia for craniotomy, to include vascular disease, cerebral tumours and posterior fossa lesions

Anaesthesia for spinal column surgery

Principles of immediate postoperative management

Neurological monitoring

**Neonatal anaesthesia**

Preoperative assessment

Recognition of common congenital anomalies requiring surgical correction at birth and their anaesthetic implications (including oesophageal atresia, diaphragmatic hernia, exomphalos, intestinal obstruction)

Principles of anaesthetic management in the neonate undergoing major surgery

Congenital pyloric stenosis

Postoperative pain management

Transport of the critically ill neonate

**Transplantation**

Principles and complications of immunosuppression

Specific anaesthetic problems associated with renal transplantation

Anaesthetic management of patients with transplanted organs

**Other specialized areas**

Anaesthesia for:

electro-convulsive therapy (ECT); radiotherapy; minimal access surgery; plastic surgery; burns

Perioperative management of a patient with sleep apnoea

## APPLIED ANATOMY

*Candidates should be able to demonstrate a good understanding of human anatomy relevant to the practice of anaesthesia. The syllabus for the Primary FRCA examination is considered core knowledge. For the Final FRCA examination, application of this knowledge to clinical practice will be explored. This will include the knowledge of anatomy as demonstrated by endoscopic and imaging techniques*

## APPLIED PHYSIOLOGY

*Candidates are expected to be able to apply the basic knowledge of human physiology*

*necessary to pass the Primary FRCA examination to the clinical practice of anaesthesia and intensive care medicine.*

*While all branches of physiology are of importance, it is recognized that clinical relevance dictates the topics selected for the examination.*

## Haematological

Anaemia

Polycythaemia

Immunity and allergy

Inflammation

Blood groups

Alternative oxygen carrying solutions

Abnormalities of coagulation and haemostasis

Abnormal haemoglobins: sickle cell disease; thalassaemia

## Muscle function

Muscle contracture and malignant hyperthermia

Disturbances in neuromuscular transmission

Myopathies

## Cardiovascular

Abnormal electrocardiogram and arrhythmias

Cardiomyopathy

Abnormal ventricular function

Heart failure

Hypovolaemia and shock

Ischaemic heart disease

Valvular defects

Hypertension

Common congenital heart defects

## Kidney and body fluids

Disturbances of fluid balance, oedema and dehydration

Management of acid–base abnormalities

Measurement of renal function

Renal failure and its management

Diuresis

Plasma electrolyte disturbances

**Liver**

Hepatic failure

Jaundice

**Respiration**

Disorders of respiratory mechanics, gas exchange and gas transport

Disorders of the pulmonary circulation

Respiratory failure and ventilatory support

Effects of changes in barometric pressure

**Nervous system**

Consciousness and sleep

Depth of anaesthesia

Consequences of spinal cord injury and deafferentation

Monitoring of spinal cord function under general anaesthesia

Mechanisms of pain: somatic, visceral, neuropathic

Control of cerebral circulation, intracranial and intraocular pressures

Disorders of the autonomic nervous system

**Gastrointestinal tract**

Nausea and vomiting

Oesophageal reflux

Obstruction

Swallowing disorders

The mucosal barrier

**Metabolism and body temperature**

Hormonal and metabolic response to trauma

Hyperthermia and hypothermia

Starvation/obesity

**Endocrinology**

Endocrine diseases of significance in anaesthesia

**Obstetrics and paediatrics**

Principles of neonatal physiology

Effects of prematurity

Development in infancy and childhood

Physiology of normal and abnormal pregnancy

## APPLIED CLINICAL PHARMACOLOGY

*This section requires a wider knowledge of drugs than in the Primary FRCA examination. In the case of drugs used in anaesthesia and intensive care medicine, candidates will also be expected to be aware of new drugs which are undergoing evaluation and whose human application has been reported in the mainstream anaesthetic journals. There will be emphasis on the practical application of pharmacological and pharmacokinetic knowledge, and upon an appreciation of the hazards and limitation of individual techniques.*

**General therapeutics. Pharmacological management of:**

Heart failure, coronary insufficiency and arrhythmias

Hypertension, including hypertension in pregnancy

Acute and chronic respiratory diseases

Hepatic and renal failure

Gastrointestinal disorders including modification of gastric contents

Musculo-skeletal problems such as rheumatoid and osteoarthritis

Myasthenia and muscle diseases

Pituitary, adrenal and thyroid dysfunction

Depression, anxiety states and schizophrenia

Epilepsy

Bacterial, fungal and viral infections

Malignant disease

Adverse reactions: Types of reactions; The yellow card system; Regulation of drug licensing

**Application of pharmacological principles to the practical management of anaesthesia:**

Premedication: The use of anxiolytics, sedatives and antisialogogues. Pro-kinetic and anti-emetic drugs. $H_2$ and proton pump antagonists

Inhalational anaesthesia: Control of alveolar tension during induction and recovery. Control of anaesthetic depth and prevention of awareness

Management of sedation techniques

Intravenous anaesthesia: Methods for achieving specified plasma concentrations. Bolus, infusion, and profiled administration

Management of neuromuscular blockade: Techniques for the use and reversal of muscle relaxants. Management of abnormal responses

Regional anaesthesia: Choice of agent and technique. Additives. Systemic effects. Avoidance of toxicity

**Application of pharmacological principles to the control of acute pain (including intraoperative analgesia and postoperative pain management) and chronic pain:**

Opioid and non-opioid drugs

Opioid infusions

Patient-controlled analgesia

Regional techniques

Inhalational techniques

Other drugs used to manage chronic pain – antidepressants, anticonvulsants, antiarrythmics, etc.

Management of severe pain and associated symptoms in terminal care

Non-pharmacological methods (e.g. TENS, acupuncture)

**Application of pharmacological principles to neurosurgery and management of head injuries:**

Effect of drugs on cerebral blood flow

Control of intracranial pressure

Control of convulsions

Management of cerebral ischaemia

**Pharmacological control of myocardial function, vascular resistance, heart rate and blood pressure**

**Anticoagulant and thrombolytic therapies. Management of coagulopathies**

**Pharmacological control of blood sugar**

**Pharmacological problems in cardiopulmonary bypass. Cardioplegia**

**Therapeutic problems associated with organ transplantation: heart, lung, liver, kidney**

**Management of malignant hyperthermia**

**Pharmacological considerations in cardiopulmonary resuscitation, major trauma and exsanguination**

**Pharmacological control of severe infections**

**Pharmacological treatment of severe asthma**

**Effects of renal or hepatic impairment on drug disposition**

## THE STATISTICAL BASIS OF CLINICAL TRIAL MANAGEMENT

*Candidates will be expected to understand the statistical fundamentals upon which most clinical research is based. They may be asked to suggest suitable approaches to test problems, or to comment on experimental results. They will not be asked to perform detailed calculations or individual statistical tests.*

Study design: Trial planning. Elimination of bias: randomization and use of controls. Determination of sample size. Statistical advice

Ethical considerations: Exclusion categories. Avoidance of ethical errors. Ethical approval procedures

Data collection: Methods. Escape procedures. Statistical endpoints

Data analysis: Statistical analytical methods. Presentation of data and analytical results-page

## CLINICAL MEASUREMENT

*The Final examination assumes knowledge of the Primary FRCA examination*

*syllabus, with the addition of more sophisticated measurements. There is an emphasis on clinical applications of clinical measurement, such as indications, practical techniques and interpretation of acquired data. Candidates will be expected to understand the sources of error and the limitations of individual measurements.*

Assessment of respiratory function

Assessment of cardiac function, including echocardiography

The electroencephalograph (EEG) and evoked potentials

The electromyograph (EMG) and measurement of nerve conduction

Principles and practice of in vitro blood-gas measurements. Interpretation of data

Interpretation of biochemical data

Interpretation and errors of dynamic pressure measurements including systemic, pulmonary arterial and venous pressures, intracranial, intrathoracic and intra-abdominal pressures

Methods of measurement of cardiac output and derived indices; limitations and interpretation

Principles of imaging techniques including CT, MRI and ultrasound. Doppler effect

Interpretation and errors of capnography, oximetry and ventilatory gas analysis

## INTENSIVE CARE MEDICINE

*Candidates should have a good understanding of the diagnosis and management of the critically ill patient and should be skilled in resuscitation to an advanced standard. An understanding of the particular problems associated with the critically ill child (excluding neonates) will be expected.*

*All candidates should be familiar with the monitoring and life support equipment used in the treatment of critically ill patients. Candidates must be able to demonstrate their knowledge of practical invasive procedures, with an understanding of the principles and hazards involved. Interpretation of data from such procedures.*

*An awareness of the importance of communication skills and interpersonal relationships will be expected.*

**Transport of the critically ill**

**Infection and multiple organ failure**

Sepsis and endotoxaemia

Nosocomial infections

Assessment and management of oxygen delivery

Antibiotics and immunotherapy

**Cardiovascular system to include**

Pathophysiology and management of cardiogenic and hypovolaemic shock

Pulmonary embolism

Investigation and management of cardiac failure

Investigation and management of arrhythmias

**Respiratory system to include**

Airway care

Ventilators and modes of pulmonary ventilation

Management of acute and chronic respiratory failure

**Nervous system to include**

Central nervous system infection

Acute polyneuropathy

Traumatic and non-traumatic coma

Encephalopathies

Cerebral ischaemia

Status epilepticus

Brain stem death

**Renal, electrolyte and metabolic disorders to include**

Diagnosis, prevention and management of acute renal failure

Fluid, electrolyte and acid–base disorders

Body temperature

**Haematological disorders to include**

Coagulopathies

Immunocompromised patients

**Gastrointestinal disorders**

Acute liver failure – diagnosis and management

Acute pancreatitis

Gut ischaemia

Gastrointestinal ulceration and bleeding

Translocation and absorption disorders

**Nutrition**

Requirements for enteral and parenteral nutrition

**Analgesia, anxiolysis and sedation**

**Trauma**

Management of multiple injuries

Near-drowning

Burns and smoke inhalation

**Management of acute poisoning**

**Organ donation**

**Scoring systems and audit**

**Ethics**

# PAIN MANAGEMENT

*A detailed knowledge of the control of acute pain in the context of postoperative and post-traumatic conditions will be expected, as will an understanding of the principles of chronic pain management in the pain clinic setting.*

Anatomy, physiology, pharmacology and basic psychology relevant to pain management

Assessment and measurement of acute pain – including special problems with children, the elderly, and patients who are unconscious or in intensive care

Assessment of patients with chronic pain and pain in patients with cancer

Use of medication for pain management; conventional analgesics and adjuvant analgesics; side-effects; problems of drug dependency and addiction

The role of and indications for neural blockade: peripheral nerve, plexus, epidural and subarachnoid blocks; techniques of sympathetic blockade; neurolytic agents and procedures; implanted catheters and pumps for drug delivery

Stimulation produced analgesia including transcutaneous techniques and acupuncture

Other treatment modalities; physical therapy, surgery, psychological approaches, rehabilitation approaches, pain management programmes

Symptom control in terminal illness

The organization of pain management services

Principles and ethics of pain research

## REGULATIONS: PRIMARY AND FINAL EXAMINATIONS FOR THE FRCA

### INTRODUCTION

The Regulations which follow govern the content and conduct of the examinations leading to the award of the Fellowship of the Royal College of Anaesthetists. They specify the requirements which must be satisfied before a candidate is eligible to apply to take the examinations. They specify the procedure to be followed in order to apply, limit the number of attempts and provide for guidance in the event of failure. They describe the procedure for making representations and provide sanctions for infringements.

These Regulations were made by the Council of the Royal College of Anaesthetists on 18th March, 21st May, 19th November 1997 and 20th January 1999.

### TRAINING: INTERPRETATION

1. (a) For the purpose of these regulations 'approved training' in the United Kingdom means, subject to regulation 1(b), training which:

(i) is appropriate to the part of the examination for which the candidate is applying to enter; and

(ii) has been approved by the College as part of a course of training which, if satisfactorily completed, may contribute to the award of a Certificate of Completion of Specialist Training.

(b) In calculating the length of any period of training for the purpose of determining eligibility to enter either part of the examination, candidates shall normally be entitled to include:

(i) training which the candidate expects to have completed by the date given in the published calendar for the examination in question on which the clinical and oral elements will probably commence; or

(ii) a period of maternity or sick leave up to a maximum of one month per full training year; or

(iii) a period of training not longer than six months and not shorter than three months spent in one locum approved training post whether a locum SHO or Locum Appointment Training (LAT) post; or

(iv) a period of training not longer than twelve months and not shorter than six months spent in one Fixed Term Training Appointment (FTTA) – a Visiting Training Number (VTN) or, after February 1998, a Fixed Training Number (FTN) should normally be provided; or

(v) a period of training not longer than twelve months and not shorter than three months spent in one honorary or supernumerary SHO post, provided that the post is within the approved maximum training capacity of the hospital; or

(vi) any combination of the preceding sub-paragraphs.

## SECTION 1: EXAMINATIONS

2. (a) The examination for the Fellowship of the Royal College of Anaesthetists (FRCA) will be in two parts. The first part will be known as the Primary FRCA examination and the second part will be known as the Final FRCA examination.

(b) There will be three sittings of the Primary FRCA examination in each academic year starting on 1st August, and two sittings of the Final FRCA examination. Council may at any time decide, subject to adequate notice, to alter the number of sittings of either or both parts in any year.

3. Each part of the examination will comprise written, oral and clinical elements. The nature and number of these, together with details of the marking system to be used and of the prizes which may be awarded, are described in the Appendix to these Regulations. The subject matter of each part of the examination is specified in the syllabus for the Primary and Final FRCA examinations published annually by the College.

## SECTION 2 : ELIGIBILITY

### Eligibility for the Primary FRCA examination

4. A person is eligible to enter for the Primary FRCA examination who:

(a) is eligible for registration with the General Medical Council (United Kingdom), whether such registration is full or limited; and

(b) is registered with the College as a post-graduate trainee in the specialty of anaesthesia, or is exempt from such registration, not being in a training post in the UK at the time of sitting the examination; and

(c) has completed one year of training in post(s) approved by the Royal College of Anaesthetists, or one year of training in the Republic of Ireland in post(s) approved by the College of Anaesthetists of the Royal College of Surgeons in Ireland; and

(d) satisfies the requirements of these Regulations with regard to application procedures and other matters; with the exception that any person who, by virtue of the number of times he or she has attempted and failed the Part 1 examination of the three-part examination for the Fellowship of the Royal College of Anaesthetists, would no longer be eligible to enter for that examination, shall not be eligible to enter for the Primary FRCA examination.

## Eligibility for the Final FRCA examination

5. A person is eligible to enter for the Final FRCA examination who:

(a) is registered with the College as a post-graduate trainee in the specialty of anaesthesia or is exempt from such registration, not being in a training post in the UK at the time of sitting the examination; and

(b) has passed, or is exempt from passing in accordance with the provisions of Regulation 6, the Primary FRCA examination; and

(c) has completed thirty months of training in the specialty of anaesthesia which satisfies the following conditions:

(i) the end of the training shall be a date not earlier than five years before the closing date of the sitting applied for;

(ii) except for a period of up to twelve months which may be completed overseas, the specified period of training shall have been completed in approved posts within the United Kingdom, or in posts in the Republic of Ireland approved by the College of Anaesthetists of the Royal College of Surgeons in Ireland; and

(d) satisfies the requirements of these Regulations with regard to application procedures and other matters.

## Exemptions

6. Subject to Regulation 18(d), a candidate for the Final FRCA examination shall be exempt from passing the Primary FRCA examination who, within the ten years preceding the closing date of the sitting applied for, and only in such years as are specified, and subject to annual renewal of approval by the Council:

(a) has passed Part 2 of the examination for the Fellowship of the Royal College of Anaesthetists, or Part II or Primary of the examination for the Fellowship of the Faculty or College of Anaesthetists of the Royal College of Surgeons in Ireland; or

(b) has obtained any of the following qualifications:

(i) Fellowship of the Faculty or College of Anaesthetists of the Royal College of Surgeons in Ireland;

(ii) Doctor of Medicine (Anaesthesiology) of the University of Colombo, Sri Lanka;

(iii) Master of Medicine (Anaesthesiology) of the University of Nairobi, Kenya, awarded in respect of success in the relevant examination taken prior to 1992;

(iv) Master of Anaesthesia of the University of Khartoum, Sudan, awarded in respect of success in the relevant examination taken in 1989, 1990, 1992, 1993 or any year after that;

(v) Master of Medicine (Anaesthesia) of the National University of Singapore awarded in respect of success in the relevant examination taken in 1991 or any year after that;

(vi) Fellowship in Anaesthesiology of the College of Physicians and Surgeons Pakistan in April 1998;

(vii) Fellowship of the Australian and New Zealand College of Anaesthetists;

(viii) Fellowship of the College of Anaesthetists of South Africa;

(ix) Certificate of the American Board of Anesthesiology;

(x) Fellowship in Anaesthesia of the Royal College of Physicians and Surgeons of Canada;

(xi) European Diploma in Anaesthesiology and Intensive Care of the European Academy of Anaesthesiology; or

(c) has obtained such other degree or qualification as the Council may from time to time accept.

## SECTION 3: APPLICATION PROCEDURES

7. Dates of examinations shall be published by the College in the Examinations Calendar, copies of which may be obtained, free of charge, from the Examinations Directorate, Royal College of Anaesthetists, 48–49 Russell Square, London WC1B 4JY.

8. Applications for admission to an examination must reach the Examinations Directorate after the commencement of the previous sitting but not later than the closing date for the sitting applied for, as shown in the Examinations Calendar. Application forms for admission may be obtained free of charge from the Examinations Directorate.

9. Applications for admission must be accompanied by the fee and the certificates required on the application form.

10. The fees payable for admission to each part shall be those fixed by the Council and published in the Examinations Calendar and should be paid by a cheque made payable to the Royal College of Anaesthetists and drawn on a United Kingdom clearing bank, or by a sterling draft or postal order, or by Eurocheques.

11. Subject to Regulations 14 and 15, a candidate withdrawing an application for admission to an examination before the closing date may receive back the full amount of the fee paid provided the withdrawal is received in writing, subject to a deduction for administrative expenses. A candidate who withdraws in any other circumstances or who fails to appear for an examination will not normally be entitled to any refund of fee.

## SECTION 4: PREGNANCY

This regulation applies only to female candidates whose pregnancy or pregnancy-related illness or condition renders them unable to attend the examination. This regulation does not apply to any other situations. This special treatment in relation to female candidates is permitted under the Sex Discrimination Act 1975.

12. Any prospective candidate should notify the Examinations Directorate as soon as possible of the fact of their pregnancy and the expected week of confinement (EWC). Such details should, where possible, be attached to the appropriate application form and fee.

13. Where the prospective candidate:

(a) has any pregnancy-related problems or illness; or

(b) whose confinement is due shortly before or around the date of the examination; or

(c) whose condition gives her sufficient discomfort for her to consider that it will have a detrimental effect upon her performance,

she must submit an appropriate medical certificate which satisfies the College.

14. In such circumstances, should such a candidate be unable to sit for the examination, withdrawal will be permitted and the examination fee will be refunded (subject to a deduction for administrative expenses).

15. Any candidate who does not inform the Examinations Directorate of her pregnancy will not normally be allowed to withdraw her application after the closing date without forfeiting her examination fee. However, when pregnancy occurs after submitting an application but prior to the examination and the candidate is subsequently unable to attend for the examination due to pregnancy-related reasons, then upon submission of an appropriate medical certificate which satisfies the College, the candidate may withdraw

from the examination and the fee will be refunded (subject to a deduction for administrative expenses).

## SECTION 5: FELLOWSHIP BY EXAMINATION

16. As stated in the Charter and Ordinances of the Royal College of Anaesthetists, a person shall be entitled to be admitted a Fellow of the College if he or she has:

(a) passed the appropriate examinations for Fellowship; and

(b) complied with such conditions as may be prescribed by the Council in the Regulations of the College.

## SECTION 6: REFERRALS AND GUIDANCE

17. A candidate who is unsuccessful in an examination may, subject to the provisions of Section 2 and Regulation 18, enter for the next or any subsequent sitting of that examination.

18. (a) No candidate may attempt the Primary FRCA examination more than twice without guidance or more than four times in all.

(b) No candidate may attempt the Final FRCA examination more than twice without guidance or more than six times in all.

(c) For the purpose of this Regulation, 'guidance' shall comprise:

(i) subject to the consent of the candidate, the provision to the College by the appropriate College Tutor of a confidential report on that candidate, and

(ii) the attendance by the candidate at a guidance session arranged by the College.

(d) No candidate who has failed the Primary FRCA examination four times will be eligible for exemption from the Primary FRCA examination under the conditions stated in Regulation 6.

19. After January 1998, a candidate in a Primary FRCA examination whose mark in the written element of the examination is such that it will be impossible for that candidate to pass the examination as a whole will forthwith be declared to have failed, and will not be allowed to attempt the remaining elements of the examination and will not be entitled to any refund of the examination fee.

20. A candidate in a Final FRCA examination whose marks in the written elements of the examination are such that it will be impossible for that candidate to pass the examination as a whole will forthwith be declared to have failed, and will not be allowed to attempt the remaining elements of the examination and will not be entitled to any refund of the examination fee.

## SECTION 7: REPRESENTATIONS AND APPEALS

21. A candidate, or any person on behalf of that candidate, wishing to make representations with regard to the conduct of an examination or to appeal against any result must address such representation or appeal to the Examinations Director in writing within two months of completing the relevant examination. In no circumstances may such representations be addressed to an examiner. Representations and appeals shall be dealt with in accordance with the Council's Examinations (Representations and Appeals) Regulations. Copies are available from the Examinations Directorate, Royal College of Anaesthetists, 48–49 Russell Square, London WC1B 4JY.

## SECTION 8: INFRINGEMENTS

22. The College's Council may refuse to admit to an examination, or to proceed with the examination of, any candidate who infringes any of the Regulations, or who is considered by the presiding examiner to be guilty of behaviour prejudicial to the proper conduct and management of the examination or who has previously been found guilty of such behaviour. If in the opinion of Council any examination success has been secured by cheating, deception or fraud of any kind whatsoever, the Council may quash that result and any qualifications resulting from it and withdraw any diploma, certificate or other award so obtained.

## SECTION 9: COMMENCEMENT AND REVOCATION

23. (a) These regulations shall come into force on 20th January 1999.

(b) These Examinations Regulations made by the Council of the Royal College of Anaesthetists supersede any previous Regulations which are hereby revoked.

## APPENDIX TO REGULATIONS

## STRUCTURE OF THE EXAMINATION

### Primary FRCA

There are four sections:

(a) 90 multiple choice questions (MCQ) – 3 hours

comprising three subsections: approximately 30 questions in pharmacology, 30 questions in physiology and biochemistry, and 30 questions in physics and clinical measurement.

(b) Objective structured clinical examination (OSCE) – 16 stations in approximately 1 hour 40 minutes comprising stations in resuscitation, technical skills, anatomy (general procedure), anatomy (local block), history-taking, physical examination, communication skills, interpretation of ECG, X-ray and biochemistry/haematology/photographs/charts, statistics, anaesthetic equipment, monitoring equipment, measuring equipment and anaesthetic hazards.

(c) Viva 1 – 30 minutes

A structured viva comprising 15 minutes in pharmacology, and 15 minutes in physiology and biochemistry.

(d) Viva 2 – 30 minutes

A structured viva comprising 15 minutes in physics, clinical measurement, equipment and safety, and 15 minutes on clinical topics (including a critical incident).

**Final FRCA**

There are four sections:

(a) 90 multiple choice questions (MCQ) – 3 hours

comprising approximately 20 questions in medicine and surgery, 40 questions in anaesthesia and pain management including applied basic sciences (mainly pharmacology and physiology), 10 questions in clinical measurement and 20 questions in intensive therapy.

(b) Short answer question (SAQ) paper (all 12 questions being compulsory) – 3 hours on the principles and practice of clinical anaesthesia

(c) Viva 1: Clinical Anaesthesia – 50 minutes

A structured viva comprising 10 minutes to view clinical material, 20 minutes of questions on the clinical material and 20 minutes of questions on clinical anaesthesia unrelated to the clinical material

(d) Viva 2: Clinical Science – 30 minutes

A structured viva on the application of basic science to anaesthesia, intensive therapy and pain management.

## THE MARKING SYSTEM

The College uses a five-point close-marking system in its examinations, the marks being:

2+   outstanding performance

2    pass

1+  fail

1   poor fail

0   veto (if a candidate fails to answer a compulsory question in the SAQ paper of the Final FRCA examination)

The following marks are required to pass both the Primary and Final FRCA examinations:

2, 2, 2, 1+ or better

In both parts of the examination, the performance of borderline candidates is reviewed by all the examiners before the final marks are awarded.

Elimination of candidates will be applied on the following criteria:

*Primary FRCA:*
Candidates who receive a mark of 1 (poor fail) in the MCQ paper. It should be noted that a candidate's performance in each of the three subsections is taken into consideration when calculating the overall mark for the MCQ. Candidates who perform very poorly in one or more subjects cannot obtain an overall pass mark in the MCQ.

*Final FRCA:*
Candidates who receive a combination of marks below a mark of 2 (pass) and 1+ (fail) in the written sections of the examination.

## PRIZES

The following prizes may, at the discretion of the examiners, be awarded to candidates who achieve particularly high marks in their examination:

*Nuffield Prize:* awarded for outstanding achievement in the Primary FRCA examination

*Macintosh Prize:* awarded for outstanding achievement in the spring sitting of the Final FRCA examination

*Magill Prize:* awarded for outstanding achievement in the autumn sitting of the Final FRCA examination

To be eligible for the award of a Nuffield, Macintosh or Magill Prize a candidate must be sitting the relevant examination for the first time and must obtain a mark of 2+ in all the sections of the examination.

## AMENDMENTS

A new edition of the regulations is currently being prepared which will include revision made by the Committee and Council.

The amendments are as follows:

1. that compulsory guidance in the Final FRCA be provided after the third unsuccessful attempt, rather than after the second attempt – Regulation 18(b), noting that those candidates who have already attended a guidance interview after two unsuccessful attempts at the Final FRCA examination will not be required to attend a guidance interview again after a third attempt

2. that failing the Primary FRCA four times should not prevent someone attempting the Final FRCA if they subsequently pass an exempting qualification – Regulation 18(d)

3. that the requirement to have been in training within the last five years to be eligible to sit the Final FRCA be removed – Regulation 5(c)(i)

4. the maximum number of attempts at each part will remain at four for the Primary FRCA (with compulsory guidance after two unsuccessful attempts) and six for the Final FRCA: Regulation 18(a) and (b).

Council also agreed that the following statement be incorporated into the Regulations:

*The college strongly recommends that candidates should only sit the Final FRCA examination when they have spent a minimum of 6 months in a LAT, FTTA or SpR post. The SHO years should be used to obtain the training necessary to be successful in the Primary FRCA examination and to provide a broad clinical base from which to enter SpR training.*

# Index